Colonoscopy

Publication of this book
has been facilitated by the generous support
of the Olympus Corporation of America

To our wives

Marlène and *Meg*

Colonoscopy

Techniques, Clinical Practice and Colour Atlas

Edited by

RICHARD H. HUNT
MB, FRCP

Surgeon Commander, Royal Navy,
Consultant Physician and Gastroenterologist,
Head, Department of Gastroenterology,
Royal Naval Hospital, Haslar,
Gosport, Hampshire

and

JEROME D. WAYE
MD

Associate Clinical Professor of Medicine
The Mount Sinai School of Medicine
of the City University of New York
and Chief, Gastrointestinal Endoscopy Unit,
The Mount Sinai Hospital, New York

LONDON
CHAPMAN AND HALL

First published 1981 by
Chapman and Hall Ltd
11 New Fetter Lane, London EC4P 4EE

© *1981 Chapman and Hall*

Printed in Great Britain at the University Press, Cambridge

ISBN 0 412 22710 X

British Library Cataloguing in Publication Data

Colonoscopy
  1. Colon (Anatomy) – Diseases
  2. Intestines – Diseases – Diagnosis
  I. Hunt, Richard, H. II. Waye, Jerome D.
  611'.347   RC803

ISBN 0-412-22710-X

Contents

Foreword   vii
Hiromi Shinya

List of Contributors   viii

Preface   xi

Acknowledgements   xii

1 The History of Colonoscopy   1
Bergein F. Overholt

PART ONE
Organization and Techniques

2 Indications for Colonoscopy   11
Richard H. Hunt and Jerome D. Waye

3 Preparing the Patient   19
Gabriel S. Nagy

4 The Endoscopy Suite   27
Yoshihiro Sakai

5 Instrumentation and Disinfection   39
Jack A. Vennes

6 The Gastrointestinal Assistant   51
Brian Wright and Anna M. Ricoma

7 Radiology of the Large Bowel   63
David E. Beckly and Giles W. Stevenson

8 Colonoscopy Intubation Techniques with Fluoroscopy   109
Richard H. Hunt

9 Colonoscopy Intubation Techniques without Fluoroscopy   147
Jerome D. Waye

10 Flexible Sigmoidoscopy   179
Stephen E. Hedberg

11 Intraoperative Colonoscopy   189
Kenneth A. Forde

12 Therapeutic Colonoscopy   199
P. Frühmorgen

13 Complications and Hazards of Colonoscopy   237
B. H. Gerald Rogers

PART TWO
Clinical Practice

14 Rectal Bleeding   267
Edwin T. Swarbrick and Richard H. Hunt

15 Emergency Colonoscopy   289
F. P. Rossini and A. Ferrari

16 The Polyp Problem   301
David W. Day and Basil C. Morson

17 Colon Cancer   327
Sidney J. Winawer

18 Inflammatory Bowel Disease   343
Robin H. Teague and Jerome D. Waye

19 Diverticular Disease and Strictures   363
Christopher B. Williams

20 Paediatric Colonoscopy   383
Angelita Habr-Gama

PART THREE
A Colour Atlas of Colonoscopy

Introduction   403

Index   405

Foreword

When I first introduced the technique of colonoscopic polypectomy in 1969, neither the medical world nor myself were aware of the far-reaching ramifications of this procedure. Colonoscopic endoscopy has developed rapidly over the past decade, with major leaps into the field of therapeutic endoscopy. The entire field of diagnostic colonoscopy is not quite 15 years old but has captured the imagination and interest of thousands of physicians throughout the world, affording a new and previously unchartered look at the entire large bowel.

The chapters in this internationally authored book are written by world-famous experts in their fields. The editors, Drs Richard Hunt and Jerome Waye, are well-known and superb colonoscopists, who have admirably managed to weave the separate chapters into a thoroughly readable and comprehensible exposition on the current state of the art of colonoscopy.

Having just completed my own book on colonoscopy, I am aware of the tremendous amount of work and effort with which these two editors have moulded each chapter to their satisfaction, while keeping the contents thoroughly representative of the international scope of this volume, and retaining the individual authors' thoughts and approaches.

The teaching of colonoscopy and colonoscopic polypectomy is especially difficult to convey by the written word alone. I highly commend the authors in their written approach to this subject, but would like to stress that mastering the technique of colonoscopy requires many hours of practice and patience. Attending seminars and lectures, observing experts in the field, and working with colon models all lend to the complete training of the fledgling endoscopist.

The colour atlas contains some of the finest colour photographs of endoscopic anatomy and pathology, as well as detailed pictures of the approaches to colonoscopic polypectomy. The addition of appropriate histological photomicrographs enhances the appreciation of the reader for the endoscopic pathology.

This multi-authored book is a true landmark in the field of colonoscopy and contains information for all colonoscopists as well as for those who wish to know about the techniques, pitfalls and applications of colonoscopy.

HIROMI SHINYA, MD
Chief, Surgical Endoscopy Unit,
Beth Israel Medical Center, New York
Clinical Associate Professor,
The Mount Sinai Medical Center
of the City University of New York

List of Contributors

Beckly, David E., MB BS MRCP FRCR
Consultant in Radiodiagnosis, Plymouth General Hospital, UK.

Day, David W., MA MB BChir MRCPath
Senior Lecturer in Pathology, University of Liverpool; Honorary
Consultant Pathologist, Liverpool Area Health Authority, UK.

Ferrari, A., MD
Assistant, Gastroenterology–Gastrointestinal Endoscopy Service,
Department of Oncology, Ospedale Maggiore di San Giovanni
Battista e della Città di Torino, Turin, Italy.

Forde, Kenneth A., BS MD FACS FACG
Associate Professor of Clinical Surgery, College of Physicians and
Surgeons, Columbia University, New York, USA; Associate
Attending Surgeon, Presbyterian Hospital, New York, USA.

Frühmorgen, P., Privatdozent Dr. Med.
Medizinische Klinik mit Poliklinik der Universität
Erlangen-Nürnberg, Erlangen, West Germany.

Habr-Gama, Angelita, MD FACS FACG
Associate Professor of Surgery, University of São Paulo, Brasil.

Hedberg, Stephen E., MD DABS FACS,
Clinical Assistant Professor of Surgery, Harvard Medical School,
Massachusetts, USA; Visiting Surgeon and Senior Endoscopist in
Gastrointestinal Surgery, Massachusetts General Hospital, Boston,
USA.

Hunt, Richard H., MB FRCP
Surgeon Commander, Royal Navy; Consultant Physician and
Gastroenterologist, Head, Department of Gastroenterology, Royal
Naval Hospital, Haslar, Gosport, Hampshire, UK.

Morson, Basil C., VRD MA DM FRCS FRCPath
Consultant Pathologist and Director of Research Department, St.
Mark's Hospital, London, UK; Honorary Senior Lecturer in
Pathology, Royal Postgraduate Medical School, London, UK.

Nagy, Gabriel S., FRCP FRACP
Lecturer in Clinical Medicine, University of Sydney;
Gastroenterologist, Royal North Shore Hospital, Sydney, Australia.

Overholt, Bergein F., MD FACP
Chief GI Lab, St Mary's Medical Center, Knoxville, Tennessee, USA.

Ricoma, Anna M., RN
Senior Clinical Nurse, Endoscopy Department, Mount Sinai Hospital,
New York, USA.

Rogers, B. H. Gerald, MD
Clinical Associate (Associate Professor) in Medicine, University of
Chicago, Pritzker School of Medicine, Chicago, Illinois, USA.

Rossini, F. P., MD
Professor, Oncology Medical School, University of Turin,
Division of Gastroenterology; Gastroenterology–Gastrointestinal
Endoscopy Service, Department of Oncology, Ospedale Maggiore di
San Giovanni Battista e della Città di Torino, Turin, Italy.

Sakai, Yoshihiro, MD DMSc
Associate Professor of Medicine, Department of Medicine, Tokyo
Medical College Hospital, Tokyo, Japan.

Stevenson, Giles W., MRCP FRCR FRCP(C)
Associate Professor in Diagnostic Radiology, McMaster University
Medical Centre, Hamilton, Ontario, Canada.

Swarbrick, Edwin T., MD MRCP
Lecturer in Gastroenterology, St. Bartholomew's Hospital, London,
UK.

Teague, Robin H., MD MRCP MRCS
Consultant Physician, Torbay Hospital, Torquay, Devon, UK.

Vennes, Jack A., MD
Professor of Medicine, University of Minnesota Medical School,
Minneapolis VA Medical Center, Minneapolis, Minnesota, USA.

Waye, Jerome D., MD
Associate Clinical Professor of Medicine, The Mount Sinai School of
Medicine of the City University of New York, USA; Chief,
Gastrointestinal Endoscopy Unit, The Mount Sinai Hospital, New
York, USA.

Williams, Christopher B., BM FRCP
Consultant Physician, St. Mark's Hospital for Diseases of the Rectum
and Colon, St. Bartholomew's Hospital, London, UK; Honorary

Consultant Physician, Hospital for Sick Children, Great Ormond Street, London, UK; Queen Elizabeth's Hospital for Children, London, UK.

Winawer, Sidney J., MD FACG
Chief, Gastroenterology Service, Department of Medicine, Memorial Sloan-Kettering Cancer Center, New York, USA; Professor of Clinical Medicine, Cornell University Medical College, New York, USA.

Wright, Brian, SRN
Chief Medical Technician, Royal Navy, Charge Nurse, Gastroenterology Department, Royal Naval Hospital, Haslar, Gosport, Hampshire, UK.

Preface

Colorectal diseases present the gastroenterologist and abdominal surgeon with much of their daily workload. Adenomatous polyps are frequently encountered throughout the Western World and colorectal cancer is amongst the most common of malignant diseases in the USA, the UK and the countries of Western Europe. Inflammatory bowel diseases are similarly widespread and also increasing in frequency, while diverticular disease is so common as to be widely accepted as an inevitable consequence of aging.

The problems of diagnosis and management of such conditions highlight the need for endoscopy in the colon. Despite this obvious role, colonoscopy has been something of a poor relation, when compared to the rapid development and widespread application of upper gastro-intestinal endoscopy. Acceptance of colonoscopy has previously been hindered by problems of preparation, the technical difficulties of intubating the colon to the caecum, and the length of time taken to perform the procedure. Initially, endoscopists were consequently reluctant to become involved. However, determination to master the skills of colonic intubation, combined with the technical advances in instrumentation, has been rewarded. The techniques of preparation, intubation, biopsy and snare polypectomy are widely applied throughout the world, and much valuable data on the role of colonoscopy in clinical practice has now become available.

The indications point to significant cost-benefit advantages of colonoscopy. Although the cost of a colonoscopic examination is greater than that of a barium enema, a definite endoscopic diagnosis may prevent unnecessary laparotomy, or alternatively identify previously undiagnosed pathology which will benefit from earlier corrective surgery. There is no doubt that colonoscopic polypectomy dramatically reduces hospitalization time, days lost from work and overall cost, when compared to surgical laparotomy and colotomy.

The international contributors to this book have all been at the forefront in establishing colonoscopy as a practical diagnostic and therapeutic procedure. Each author brings a unique regional knowledge and personal approach to the field of colonoscopy, yet we have attempted to keep the framework applicable to all colonoscopists wherever they practice. In each chapter we have attempted to maintain the individuality of the author, while still maintaining a unity of approach which is usually only seen in single author texts.

The production has been a truly collaborative and equal effort between us, from the conception and planning, through the editing and re-editing of the manuscripts, each of which crossed the Atlantic many times between telephone discussions, before finalization. The combined efforts of authors and editors has resulted in a book which we believe to be unique in its field. The first section, on Organization and Techniques, is principally technical and intended for the colonoscopist both experienced and novice and includes chapters on flexible sigmoidoscopy for those planning to use the short instruments and on the nurse assistant to whom much of this first section should prove invaluable.

The second section, on Clinical Practice, is intended to identify the exact part that colonoscopic procedures can play in the wider context of patient management and should be of value to all clinicians, histopathologists and radiologists, in addition to the endoscopist.

The Colour Atlas of Colonoscopy contains the most comprehensive collection of photographs of colonoscopic pathology yet assembled. These views will undoubtedly help all colonoscopists of varying skills to recognize the variety of intracolonic pathology and will, we hope, also be of interest and value to others, especially pathologists.

Over the past ten to fifteen years colonoscopy has revolutionized our approach to the diagnosis and management of colonic disease and is now a firmly established procedure. Awareness of the indications and problems of colonoscopy, combined with a knowledge of its potential, coupled with skilled techniques, can lead to earlier diagnosis and more effective treatment. We hope that the contributions which have been gathered in this book will help, at least in some way, to further these aims.

Acknowledgements

We are grateful to all our colleagues, staff and patients who have made this book possible.

April 1981

RICHARD H. HUNT
Haslar

JEROME D. WAYE
New York

CHAPTER ONE

The History of Colonoscopy

BERGEIN F. OVERHOLT

At any one moment in time, society in general and perhaps physicians in particular take for granted the excellence of what is placed at their disposal. Can this be more true than in the field of colonoscopy, where the endoscopist demands and has available a highly sophisticated flexible instrument providing directional controls, a lens-washing facility, air or CO_2 insufflation, and channels for biopsy, cytology and polypectomy? Photographic reproduction and TV imaging are readily available. Special facilities and trained ancillary personnel are now considered routine. We look forward with optimism to future developments, yet ten years ago colonoscopy was in its infancy, and it is less than twenty years since the first efforts at instrument design emerged.

Endoscopy owes its primitive beginning to Bozzini who, in 1806, developed his endoscope, a 'light transmitter', using candle light reflected down an endoscope to view various physiologic orifices, including the rectum (Schindler, 1966; Bush *et al.*, 1974). Although better external light sources continued to be developed, it was not until the early 1900s that the miniature Edison electric bulb was used in instruments to examine the rectum. In 1902, Tuttle made the earliest proctoscope with an electric light carrier as an integral part of the instrument (Tuttle, 1903). A further advance in lighting occurred about 1960, when Welch-Allyn of New York introduced its rigid sigmoidoscope, incorporating fixed fibreoptic bundles in the instrument wall to transmit light.

Meanwhile, other technological advances were occurring. In 1952, Hopkins and Kapany in England, and Van Heel in Holland began their independent work on flexible fibreoptic glass bundles for light transmission (Kapany, 1958; Hopkins and Kapany, 1954; Van Heel, 1954). This information found its way to Dr H. M. Pollard and Dr Basil Hirchowitz at the University of Michigan in Ann Arbor, where they formed a team with C. Wilbur Peters, an assistant professor of physics, and Lawrence E. Curtiss, a physics student, to fabricate a flexible optical bundle for image transmission (Overholt, 1968;

1

Hirschowitz, Peters and Curtiss, 1957; Hirschowitz *et al.*, 1958). In a fascinating description of the development of fibre bundles, involving individual fibre coating and orientation, Hirschowitz has detailed the development of these bundles and their eventual application to the gastroscope used first by himself at the University Hospital in Ann Arbor in February, 1957 (Hirschowitz *et al.*, 1957; 1979). Subsequent clinical experience was further detailed in his landmark article of 1961 (Hirschowitz, 1961).

As advances in fibregastroscopy were occurring, the birth of fibresigmoidoscopy and colonoscopy took place in the spring of 1961. Dr B. F. Overholt, then an intern at the University of Michigan, was being interviewed for a position in the Public Health Service by Dr G. Howard Gowen, who had that very day been the recipient of an uncomfortable rigid sigmoidoscopy. Overholt, who had reviewed an article on flexible fibreoptics in *Life* magazine, commented on the need for a 'flexible sigmoidoscope'. Developments were rapid, with the first grant by the Public Health Service being awarded to Optics Technology Inc. of California, whose President was the previously mentioned N. S. Kapany. The initial attempts at instrument design and development were unsuccessful and it became apparent that more information on the anatomy of the colon was needed for engineers to develop instrument prototypes. This need was met when Dow-Corning Aid to Medical Research provided Dr Overholt with a silastic foam enema (Fig. 1.1). This material with an added catalyst was injected into the rectum using a technique similar to that of barium enema. The foam quickly solidified into a soft spongy cast

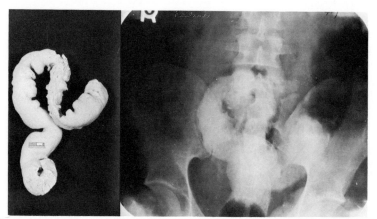

Fig. 1.1 Silastic foam enema of rectum and sigmoid colon expelled from the distal colon with corresponding X-ray.

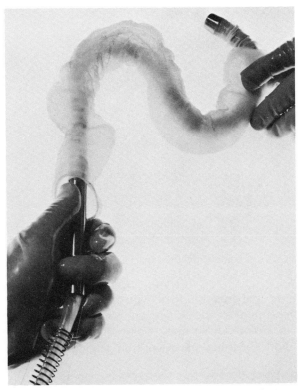

Fig. 1.2 Reverse silastic mould of rectum and sigmoid colon with inserted prototype instrument.

of the rectum and sigmoid colon which was then expelled. A reverse mould provided the required anatomical model (Fig. 1.2). The tip deflection mechanisms which were developed during those early years are remarkably similar to present designs.

Although many companies became interested in this new field, it was the Illinois Institute of Technology Research Institute and the Eder Instrument Company that developed the first successful prototypes of the flexible fibreoptic sigmoidoscope. After somewhat difficult trials in animals, clinical experimentation began.

The flexible fibresigmoidoscope (Fig. 1.4) was successfully used clinically in 1963 (Overholt, 1970), but Overholt (1968) first visually confirmed the presence of a radiographically suspected sigmoid cancer in February 1966, at the Veterans Hospital in Ann Arbor, Michigan.

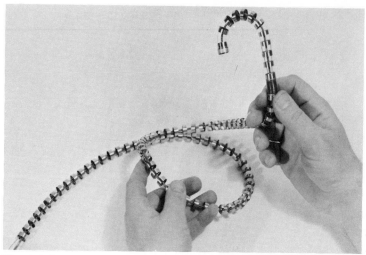

Fig. 1.3 Series of oval metal segments with interspaced connecting and control wires.

The first series of 40 patients studied with the flexible fibre-sigmoidoscope was presented to the American Society for Gastrointestinal Endoscopy in Colorado Springs, Colorado, in May 1967 (Overholt, 1968b). As with the initial phases of fibregastroscopy, there

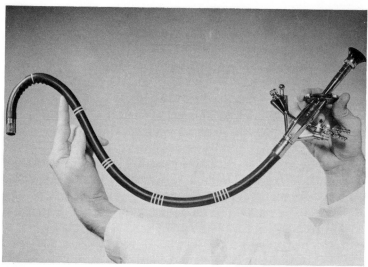

Fig. 1.4 Phase 2 clinical fibresigmoidoscope developed by Eder Instrument Company.

was much speculation about the value of the procedure. Nonetheless, the birth of flexible fibreoptic sigmoidoscopy, and subsequently colonoscopy, had occurred and the revolution in the diagnosis and management of diseases of the rectum and colon had begun; its progress from that point is well documented.

In Japan, Oshiba and Watanabe working with the Machida Instrument Company developed their first colon fibrescope prototype in 1963 (Oshiba and Watanabe, 1965). Niwa (1965) and Kanazawa (Kanazawa and Tanaka, 1966) likewise developed prototype instruments with the Olympus Corporation shortly after that. The early instruments were gradually improved, but it was not until American Cystoscope Makers Inc. (ACMI) of New York entered the field in the late 1960s that colonoscopy began to flourish. Although others (Lemire and Cocco, 1966) had viewed the descending colon with flexible gastroscopes, it was ACMI that developed the first true colonoscope. Technical advances in instruments and improvements in both intubation techniques and accessories occurred in rapid succession. Pioneer colonoscopists sprang forward in the late 1960s: Overholt, Waye, Shinya and Sugarbaker in the United States; Niwa, Oshiba, Kanazawa, Yamagata and Sakai in Japan; Fox, Salmon, Teague and later Williams in England; Dehyle and Classen in Germany; Provenzale and Revignas in Italy, and Hansen in Denmark.

The era of therapeutic colonoscopy began in the early 1970s, when Dr Hiromi Shinya made the outstanding contribution of polypectomy using an expandable wire-loop snare inserted through a channel of the colonoscope. Shinya was able to remove polyps safely, thus avoiding the necessity of repeated barium enema observation and transabdominal colotomy for polypectomy (Wolff and Shinya, 1971). To Williams in England can be given most of the credit for teaching the technique of colonoscopy to hundreds of physicians who recognized the value of the procedure (Williams, Overholt and Sakai, 1973; Williams, 1973; Cotton and Williams, 1980).

A decade of slow erratic growth, beginning in 1961, was thus followed by a decade of remarkable accomplishments in technology as well as in intubation techniques, colonoscopic diagnosis and management (Overholt, 1975; Cotton and Williams, 1980). Instruments now provide the trained and experienced colonoscopist with the capability to reach the caecum in over 90% of cases. Physicians, engineers, private industry and federal governments have co-operated to develop both the instruments and the techniques of colonoscopy which have revolutionized both the diagnosis and treatment of diseases affecting the large bowel.

References

Bush, R. B., Leonhardt, H., Bush, I. M. and Landes, R. R. (1974), Dr Bozzini's Lichtleiter. A translation of his original article (1806). *Urology*, **3**, 119–23.

Cotton, P. B. and Williams, C. B. (1980), *Practical Gastrointestinal Endoscopy*. Blackwell Scientific Publication, London, pp. 86–141.

Hirschowitz, B. I. (1961), Endoscopic examination of the stomach and duodenal cap with the fiberscope. *Lancet*, **1**, 1074–8.

Hirschowitz, B. I. (1979), A personal history of the fiberscope. *Gastroenterology*, **76**, 864–9.

Hirschowitz, B. I., Curtiss, L. E., Peters, C. W. and Pollard, H. M. (1958), Demonstration of a new gastroscope, the 'Fiberscope'. *Gastroenterology*, **35**, 50–53.

Hirschowitz, B. I. Peters, C. W. and Curtiss, L. E. (1957), Preliminary reports on a long fiberscope for examination of the stomach and duodenum. *Univ. Michigan Med. Bull.*, **23**, 178–80.

Hopkins, H. and Kapany, N. W. (1954), A flexible fiberscope using static scanning. *Nature*, **173**, 39–41.

Kanazawa, T. and Tanaka, M. (1965), Endoscopy of colon. *Gastroenterol. Endosc., Tokyo*, **7**, 398–400.

Kapany, N. W. (1958), Fiber optics, In: *Strong Concepts of Classical Optics*, Freeman, San Francisco, pp. 553–96.

Lemire, S. and Cocco, A. E. (1966), Visualization of the left colon with the fiberoptic gastroduodenoscope. *Gastrointest. Endosc.*, **13**, Nov. 29–30.

Niwa, H. (1965), Endoscopy of colon. *Gastroenterol. Endosc., Tokyo*, **7**, 402–8.

Oshiba, S. and Watanabe, A. (1965), Endoscopy of colon. *Gastroenterol. Endosc., Tokyo*, **7**, 400–2.

Overholt, B. F. (1968), Clinical experience with the fibersigmoidoscope. *Gastrointest. Endosc.*, **15**, 27.

Overholt, B. F. (1970), Description and experience with flexible fibersigmoidoscopes. *Proc. Sixth Nat. Cancer Conf.* (1968). J. B. Lippincott Company, Philadelphia, pp. 443–6.

Overholt, B. F. (1975), Colonoscopy: A review. *Gastroenterology*, **68**, 1308–20.

Overholt, B. F. and Pollard, H. M. (1967), Cancer of the colon and rectum: current procedures for detection and diagnosis. *Cancer*, **20**, 445–50.

Schindler, R. (1966), *Gastroscopy* (2nd ed), Hafner Publishing Company, New York, p. 2.

Tuttle, J. P. (1903), *A Treatise on Diseases of the Anus, Rectum and Pelvic Colon*. Appleton & Company, New York.

Van Heel, A. C. S. (1954), A new method of transporting optical images without aberration. *Nature*, **173**, 39.

Williams, C. (1973), *Endoscopic Polypectomy*. Stewart Hardy Films, Ltd, London, England.

Williams, C. B., Overholt, B. F. and Sakai, Y. (1973), *Colonoscopy. Principles and Techniques*, Stewart Hardy Films, Ltd, London, England.
Wolff, W. I. and Shinya, H. (1971), Colonofiberoscopy. *J. Am. Med. Ass.*, **217**, 1509–12.

PART ONE

Organization and Techniques

CHAPTER TWO

Indications for Colonoscopy

RICHARD H. HUNT and JEROME D. WAYE

The development of fibreoptic endoscopy has transformed our approach to gastrointestinal disease, and this is no more true than in the colon. The ability to examine, detect and biopsy any segment of the entire colon, from the anus to the pole of the caecum (and frequently to visualize and biopsy the terminal ileum), has great advantages over conventional proctosigmoidoscopy and barium enema examination, as is amply discussed elsewhere in this book. Clinicians commonly experience situations where the history, physical examination, digital anorectal, proctosigmoidoscopy and double contrast barium enema examinations have all failed to confirm or exclude a definitive diagnosis. At this point, colonoscopy should be considered. A list of absolute indications from our own experience and collected from the literature (Christie and Shinya, 1975; Cotton and Williams, 1980; Frühmorgen, 1980; Overholt, 1975; Rossini, 1975; Waye, 1977) is shown in Table 2.1.

2.1 Evaluation of barium enema abnormalities

The barium enema remains the mainstay in investigating colonic disease because of its relative ease and simplicity (Editorial, *Lancet*, 1974). The colonoscopist, however, is frequently requested to examine a patient who has a stricture or constant filling defect reported on the barium enema films. The majority of abnormalities are in the sigmoid colon or the caecum, which are less easy areas to display radiologically. At colonoscopy, no pathology may be found, or alternatively the lesion may turn out to be a carcinoma, polyp or an area of segmental inflammatory disease. Poor bowel preparation for the barium enema is responsible for many such 'filling defects', and timely colonoscopy may avoid unnecessary laparotomy and colotomy. The wise colonoscopist will review all such films with the radiologist to avoid unnecessary colonoscopies and to improve co-operation between disciplines, for colonoscopy is complementary to radiography in most instances (Chapter 7).

Table 2.1 Indications for colonoscopy

Evaluation of a barium enema abnormality
Unexplained rectal bleeding
Inflammatory bowel disease
  Differential diagnosis
  Extent of disease
  Evaluation of strictures
  Dysplasia surveillance
Therapeutic procedures
  Polypectomy
  Fulguration of bleeding site
  Removal of foreign bodies
Postoperative endoscopy
  Evaluate a surgical anastomosis
  Percolostomy before reconnection
Surveillance
  High-risk groups
  Follow-up after removal of polyps or cancer

2.2 Unexplained rectal bleeding

Symptoms suggestive of colonic disease, such as lower abdominal pain, diarrhoea and rectal bleeding, are commonly encountered. Frequently, the entire preliminary investigations including barium enema do not reveal the cause of a patient's symptoms. Colonoscopy is usually unrewarding in patients with unexplained abdominal pain or diarrhoea, but the symptom of unexplained persistent rectal bleeding should always prompt a request for total colonoscopy. In this group of patients (Chapter 14), a significant number will have specific pathology discovered at endoscopy, such as carcinoma, polyps, inflammatory bowel disease or a vascular abnormality. Diverticular disease rarely bleeds in a chronic persistent manner, and this symptom must be investigated and should not be readily attributed to diverticulosis (Chapter 19).

Massive rectal bleeding poses a difficult problem for diagnosis. Radioisotope scanning (Alavi, Dann and Baum, 1977; Winzelberg, McKusick and Strauss, 1979), or mesenteric angiography can be of great value in identifying the site of ongoing haemorrhage when colonoscopy may be difficult or even impossible. Such massive colon bleeding, however, is usually intermittent and subsides spontaneously. Immediately following cessation of active bleeding, semi-elective colonoscopy can be particularly helpful. A tap water or disposable phosphate enema may be given before proceeding, and clots should be removed from the rectum through a sigmoidoscope. Bleeding may be seen to arise from a specific site, such as a polyp, carcinoma, or perhaps a diverticulum. Even if a lesion is not seen, the segment of involvement may frequently be identified. The subject of emergency colonoscopy is more fully discussed in Chapter 15.

Screening for colorectal cancer using the faecal occult blood test (Hemoccult) has been widely advocated (Chapter 17), especially in the United States (Winawer *et al.*, 1980) and West Germany (Frühmorgen and Demling, 1980). In patients who have a positive Hemoccult test and negative sigmoidoscopy and barium enema, colonoscopy may be used to examine the bowel to detect small carcinomas or polyps which have been missed. The Hemoccult test has a false positive rate of about 5%, and it has not been determined whether this will place too heavy a demand upon colonoscopy services for too little return.

2.3 Inflammatory bowel disease

The majority of patients with inflammatory bowel disease will not require colonoscopy, but it may help in differentiating between Crohn's disease and ulcerative colitis in the difficult case or identifying one of the less common forms of inflammatory bowel disease. Colonoscopy with multiple biopsies may also be used to assess the extent of involvement, especially when the patient is less well than expected on the information available from sigmoidoscopy, rectal biopsy and double contrast barium enema. The barium enema frequently underestimates the extent of inflammatory bowel disease and colonoscopy used in this way may assist the surgeon in preoperative planning.

Patients with ulcerative colitis who develop strictures should be submitted to colonoscopy with biopsy and cytology to exclude the possibility of malignancy. Useful information may be obtained even if the stricture cannot be intubated. The development of small-calibre colonoscopes will ensure that the majority of colonic strictures can be passed and a more positive assessment given. The increased risk of malignancy in patients with total ulcerative colitis becomes apparent after seven years and rises thereafter. It is useful to carry out regular colonoscopy and biopsy in these patients in the search for dysplasia. It is not yet clear, however, what frequency interval is most suitable. At the present time, most centres perform total colonoscopy every one to two years, but until more data is available it is difficult to make firm recommendations. The subject of inflammatory bowel disease is discussed more fully in Chapter 18 and the risk of malignancy in ulcerative colitis in Chapter 17. It may be useful after surgery (p. 354).

2.4 Therapeutic endoscopy

The ability to remove colon polyps is one of the most widely recognized advantages of colonoscopy, and several large series have been reported. The techniques of polypectomy are discussed in detail in Chapter 12, and the polyp problem and colonic cancer in Chapters 16 and 17, respectively. Colonoscopic polypectomy has now replaced laparotomy and colotomy for polyp removal, thus avoiding their associated risks and that of general anaesthesia. Total colonoscopy should properly be performed at the time of polypectomy to rule out any synchronous lesions which might have been missed at the barium enema examination.

Because of the cumulative risk of malignancy with increasing size of polyps over 1 cm in diameter, it is wise to remove and retrieve these where it is technically possible. Virtually all pedunculated and most sessile polyps can be removed at colonoscopy, although this depends on the experience and judgment of the endoscopist. Close cooperation between the colonoscopist and histopathologist is important, especially when the head of a transected polyp is found to contain invasive carcinoma. This problem is discussed more fully on p. 316 in the Polyp Problem (Chapter 16). Since factual data are not yet available, the decision not to resect the colon in this circumstance should be reached by a team, including endoscopist, pathologist and primary physician, with strong consideration given to the physical condition and the desires of the patient at risk.

Recently, diathermy techniques have been successfully applied to small angiodysplasia regions and these are discussed on p. 281. Foreign bodies in the colon, such as swallowed dental bridges attached to the mucosa, pens or mechanical vibrators, may be removed with the colonoscope.

2.5 The postoperative colon

The barium enema may display the region of an anastomosis clearly, but nodulation or irregularity may require further definition. Colonoscopy is invaluable to inspect the anastomotic area after surgery for cancer or in the postoperative patient who develops symptoms. Recurrent cancer following colon resection does not necessarily occur at the suture line, but most commonly in the mesenteric nodes and the liver. A negative colonoscopy does not, therefore, completely exclude tumour recurrence. Evaluation of the anastomosis is especially valuable in patients with Crohn's disease who have a resection, discussed more fully on p. 354. Good visualization is usually obtained unless the region has narrowed, although biopsies can invariably be taken.

In patients who have had a defunctioning colostomy for inflammatory disease, diverticular disease or acute bowel obstruction, endoscopy either *per rectum* or through the colostomy enables biopsies to be taken which may help the surgeon to decide on whether a reconnection or resection should be made.

2.6 Colonoscopy surveillance

2.6.1 *High-risk groups*

Neither the barium enema nor colonoscopy lend themselves to a widespread application for screening for colorectal cancer or polyps because of both the complexity and cost of these procedures. However, there are certain situations in which colonoscopy may be particularly useful: a number of individuals over 40 years of age can be identified as being at risk for colorectal cancer, and these include women who have had previous breast or genital cancer, those with a family history of colorectal cancer or polyps, and patients with long-standing ulcerative colitis. This subject is discussed in more detail in Chapter 17, but any patient who fits into these groups and has suspicious symptoms should be considered for colonoscopy. In addition, it is often possible to identify a patient with familial polyposis or the polyps of Gardner's syndrome at an early stage before they may be seen at sigmoidoscopy or barium enema. Early diagnosis can allow a clear strategy of management to be planned; however, the exact place of colonoscopy remains to be defined.

2.6.2 *Follow-up of colorectal cancer and polyps*

The patient with a colorectal cancer or polyp has a one in five chance of having a synchronous lesion present in the colon at the time of diagnosis of the index lesion. Although most patients have their index lesion discovered by barium enema, each patient undergoing surgical resection for carcinoma should have total colonoscopy either prior to definitive surgery or, should total colonoscopy not be possible (for example, because of a stenosing carcinomatous stricture), the colon may be inspected postoperatively. The postsurgical examination should properly be performed between six and nine months after the operation, so that the anastomosis can be inspected at a time of greatest likelihood of anastomotic tumour recurrence. These patients are also at risk of developing a metachronous lesion, either carcinoma or polyp, during the years following surgery (Eklund and Pihl, 1974). Colonoscopy performed every two to three years ensures follow-up, and any polyps which may have developed can be removed during that examination. Again, the role of colonoscopy in these patients has not yet been clearly defined.

The co-ordinated approach to diagnosis using the index of high-risk groups, screening tests such as Haemoccult, and careful sigmoidoscopy (including fibreoptic sigmoidoscopy), combined with double contrast barium enema and colonoscopy, should allow an earlier diagnosis of colonic cancer in the majority of patients, with a consequent improvement in their prognosis.

2.7 Limitations of colonoscopy

Intubation and examination of the colon may be limited by either lack of experience and technical expertise of the endoscopist or by such factors as poor bowel preparation, strictures, severe diverticular disease and adhesion from previous pelvic surgery or radiation. As skill is acquired and instrumentation improves, many of these limitations present less of a problem.

2.8 Contraindications to colonoscopy

There are relatively few situations in which colonoscopy is inadvisable. The most obvious include a recent myocardial infarction or pulmonary embolism, but chronic cardiorespiratory disease need be no bar, providing that care is taken to assess the patient beforehand and to provide careful monitoring during both the preparation and the procedure (Table 2.2).

Abdominal problems are only a contraindication if cathartics are themselves contraindicated, and these conditions include intestinal

Table 2.2 Contraindications to colonoscopy

General medical conditions
    Recent myocardial infarction
    Pulmonary embolus
Acute colitis
Acute diverticulitis
Peritonitis

obstruction, peritonitis, acute colitis of any cause, acute diverticulitis, suspected perforation or recent bowel surgery.

An uncooperative patient may constitute a relative contraindication, but it is unusual for a patient to be unable to tolerate the procedure. Careful explanation and adequate medication will usually circumvent this problem, which is less common to colonoscopy than upper gastrointestinal endoscopy.

It is wise to postpone colonoscopy in those patients who have abdominal pain, fever, tenderness or distension, and those who have had a hypotensive episode during bowel preparation. Common sense will normally decide when to proceed, and this seldom poses a problem for the experienced colonoscopist. In the infancy of colonoscopy, physicians taught themselves the technique. Newer technology has made instrumentation safer, but there is no substitute for the skill and knowledge gained from an adequate training programme in colonoscopy.

2.9 Conclusion

Although there are clear indications for colonoscopy, these are likely to broaden as our total experience increases, and the indications listed in Table 2.1 will become more clearly defined. As experience with the procedure increases and greater skill is achieved a higher number of total colon intubations results, patient discomfort decreases, and the risk of perforation decreases. It is important for the endoscopist to learn to evaluate the findings carefully, constantly assessing the value of the procedure in order to apply endoscopic talents for the greatest benefit of the patient.

References

Alavi, A., Dann, R. W. and Baum, S. (1977), Scintigraphic detection of acute gastrointestinal bleeding. *Radiology,* **124**, 753–62.

Christie, J. P. and Shinya, H. (1975), Indications for fibreoptic colonoscopy. *South. Med. J.,* **68**, 881–86.

Cotton, P. B. and Williams, C. B. (1980), In: *Practical Gastrointestinal Endoscopy*, Blackwell Scientific Publications, London.

Ekelund, G. and Pihl, B. (1974), Multiple carcinomas of the colon and rectum. *Cancer,* **33**, 1630–34.

Editorial (1974), *Lancet,* **1**, 1265–66.

Frühmorgen, P. (1980), Colonoscopy. In: *Gastroenterology. Techniques and Indications* (Ed. P. Frühmorgen and M. Classen), Springer-Verlag, Berlin, pp. 87–99.

Frühmorgen, P. and Demling, L. (1980), Early detection of colorectal cancer with a modified guaiac test – a screening examination in 6000 humans. In: *Colorectal Cancer: Prevention, Epidemiology and Screening* (Ed. S. Winawer, D. Schottenfield and P. Sherlock), Raven Press, New York, pp. 311–15.

Overholt, B. G. (1975), Colonoscopy. A review. *Gastroenterology,* **68**, 1308–20.

Rossini, F. P. (1975), In: *Atlas of Colonoscopy.* Piccin Medical Books, Padova, Italy.

Waye, J. D. (1977), Colonoscopy: guidelines and techniques for diagnosis and therapy. In: *Progress in Gastroenterology*, Vol III (Ed. G. B. J. Glass), Grune and Stratton, New York, pp. 991–1013.

Winawer, S. J., Andrews, M., Miller, C. H. and Fleisher, M. (1980), Review of screening for colorectal cancer using fecal occult blood testing. In: *Colorectal Cancer: Prevention, Epidemiology and Screening* (Ed. S. Winawer, D. Schottenfield and P. Sherlock), Raven Press, New York, pp. 249–59.

Winzelberg, G. G., McKusick, K. A. and Strauss, H. W. (1979), Evaluation of gastrointestinal bleeding by red blood cells labelled *in vivo* with technetium-99M. *J. Nucl. Med.,* **20**, 1000–06.

CHAPTER THREE

Preparing the Patient

GABRIEL S. NAGY

The success of colonoscopy is by no means entirely dependent on the skill of the endoscopist. The patient's understanding of the procedure and therefore tolerance and co-operation as well as a satisfactory bowel preparation are of major importance.

If colonoscopy is carried out with sedation and/or analgesic cover, the procedure should only take place in an environment where adequate facilities for resuscitation are at hand and any necessary additional medical personnel are available, but one should aim for it to be regarded as an ambulant, outpatient procedure not requiring hospital admission.

Under such circumstances it is important that the patient's psychological preparation should not be overlooked while the bowel preparation is rightly emphasized.

3.1 General preparation

The patient should have the reasons for performing the colonoscopy fully explained and be given an ample description of the technique in understandable terms. While it is reasonable to highlight the potential benefits, the patient should also be informed of the anticipated discomfort associated with both the bowel preparation and the actual procedure.

Whereas the incidence of morbidity or mortality associated with colonoscopy is indeed exceptionally low when performed by an experienced endoscopist, it is wise to inform the patient that, as with any invasive procedure, the risk of complications does exist and has to be weighed against the expected benefits. It is advisable to obtain a signed informed consent which will confirm the patient's understanding and acceptance of the procedure.

Experience has shown that well-informed patients who fully comprehend the implications and circumstances of their colonoscopy show less apprehension and are more tolerant with less anxiety during the examination. Indeed the confidence imparted by the colonoscopist through honest, factual information and firm supportive assurance is essential for a successful colonoscopy.

A proper history should be obtained, including cardiorespiratory conditions and current medications, as well as any adverse reactions to drugs. Any bleeding tendency should be looked for, as colonoscopy may involve biopsy and polypectomy.

3.2 Bowel preparation

The importance of the bowel preparation can hardly be overemphasized. Total inspection of the colon is essential for absolute success and the presence of faecal material can cover or mask a mucosal lesion. Faecal fluid can be sucked out but excess mucus can still obscure vision and at times can be too viscous for suction. Similarly solid faecal lumps will not only totally obstruct vision, but may block the suction channel.

To obtain the best result in bowel preparation, it is essential to assess first the patient's general state of health with due regard for age and any debilitating coexisting illness.

It is important to be aware of the patient's bowel habit so that the preparation may be adjusted to the individual's need. Those suffering from severe constipation will undoubtedly need a more vigorous regime, where the existence of diarrhoea may justify some adjustment although it will not, contrary to some belief, obviate the need for effective bowel preparation.

Colonoscopists throughout the world use a variety of bowel preparations and this fact alone clearly suggests that an ideal regime has not yet been established. Each of the methods practised offer both advantages and disadvantages either to the patient or to the endoscopist.

Whatever bowel preparation regime is recommended the instructions must be in writing and clearly outline each phase of the preparation including explicit advice on diet. The need for adequate fluid and electrolyte intake must be stressed, especially to the elderly. Stress must also be laid on the need to adhere strictly to the instructions, warning the patient of the risk of failure of the examination if the preparation is inadequate. The patient should be asked to report if effective catharsis has not been obtained.

Certain medications should be avoided: iron-containing preparations should be stopped four or five days before endoscopy where aspirin and anticoagulants may only have to be omitted 24–48 hours prior to colonoscopy.

The ideal bowel preparation requires that the colon is entirely free of any faecal matter, or significant amounts of mucus or fluid and there are a variety of methods by which bowel clearance can be achieved. A combination of these are usually incorporated in the standard regimens for colonoscopy.

3.2.1 *Cleansing agents*

(a) *Chemical cathartics*

Most commonly used are castor oil (30–60 ml), sennosides (senna syrup, X-Prep Senokot equivalent to 140 mg of sennosides), bisacodyl (Durolax or Dulcolax) (Classen, 1971; Waye, 1975; Williams and Teague, 1973).

(b) *Osmotic aperients*

Magnesium sulphate (125–250 ml of 25% solution) taken during the day before the examination.

An equivalent amount of magnesium citrate can also be used.

Mannitol 500 ml of 10–20% solution followed by 500–1000 ml water ingested 4–5 hours before the procedure (Waye, 1975; Williams and Teague, 1973).

3.2.2 *Mechanical cleansing*

In recent years the introduction of whole gut irrigation has achieved some popularity by its most effective results. However, the regime demands hospital admission, and adequate space and staff, which in itself places some limitations on its application.

The regime consists of ingestion or instillation through a nasogastric tube (Salem double lumen tube, size 14), of a solution composed of sodium chloride 6.5 g/l, sodium bicarbonate 2.5 g/l and potassium chloride 0.75 g/l at 37°C. Some workers use isotonic saline solution alone. Intramuscular injection of metoclopramide 10 mg helps to eliminate nausea and abdominal discomfort. The administration of a parenteral diuretic (furosemide, Frusemide (Lasix) 40 mg) may be advisable for patients with the potential risk of circulatory decompensation. Prior administration of an osmotic aperient may reduce the volume of irrigation needed. The ingestion or instillation rate is regulated to the maximum tolerated, which is usually about 2 l/h. The patient is seated on a commode and the procedure terminated when the anal effluent is clear.

One must regard the following as contraindications to the above procedure: (1) serious illness or debilitation; (2) aged patients or children; (3) medical conditions requiring salt restriction; (4) impaired renal function; (5) dysphagia; (6) mental disorder; (7) obstructive or inflammatory bowel disease.

Provided the patient is under adequate nursing surveillance, whole gut irrigation is safe and effective (Levy *et al.*, 1976).

In contrast to whole gut irrigation the use of cleansing enemas is universal. The earlier claim for cleansing enemas given the day before colonoscopy is no longer accepted and is regarded to be of little value. Nevertheless, enemas given 1–3 hours prior to the procedure are now routine and some advocate repeated tap water enemas until the return is clear. Others use a single tap water enema of varying volume between 500–1500 ml, while the use of oxiphenisatin (Veripaque 3 g in 1500 ml water), or bisacodyl, or small volume (100 ml) hypertonic saline enemas have also been frequently mentioned. It is claimed that with the oxyphenisatin enema there is no risk of hepatotoxicity, which can occur with oral administration of the compound.

3.2.3 *Dietary regimes*

In addition to cathartics and other cleansing methods various dietary restrictions are usually also advocated. These dietary restrictions frequently require the intake of clear fluids only for 24–48 hours and may even be extended to a low residue diet for a further 24 hours prior to the day on clear fluids. Stress is laid on the advice to increase fluid intake to counteract the inevitable fluid loss with purging.

Bowel cleansing can also be achieved over a period of 3–4 days without any preparation with a non-residue diet (Vivonex). This method can be effective but is limited by cost. Nevertheless its use should be considered in patients where special conditions make the use of powerful cathartics inadvisable.

3.2.4 *Critical assessment of preparation regimes*

The results of bowel preparations have an inverse relationship from the patient's and colonoscopist's point of view. It is clear that the more drastic the cleansing procedure, the greater the endoscopist's satisfaction but the greater the patient's discomfort during the preparation period (Downing *et al.*, 1979).

The divergent interest of the active and passive protagonists will demand some compromise and even at best there will be at least a 10% poor result.

Aperients such as castor oil, senna and magnesium salts if given in doses to produce purging are often distasteful to ingest and may produce troublesome cramping abdominal pain. Mannitol if taken chilled and flavoured with some lemon or lime juice is more acceptable but may also cause some nausea or vomiting. This can be overcome by giving oral metoclopromide 10–20 mg. The drawback of the mannitol preparation is the frequent presence of excessive fluid in the colon. Recently an intracolonic explosion has been reported during the application of diathermy current (Bigard, Gaucher and Lassalle, 1979) following preparation with Mannitol.

Hydrogen and methane, two explosive gases, may, under certain conditions be present in combustible concentrations in the colon. Such situations present a risk during electrocautery procedures.

The combined effect of a clear fluid diet, effective purging, the use of enemata and insufflation of air during colonoscopic examination will undoubtedly eliminate the risk of an explosion occurring within the bowel due to a spark emitted during the use of diathermy. The risk of explosion, nevertheless, however low, may exist when using mannitol, an oligosaccharide, the bacterial degradation of which can produce a high concentration of hydrogen and methane. Recently, Taylor and Keighley (1981) have shown that the use of metronidazole and tetracycline given together orally for 48 hours before mannitol reduces the viable bacterial count to very low levels with a concomitant reduction of both hydrogen and methane to insignificant levels. Should mannitol be used for bowel preparation, the insufflation of CO_2 gas prior to the use of diathermy is recommended but the routine use of CO_2 gas insufflation in a well-prepared patient seems unnecessary (Bigard, Gaucher and Lassalle, 1979; Bond and Levitt, 1979; Ragins, Shinya and Wolff, 1974).

All the bowel cleansing regimes so far mentioned combine the use of purgation, dietary change and the administration of one or more enemas and involve the patient in one to three days of preparation with its associated discomfort.

From the point of view of the colonoscopist the above methods of preparation are eminently successful provided the patient strictly adheres to the regime but prior to the colonoscopy there is no means to assess the patient's compliance with the instructions. Undoubtedly some of the preparation failures are due to a lack of patient co-operation.

The use of whole gut irrigation certainly overcomes any problems caused by lack of co-operation by the patient over diet or taking purgatives and thus eliminates any active involvement in preparation prior to the day of the examination, but does require hospital admission. From the patient's point of view it may be associated with the discomfort of nasogastric intubation, sitting on a commode over a long period of time and the boredom associated with this procedure. The risk of overloading the circulation and fluid retention limits its use in all instances where this could constitute a hazard. Its application demands special facilities and staffing in the hospital environment and could not be applied universally where many colonoscopies are undertaken in a single session.

The no-residue diet may be reasonably acceptable to the patient but is relatively expensive and may not on its own offer the degree of cleansing that one would like to achieve.

3.2.5 *Recommendations for routine bowel preparation*

Intake of oral iron preparations should be omitted for five days before colonoscopy; aspirin and anticoagulants should be stopped during the preparation period. The second night before the procedure a laxative such as two tablets of Senokot or bisacodyl should be taken.

On the day before the examination the intake of clear fluids only is permitted. Instructions should specify that at least 200–250 ml of oral fluids should be consumed hourly consisting of water, black tea or coffee; clear soups, e.g. beef tea, 'stock cube' soups, strained broth; cordials, e.g. orange, lemon and glucose added to the drinks is useful; soft drinks, e.g. lemonade, ginger ale, non-alcoholic apple cider; strained fruit juices, e.g. orange, grapefruit, apple; or jelly.

The consumption of boiled sweets and lollies, e.g. barley sugar, is encouraged.

During the afternoon or evening of the day preceding the colonoscopy, castor oil 30 ml is taken. This may be substituted by magnesium sulphate 125 ml (or preferably citrate 25% solution) or Sennokot, four tablets. Ample fluid intake is encouraged until the examination is imminent (Burbige, Bourke and Tarder, 1978).

The patient is warned to expect some abdominal rumbling, followed by extremely loose bowel actions within 2–3 hours. The endoscopist should be advised before the procedure if this expected response has not occurred.

Routinely, 1–2 hours before the procedure a warm (37°C) tap water enema of 1500 ml volume is given. If the response to the aperients seems inadequate, the enema may have to be repeated until a clear return is obtained.

The preparation regime which has been described will produce satisfactory results in the majority of patients.

3.2.6 *Special preparations*

Chronic constipation
For those suffering from chronic constipation it is advisable to extend the clear fluid intake to include a second day as well as to double the

dose of castor oil, magnesium salt or senna preparation, whichever is selected.

Chronic diarrhoea
Patients presenting with frank diarrhoea should reduce the dose of purgative and it helps then to substitute an extra day of clear fluid. Should diarrhoea be a major problem the whole gut irrigation regime may be preferable to the use of strong purgatives.

Diverticulosis
In addition to the routine preparation the period of clear fluids should be extended to 48 hours and two enemas should be given 3 and 1 hour before the procedure because cleansing of the diverticular segment, with impacted faecal matter protruding from the diverticular openings, can be exceedingly difficult.

Colostomy
Preparation is often surprisingly difficult and extra attention as in chronic constipation is required. These patients may also be better served by whole gut irrigation and with a catheter inserted into the colostomy, during the preparation period.

Inflammatory bowel disease
In cases of chronic inflammatory bowel disease the routine regime is recommended.

For those with moderately active disease the dose of purgatives should be reduced and the dietary restrictions prolonged as previously suggested for patients with diarrhoea (Williams and Waye, 1978).

Finally patients with more than three or four loose bowel motions daily may be best prepared by no-residue diet (Vivonex) for 3–4 days followed by an enema 1–2 hours before colonoscopy.

Colonic obstruction
Bowel preparation in these patients is especially difficult and may be hazardous. Strong purgation is contraindicated. The best results are probably obtained by the combined use of a no-residue diet and repeated tap water enemas.

3.2.7 Fibre sigmoidoscopy

In situations where an examination of the left side of the colon alone is contemplated, and time is of the essence, the examination can be undertaken with reasonable expectations of a clean colon by using only 200 ml of a disposable hypertonic enema (e.g. Traval, Klyx etc., ready-to-use enema containing sodium dihydrogen phosphate 13.9 g, disodium hydrogen phosphate 3.18 g, and benzoic acid 0.1 g/100 ml).

3.3 Conclusion

It is clear from the foregoing discussion that there is no ideal, single, clear cut bowel preparation regime. The best results are obtained if the basic procedure is adjusted to the needs of each individual patient. With due attention the risk of failure due to poor bowel preparation can be kept very low indeed.

References

Bigard, M., Gaucher, P. and Lassalle, C. (1979), Fatal colonic explosion during colonoscopic polypectomy. *Gastroenterology*, **77**, 1307–10.

Bond, J. H. and Levitt, M. D. (1979), Colonic gas explosion – is a fire extinguisher necessary? *Gastroenterology*, **77**, 1349–50.

Burbige, E. J., Bourke, E. and Tarder, G. (1978), Effect of preparation for colonoscopy on fluid and electrolyte balance. *Gastrointest. Endosc.*, **24**, 286–7.

Classen, M. (1971), Progress report – fibre-endoscopy of the intestine. *Gut*, **12**, 330–8.

Downing, R. *et al.* (1979), Whole gut irrigation; a survey of patient opinion. *Br. J. Surg.*, **66**, 201–2.

Levy, A. G. *et al.* (1976), Saline lavage: a rapid, effective, and acceptable method for cleansing the gastrointestinal tract. *Gastroenterology*, **70**, 157–61.

Taylor, E. W. and Keighley, M. R. B. (1981), The explosive potential of colonic gas with three bowel preparation regimes. *Gastroenterology*, in press.

Waye, J. D. (1975), Colonoscopy: a clinical review. *Mt Sinai J. Med.*, **42**, 1–33.

Williams, C. B. and Teague, R. H. (1973), Progress report – colonoscopy. *Gut*, **14**, 990–1003.

Williams, C. B. and Waye, J. D. (1978), Colonoscopy in inflammatory bowel disease. *Clinics Gastroen.*, **7**, 701–17.

Ragins, H., Shinya, H. and Wolff, W. (1974), The explosive potential of colonic gas during colonoscopic electrosurgical polypectomy. *Surgery Gynec. Obstet.*, **138**, 554–6.

CHAPTER FOUR

The Endoscopy Suite

YOSHIHIRO SAKAI

A wide range of locations is currently used by clinicians performing colonoscopy. An examination which uses a fully prepared endoscopy suite is generally the most efficient and the most satisfactory for both the patient and the examiner (Salmon, 1974). The well-equipped endoscopy unit will be purpose-designed and built, with fluoroscopy and television monitoring, although the examination may also be performed at the patient's bedside. In between these two extremes a wide range of acceptable endoscopic locations is used which includes the specialist's consulting room, an operating room for intra-operative colonoscopy, and the X-ray department. In any hospital setting, a specific area should be designated for colonoscopy and, ideally, the instruments and accessories should be stored at that location. Transportation of these delicate instruments is often associated with damage and shortens the useful life of the instruments. Replacement of a carelessly damaged instrument is wasteful in terms of both time and money. It is not recommended that the routine examination be performed in an operating theatre, since faecal contamination of the area may occur. Facilities which are used for colonoscopy may also be used for upper gastrointestinal endoscopic procedures.

4.1 The colonoscopy room (Fig. 4.1)

The minimum requirements for a colonoscopy room include space for an examination table, an adequate area for the endoscopy team and for the light source, suction pump and instruments. The minimum floor space which is required is 5 m × 4 m and in general, the room should be slightly more than five times the area of the endoscopy table but the endoscopy room should not be too large, or efficiency will be wasted by needless and repetitive walking to obtain the necessary accessories and equipment during the procedure. Consequently, the siting of equipment becomes of considerable importance for ease of operation by both the endoscopist and the ancillary staff. However, with the continued development of both instruments and accessories,

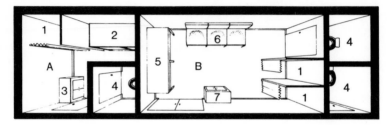

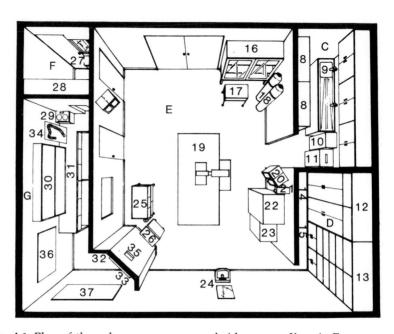

Fig. 4.1 Plan of the colonoscopy room and side rooms. *Key*: A: Enema room; B: waiting room; C: cleansing room; D: storage room for endoscopy and accessories; E: examination room; F: reception; G: discussion room; 1. dressing area; 2. bed for enema; 3. medicine cabinet; 4. lavatory; 5. stretcher; 6. chairs; 7. locker for patient; 8. linen cabinet; 9. sink; 10. suction pump; 11. trash can; 12. cabinet for storage of colonoscopes; 13. cabinet for storage of accessories; 14. trolley storage area; 15. light source storage area; 16. medicine cabinet; 17. trolley for nursing staff; 18. O_2 gas cylinder; 19. X-ray table; 20. TV monitor; 21. TV camera; 22. high voltage X-ray transformer; 23. endoscopy TV transformer; 24. wash stand; 25. trolley including suction pump and coagulator; 26. light source; 27. reception counter; 28. cabinet for papers; 29. tape recorder; 30. X-ray viewing box; 31. table; 32. X-ray film storage; 33. X-ray control table; 34. model of the colon; 35. observation window; 36. white board; 37. panelled pictures and figures. The following

increasing space is required and forward planning should anticipate possible changes in layout. Additional space is also desirable to accommodate any observers, especially doctors or nurses in training who are frequently present whenever colonoscopy is being performed.

4.2 Colonoscopy team position (Fig. 4.2)

4.2.1 *Two-person technique*

During the description of this technique, it will be assumed that the patient is examined in the supine position. With a two-person team for the performance of colonoscopy, the examiner stands at the foot of the patient (Sakai 1977). The space required by the examiner is relatively small, since the examiner concentrates on manoeuvring the tip deflection of the colonoscope and performing endoscopic observation, while the second member of the endoscopy team controls the X-ray equipment, insertion, withdrawal and rotation of the colonoscope, as advised by the examiner. The assistant also inserts a stiffening tube, if one is to be used during the examination. The position of the assistant is beside the patient, on the patient's right-hand side (with the patient supine), since the C-arm of the X-ray apparatus is on the opposite side of the table. The space required by the assistant is larger than that for the examiner since, during a two-team examination, the assistant must move from the examination table to various instruments and accessories.

4.2.2 *One-person technique*

During the description of this technique, the patient is examined in the left lateral position. The examiner stands behind the patient near the buttocks. The endoscopic nurse/assistant is positioned on the other side of the examination table opposite the examiner. This position permits the assistant to observe and monitor the patient, as well as to pass the necessary accessory equipment to the examiner.

---

requirements for the endoscopy room should be observed: (a) permanent area should be designated; (b) minimum floor space of 5 m × 4 m; (c) soft green colour; (d) adequate suction mandatory; (e) resuscitation equipment available; (f) lavatory facilities adjacent.

Colonoscopy examination table. (a) Flat surface necessary; (b) adjustable to examiner's midthigh level; (c) no necessity for tilting; (d) fluoroscopy table may be used.

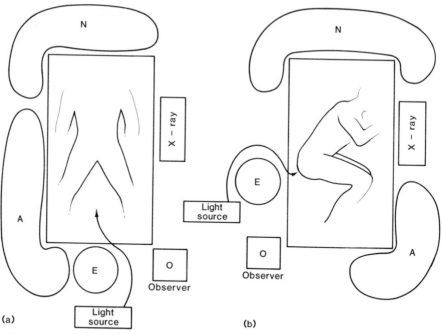

Fig. 4.2 The position of the colonoscopy team in two-man method (a) and in one-man method (b) during the procedure. *Key*: E, examiner; A, assistant; O, observer; N, nursing staff; P, clear area for the patient's passageway.

4.2.3 *Nurse*

The position of the nurse is at the head of the table during the two-person technique to observe the patient's condition during examination, and across the table from the examiner in the one-person technique. Within easy reach of the nurse should be the resuscitation equipment, including a resuscitation bag (Ambu-bag) and oxygen, as well as any medications which are likely to be used during the endoscopic procedure. The territory of the nurse should not overlap that of the examiner and ideally, access to the waiting and cleansing rooms should be close to the nursing position.

4.2.4 *Observers*

The presence of observers in the examination room can often complicate matters. They are best positioned at the foot of the patient to the right of the examiner when a two-person technique is used. In that position, they can easily observe the examiner and the assistant, as well as the patient's reaction, fluoroscopic findings (if X-ray screening is used during the examination), and the endoscopic findings. If a one-person technique is used, the observer is positioned to the examiner's left, behind the patient's shoulders. When the teaching attachment is connected to the colonoscope, only one observer at a time can see the intraluminal view, and if many observers are present, they must either share the teaching attachment, or view the examination on an endoscopic television system which can be the best answer to the teaching problem. However, factors such as the size and price of the equipment, as well as the quality of the television picture, must be considered. When both endoscopic closed-circuit television (CCTV) and X-ray television monitoring are available, observers may remain in an adjacent teaching or conference room away from the patient. In a modern teaching hospital, it is possible with these facilities to decrease the number of observers in the examination room and achieve a quieter and more peaceful procedure. Under the most ideal circumstances, a second conventional TV camera placed in the examination room can transmit detailed views of the intubation and handling techniques to observers in the teaching room.

4.3 Equipment

A passageway for moving the patient in and out of the endoscopy suite must be kept clear of light sources, instruments, TV monitors and connecting leads. There are no tables designed exclusively for colonoscopy, and it is of course possible to perform the procedure using the patient's bed, but an examination table will be helpful when many patients are examined by the same endoscopist. The table should be adjustable in height and set to the examiner's hip level, about 2 m in length, and 60–70 cm in width. There is no need to tilt the table during colonoscopy, and a stationary table is entirely adequate. Since the performance of colonoscopy is completely different from that of rigid proctosigmoidoscopy, the knee-chest position and its modifications are not recommended. A desirable feature for an examination table is firmness of the patient platform, since a soft mattress or a hammock-type trolley may permit the patient to slide away from the examiner during the procedure which can create difficulty with manipulation of the endoscope shaft.

The ideal table for colonoscopy should allow the examiner to use X-ray fluoroscopy to identify the configuration and position of the colonoscope and many colonoscopists choose to use an X-ray table. Unfortunately, accessories on the conventional X-ray table may interfere with the manipulative procedures required during colonoscopy, and a purpose-built table and screening unit is desirable where a mobile X-ray C-arm can be inserted under the examination table (Fig. 4.3). However, positioning such equipment may be cumbersome, and the field of view is often limited.

The light source should be positioned behind the examiner, either to the left or right, depending on the examiner's preference. When a two-person colonoscopy team performs the procedure, a trolley with all the necessary ancillary equipment should be within easy reach of the assistant, who normally handles the shaft of the instrument. During the one-person technique, when the endoscopist performs both the endoscopic observation, and manipulates the shaft of the instrument, an accessory trolley should be within reach of the assistant, who can provide the biopsy forceps, snares etc., upon request.

The endoscopy unit should be planned so that, if only one light source is available in the endoscopy unit, it should be strategically situated so that it may also be used to supply air and water/washing

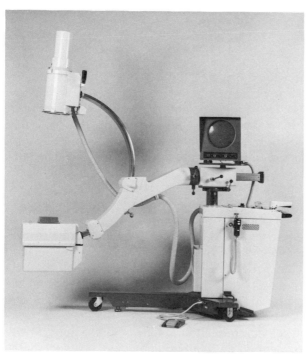

Fig. 4.3 Portable X-ray equipment with TV monitor (Model SX-6, Toshiba).

facilities when the assistant is cleaning the endoscope at the end of the procedure. Water and cleaning solutions may be brought in buckets to the instrument and light source, or the instrument and light source should be on a trolley so that they can be easily moved to the sink area.

4.3.1 *Fluoroscopy apparatus*

It is possible to perform colonoscopy without fluoroscopy when the examiner has considerable experience (Chapter 9). However, as discussed, all examinations can be easily conducted on an X-ray table in the fully equipped endoscopy suite. During fluoroscopy, protection from radiation exposure is a problem for the patient, the examiner and the ancillary personnel, as well as the colonoscope itself. Recent improvements in the design and construction of colonoscopes have resulted in easier insertion of the instrument, and there is less reliance on fluoroscopy. Consequently, now that the colonoscope is subjected to less radiation exposure, there is less 'yellowing' of the glass fibres of the instrument and radiation to the endoscopist and his team is also minimized. Although the examiner must attempt to keep exposure to a minimum, some patients with very complex bowel configurations may still require fluoroscopy (Chapter 8). Improvements in the sensitivity of X-ray equipment have also resulted in reduced radiation exposure when compared to the conventional type of fluoroscopic equipment. X-ray television systems, combining intermittent exposure with a videodisc to retain the image, can further reduce the X-ray exposure. This equipment is known as the X-ray exposure decreasing system (Sakai, 1974).

A radiographic control unit should be present in the examination room or in the adjacent conference room. Although it is unusual to need a plain X-ray during colonoscopy, it may be required and the facility should be readily available.

4.3.2 *Ventilation and lighting*

A pleasant ambient atmosphere is an important consideration for the comfort of both the patient and the colonoscopy team. A forced ventilation system is desirable, since colonoscopy is usually performed in a small confined space and odours associated with a poorly prepared bowel may linger in a confined space for several hours. After several examinations, of even well-prepared patients, there may be an unpleasant odour made worse by poor ventilation. A useful trick is to add a few drops of oil of peppermint to the collection bottle of the suction pump or into the water bottle attached to the light source so that this can help to mask any unpleasant smells (Williams and Teague, 1973). Air conditioning may be helpful to dissipate the considerable heat generated by the light source, accessories, the endoscopy team and other occupants of the room.

It should be possible to vary the intensity of illumination of the endoscopy room. Observation of the patient is required during the entire endoscopic examination, especially if any medication has been used which may depress respiration. The examination is, therefore, not performed in a darkened room, even when X-ray screening is used. It is, however, preferable during the examination to have the room slightly darkened to help the endoscopist to see transmitted light through the abdominal wall. The room lights should be turned up when biopsies and operative manoeuvres are being performed, to help the assistant organize snares for polypectomy or change settings on the diathermy unit, etc. A greenish colour is recommended for the endoscopy room because muted green colour tends to decrease any chance of ocular exhaustion of the examiner, who may spend long hours concentrating on very bright images.

4.3.3 *Ancillary equipment in the examination room*

A medication cabinet is necessary, which should contain injectable medications, needles, syringes, an emergency kit, resuscitation breathing equipment, etc. Although resuscitation is rarely necessary during an endoscopic examination, the apparatus should be readily available during every endoscopic procedure. Because the majority of complications which occur during colonoscopy are related to sedative medications which cause respiratory depression, cardiorespiratory support may be necessary until the resuscitation team arrives to deal with the emergency situation.

As much equipment as possible should be suspended from the ceiling, since the light sources and other equipment in the room may require many electrical wires and much tubing on the floor. Unless electrical sockets are located close to major items of equipment, the number of wires, etc. may create difficulty in moving apparatus, as well as constitute a hazard to personnel and patients. The fluoroscopy screen, TV monitor, TV camera, etc. may all be suspended from the ceiling.

4.4 Storage room

Colonoscopic accessories should be stored adjacent to or in the examination room. Frequently, selection of an appropriate colonoscope depends on the conditions found at colonoscopy, the purpose of the procedure, the presence of a stricture, etc., and the endoscope may have to be changed during the examination. If this is required, it is most convenient when the storage cupboard is either close to or in the endoscopy room. Colonoscopes should be stored separately from upper gastrointestinal instruments, and their accessories stored accordingly.

The storage space should be large enough to accommodate various light sources, suction pumps, diathermy units, and the trolleys used during examination.

4.5 Dictating/conference room

Following the endoscopic procedure, the endoscopist will wish to dictate a report, talk to the referring physician on the telephone, or discuss the case with any observers. It is best not to do this in the presence of the patient, and a separate room is essential. The conference room, which is indispensable for educational purposes, is also useful for reviewing the X-rays and the patient's notes before the procedure and conducting any discussions away from the patient. A lead-glass window and two-way (magic) mirror between the conference and examination rooms is recommended to enable observers to watch the procedure.

In the conference room, an X-ray viewing box is required, preferably one which is capable of taking 8–10 X-ray films simultaneously. A drawing board with markers or chalk is most helpful, and, for teaching purposes, a model of the bowel and anatomical charts which explain the techniques and demonstrate endoscopic findings. Video-tapes, tape-slide lectures and a library are also invaluable for teaching purposes. Various office supplies and forms should be kept in this room, as well as recording equipment for dictation of reports and letters (Cotton and Williams, 1980).

4.6 Cleaning room

An essential procedure before and after every endoscopic examination is the cleaning of equipment. Automatic washing machines have been developed but are not completely effective, and therefore, the assistant must wash the instruments by hand. Although the colonoscope is flexible, it should be bent as little as possible. If the endoscope is bent, the angulations should be gentle, with a large loop, and since the working length of a long colonoscope is 170–180 cm, a sink at least 1.5 m in length is required to accept the entire length of the contaminated insertion tube. It should be possible to have this in the endoscopy room, but the best design is to have a separate room. Cupboards in this room can also be used to store the patients' examination gowns, sheets, cleaning equipment, basins, swabs, etc. and solutions which are necessary for the cleansing procedures.

4.7 Waiting/recovery room and lavatory

The size of the waiting room depends on the anticipated number of cases which the unit will endoscope each day, but it should be able to accommodate at least three patients. Both inpatients and out-patients for colonoscopy should be escorted to the waiting room by a receptionist. The waiting room may serve as a dressing area and should have sufficient space for patients who are transferred by stretcher or wheelchair from their hospital beds. A lavatory close to the waiting room is essential for bowel evacuation in patients who have had recent enemas or purgation in preparation for the examination. If an enema or fluid wash-out is to be performed in the endoscopy area, a separate room with another lavatory is essential. The waiting room should be separate from the colonoscopy room and, ideally, should be on the other side of the corridor to reduce the possibility of a waiting patient hearing any sounds of discomfort from a patient undergoing colonoscopy. The decor of the waiting room should be similar to that of the colonoscopy room to allow the patient to adapt easily to the surroundings. For ambulatory patients, a separate recovery room should be available for the patient to rest until the effect of medication has worn off and this area may also be used for hospital patients to recover until transportation to their hospital ward is arranged.

4.8 Secretarial support

The presence of a receptionist/secretary can greatly increase the efficiency of an endoscopy unit and the office should be located adjacent to the dictation/conference room. The receptionist/secretary should make appointments for examinations, explain the preparation to the patient, organize for the notes and X-rays to accompany the patient, collect data from the endoscopies performed, and prepare reports for the medical records and referring clinicians.

Endoscopy films and examination reports should be kept in the receptionist's room and separate from the examination area. All the reports and endoscopic data need to be filed and should be carefully preserved and the endoscopy area should be clean and free of collections of report forms, charts, paperwork, etc.

4.9 Summary

A designated area for the performance of colonoscopy is essential in any hospital where endoscopy is performed. An ideal purpose-designed unit has been described, but the siting of equipment will differ between various endoscopy teams and the variations in techniques which they use. An experienced colonoscopist should be consulted prior to the design of any endoscopic facility to advise on the individual requirements of the particular hospital and the likely future demands which may be made on the endoscopy unit and changes which may be required as a consequence of advances in both diagnostic and therapeutic colonoscopic procedures.

Acknowledgement

Grateful acknowledgement is made to Mr M. Hata and Miss K. Kobayashi for their drawing the sketch of the colonoscopy room.

References

Cotton, P. B. and Williams, C. B. (1980), The Endoscopy Unit; Documentation and teaching, In: *Practical Gastrointestinal Endoscopy*, Blackwell Scientific Publications, Oxford.

Sakai, Y. (1974), Further progress in colonoscopy, *Gastrointest. Endosc.*, **20**, 143–7.

Sakai, Y. (1977), Current concepts concerning colonoscopy, *Mater. Med. Polona*, **30**, 65–69.

Salmon, P. R. (1974), *Fiber-optic Endoscopy*, Pitman Medical Publishing Co. Ltd, London.

Williams, C. B. and Teague, R. H. (1973), Colonoscopy, *Gut*, **14**, 990–1003.

CHAPTER FIVE

Instrumentation and Disinfection

JACK A. VENNES

Instruments which are well designed and working flawlessly cannot substitute for the skills of the endoscopist but do contribute to the successful result of any colonoscopy. Colonoscopes are built to contend with the unique features of the large bowel which is longer, has sharper turns and is not as fixed as the upper intestinal tract.

A large number of instruments are currently available for colonoscopy. Although initial cost is an important consideration, only minor differences exist between instruments. Length of the endoscope is not an economic consideration, as the cost for manufacture of a 160-cm instrument is approximately the same as that of a 180-cm model. The longer-range costs of service will be discussed.

5.1 Length

Total intubation of the colon should be the goal of any colonoscopy. This will be achieved with the highest frequency by the use of a long colonoscope. The difference between an instrument length of 165 or 185 cm is not important, but the ability to reach the caecum decreases with shorter instruments, although there has been a report of total intubation in 90% of patients using the 140-cm colonoscope (Gulbis and Lammens, 1980). Most endoscopists do not expect to visualize the ileocaecal valve with a 110-cm instrument, although some may achieve this regularly. During examinations with the intermediate or short-length colonoscopes, the endoscopist uses most of the available shaft during intubation, requiring close approximation of the endoscopist to the patient's buttocks. Although this technique is feasible, instrument torque must be accomplished by turning the head of the instrument, together with the head and trunk of the endoscopist to keep the image in proper spatial alignment. These manoeuvres are rarely necessary with the long colonoscopes, since a sufficient portion of shaft is available between the rectum and the eyepiece to absorb rotational torque applied to the insertion tube, so that the instrument control head does not need to be similarly rotated. The extra length of the long colonoscope does not demand its total insertion, and the amount of the shaft remaining outside the patient can be easily managed by the endoscopist.

5.2 Diameter

The adult rectum readily accepts a rigid sigmoidoscope introduced with an obturator. However, the anal sphincter muscles will not permit entry of the blunt tip of the metal tube itself. Similarly, the diameter of a flexible colonoscope is not limited by the size of the colon but by the width accepted by the anus in the absence of an introducer. All colonoscopes currently available can be accommodated by the adult colon, and the present technology does not require any increase in diameter. As optical engineering advances, colonoscopes are becoming thinner and less bulky. Concomitant with this decrease in calibre is a change in the shaft flexibility and the transmission of forces around colon loops (variable vectoring). The insertion tube must be flexible enough to negotiate all the colon bends without patient discomfort, yet have sufficient resistance to deformation, so that a directional force applied by the operator's hand is transmitted to the flexible controllable tip. The flexible tube wastes energy with each curve, tending to direct more force straight ahead and less around each bend. If the insertion tube is too rigid (and perhaps too thick), patient discomfort results because curves in the colon are stretched during instrument advance to conform to the course of the colonoscope. Conversely, if the shaft is too flexible, directional force from the operator's hand is inefficiently transmitted to the scope tip, which results in coiling rather than forward motion. Even though various instruments have inherent flexibility characteristics, individual touch and technique are also important. Some examiners may do a more comfortable, expeditious colonoscopy with a more rigid scope, while others obtain similar results with a thinner more pliant shaft. Most manufacturers build progressive proximal stiffness into the insertion tube for better transmission of forward force to the tip. This aims to achieve less coiling in the sigmoid region while maintaining the desired flexibility of the forward sections.

5.3 Tip flexion

There is variability in maximal tip flexion between colonoscopes of the various manufacturers, although all flex in one vertical plane to at least $180°$ when outside the colon. The degree of tip deflection may be markedly attenuated when the scope has been inserted deep in the colon

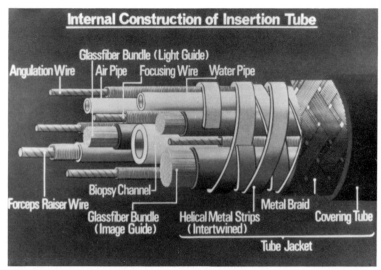

Fig. 5.1 Contents and construction of a typical endoscope insertion tube. The conduits through which precisely adjusted control wires pass are usually the structures permanently damaged with use or abuse. The helical metal strips result in a balance between flexibility and transmission of rotational (torque) control. Focusing control wire is not part of colonoscope controls.

after negotiating several bends. Deflection wires are stretched at each scope bend; wire stresses, which are insignificant in a straight instrument, increase markedly after four to five turns. Broken and stretched control wires (or distortion of the wire conduits) have been a major cause of colonoscope repairs (Fig. 5.1). Conscious efforts to straighten the instrument must be made during insertion, since cable damage is reduced, and complete tip deflection is restored as loops are removed.

5.4 Rotational (torque) stability

Rotation about the axis is another feature of colonoscope control. During colonoscopy, the insertion tube is held near the anus and rotated until the desired image occurs. Torque integrity, or the ability to transmit rotational force from the rectum to the tip around several bends, is a quality built into the instrument design. This desirable characteristic is obtained by a spiralled flat wire reinforcement of the insertion tube. Because of the configuration of this coil, a slight clockwise torque of the shaft during advancement tends to stiffen the scope and resists the inherent tendency of the straight colonoscope to bend.

5.5 Visual image

The angle of view, or width of the visual field, has been enlarged in the newer endoscopes. Although more of the colon can be seen, some negative features occur, as with any wide-angle lens: decreased illumination with a tendency to spherical aberration, image distortion, and loss of ability to judge the depth of field may all occur. Depth distortion becomes important when attempting to place precisely a snare over a polyp or to biopsy a lesion. A wide view, however, reduces the blind areas beyond sharp curves and always facilitates identification of the lumen.

The focal distance of lens systems used in colonoscopes is fixed and short, ensuring high quality of close-up viewing. The correlated depth of field, as individually determined by manufacturers, varies from 3–120 mm from the tip. Within these limits, the closely approximated lines on a test chart are separable and in acceptable focus. Variations of depth of field between instruments are minor, however. There is a direct relation between the angle of view and depth of visual field. The wide-angle lens presently used in colonoscopes has a wide and deep field; although a fish-eye type of distortion is not noted clinically, accessories such as snares may appear distortedly large when close and small when farther away. A magnification lens increases the image size 10–12 times, with a nearly life-size view at about 2 cm from the distal lens. Zoom lenses have been tested, but there appears to be no need for this optically complex addition. Optical magnifiers have been used to enlarge the proximal eyepiece image, but this does not result in a magnified mucosal view, nor in an altered visual field. All instruments have a focusing ring which offers the imperfect human eye the addition of either minus or plus diopters to bring the image into focus.

5.6 Photography

Good quality colonoscopic photographs can be an important part of a clinical record and are crucial to endoscopic learning. Serial observations of inflammatory bowel disease, and appraisal of benign versus malignant characteristics of polypoid lesions, or visual documentation of polyps prior to removal are clinical examples of the desirability for photographic records. The illuminated colonic image is focused through a series of lenses on to the tip of the fibre bundle (Fig. 5.2). The image is transmitted to the proximal end of the fibre bundle, and viewing only requires a magnifying lens. The illuminated image is focused on the film plane in some instruments by physically moving lenses in the eyepiece with a mechanism coupled to the attachment

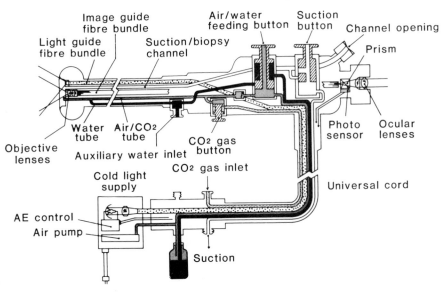

Fig. 5.2 Schematic cutaway diagram of a fibreoptic colonoscope. Both mechanics and function are illustrated.

and rotation of a camera adapter. In this system no camera lens is needed, since the endoscope eyepiece is used to focus the image correctly. Another method is to attach a standard camera and lens in front of the endoscope lens.

Automatic controls routinely correct for exposure within the limits of the film. In the head of some endoscopes, the light beam is split by a small prism. The shutter is in the light source, and shutter speed is dictated by the amount of light delivered to a photocell by the beam splitter and varies in response to image illumination. Using an automated exposure system, the camera shutter is set open at 1/4 s, while the automated shutter of the light source determines the proper speed for correct exposure. When attempting to photograph a lesion far from the colonoscope tip, illumination may be insufficient for proper exposure, since the amount of light reaching the object diminishes in proportion to the square of the distance from the source. Even the slowest shutter speeds may result in a dark picture, in spite of the manual Exposure Index Controls that permit the operator some adjustment.

Successful endoscopic photography requires attention to some very practical considerations. The distal cover glass must be clean before inserting the scope and must be flushed as needed. The film must match the light source; tungsten film should be used with tungsten filament lights, and daylight film with xenon light. A sharper picture may result if the colonic image is still – for example, have the patient momentarily stop breathing, choose a moment when motility is absent, etc.

Different conditions pertain to obtaining satisfactory videotape or 16-mm movie imaging, since the film used is slower, and light requirements change widely and quickly when filming a moving object. Available light must, therefore, automatically change rapidly to maintain a constantly illuminated picture (this is not required during routine endoscopy, since the human eye adjusts instantaneously to variations of light in the mid-ranges). This requires a photocell within the camera system or a beam-splitter with continuous feedback to the light source for movement of an apertured disc in and out of the light beam. As with still photography, video equipment does not function well when attached via a teaching adapter (lecturescope), as the split light beam is of insufficient brightness for imaging. Special beam-splitters or articulated lens systems are available for overcoming some of the coupling problems encountered in a fibreoptic interface system.

Instant development film systems have been an attractive idea for several years, with the promise of supplying an immediate clear colour picture for the patient's record or the referring physician's files. At this time, available film is still too slow to use with available light sources; since the final photographic image is real and not enlarged, much more light is required than for conventional small-image still photography.

5.6.1 *Light sources*

The smaller, least expensive light sources have a filament temperature of 5400 K in the 100-watt tungsten-halogen bulb. Bulb rating in watts varies from 75 to 150, but is an imprecise measurement as the same power passed across a 75 or 100-watt bulb may result in the same visual energy (light), though the 75-watt bulb burns out faster. In the larger xenon sources, light is produced by arcing between electrodes in a glass tube filled with gas mixtures. The resulting light is brighter than that emitted from a tungsten filament, with a whiter (more blue) spectrum resembling daylight, hence, the need for daylight film when photography is to be used with these more expensive machines.

5.7 Electrocautery

Power sources of radio frequency current for use in electrocoagulation will not be covered in any detail in this chapter. Colonoscopic needs are more nearly defined by using a coagulation setting with cutting occurring secondarily. The precise characteristics of 'coagulation' versus 'cutting' current are not completely known but wave form, duty cycles and frequency variations are factors, and the total power delivered is also a determinant of the subsequent tissue effects.

5.8 Accessories

5.8.1 *Biopsy forceps*

The spike-biopsy forceps are useful for impaling mucosa, and prevent the open biopsy forceps from skidding along the colonic wall. The needle-like spike in the middle of the biopsy forceps also assists in tissue orientation once the biopsy has been retrieved.

5.8.2 *Snares*

Variations of basic colonoscopic accessories are offered by each manufacturer. A high degree of individual preference is evident in the choice of snares; it is probable that personal experience and skill with a given snare have more to do with preference than specific or innovative characteristics. Snares are made to open in oval, hexagonal and crescent shapes. In the popular crescent model, with extrusion of the wire, the snare opens asymmetrically by flexion of one side of the wire loop, while the other wire remains straight. Rotatable snares are an attractive idea but require further development. Snares made with braided wire are less stiff and last longer than those with single strands but coarse braiding may lead to the snare embedding in a polyp stalk, especially at low power settings. Wire diameters are properly rather uniform, for making them too thin can result in unpredictable mechanical cutting as the loop is tightened. The amount of energy applied to tissue is a function of the total wire–tissue contact area, which varies directly with the circumference and length of wire in tissue contact. A finer wire will permit tighter encirclement of a polyp stalk with a resulting smaller loop diameter than a thicker wire. If the same power setting is used with both wires, polypectomy will be more quickly accomplished with a fine wire which may not be desirable under special circumstances, such as the thick stalk that tends to bleed with transsection.

5.8.3 *Stiffening tube*

Stiffening tubes are used to maintain the sigmoid in a straight configuration. The differential stiffness of newer colonoscopes has partially obviated the need for such devices.

5.9 Care of endoscopes

5.9.1 *Service*

Maintenance and service of endoscopes determines the clinical usefulness of instruments and their availability. The manufacturers' or agents' ability to offer prompt service and repair may be locally variable. Apart from instrument durability and repair availability, many factors that keep an instrument in service are controlled by the endoscopist and nurse assistant (Chapter 6). The skill and attention to detail in the care of instruments by a well-trained gastrointestinal assistant are of primary importance. If at all possible, an endoscopist or endoscopy unit should work with only one or two assistants and provide for their adequate training, so that the best possible care of patient and instruments will result.

5.9.2 *Cleaning*

Colonoscopes perform their everyday functions in a bacterial world. Pathogenic bacteria are occasionally present in the colon but the frequency is unknown. Methods of cleansing endoscopes vary, and it has been a natural concern that colonoscopes might transmit disease, either bacterial or viral. Fortunately, experience in the first fibreoptic decade has been reassuring. In an unpublished survey of 277 responding American endoscopy units by Pfeiffer and Geenen for the Society of Gastrointestinal Assistants, only seven instances of proven or probable endoscopic disease transmission were reported in both upper and lower examinations. Published case reports have been similarly few and anecdotal (Chmel and Armstrong, 1976). Although this is reassuring, the possibility of disease transmission via the colonoscopes still exists, and disciplined routine cleansing methods are indicated to ensure patient safety.

The need for routine disinfection or sterilization of all colonoscopes has not been demonstrated, given the low incidence of disease transmission. However, in the survey by Pfeiffer and Geenen, the majority of respondents routinely used disinfecting solutions on gastrointestinal endoscopes – chiefly iodophors or glutaraldehyde, – as added precautions. In 1978, guidelines for endoscopic infection control were drawn up by a working party including hospital epidemiologists, infection control specialists, nurses, endoscopists and bacteriologists. They concluded that insufficient data exist regarding infectious complications from endoscopic instruments to make any final recommendations, but they did suggest the following guidelines (Hedrick, 1978):

1. Scrupulous mechanical cleansing of the insertion tube and channels immediately after use.
2. Inspection of equipment for damage at all stages of handling.
3. Disinfection of the insertion tube and channels is desirable. This should be performed with a chemical substance having disinfecting action sufficient to kill all micro-organisms except bacterial spores (the definition of disinfection). Certain iodophors and glutaraldehyde can be used.
4. Adequate rinsing should follow such disinfection.
5. The insertion tube and inner channels should be immediately air-dried after cleaning and prior to storage.
6. Instruments should be stored according to manufacturers' recommendations.
7. Ethylene oxide is not generally practical for fibreoptic endoscopes. If it is used, meticulous cleansing must be accomplished, first, and it must be followed by adequate aeration.
8. Accessories, such as snares, biopsy forceps and cytology brushes, are difficult to clean and disinfect. Following immediate cleansing after use, either steam under pressure or gas (ethylene oxide) sterilization is advisable. Heat treatment should be applied only to accessories, not to fibreoptic devices.
9. Diagnosis of suspected infections, including hepatitis B infections, is not considered a contraindication to endoscopy. Endoscopes are used on patients with both recognized and unrecognized infections and should be cleaned and disinfected in the same manner after each use.

5.9.3 *Cleaning material*

To fulfill the above recommendations, the following equipment is needed:

(a) cotton tip applicators
(b) 4 × 4 in cotton gauze pads
(c) 70% alcohol
(d) cleaning brush and toothbrush
(e) iodophor solutions (Betadine, Hibitane)
(f) glutaraldehyde
(g) suction equipment
(h) soaking basin

5.9.4 *Cleaning procedure*

1. Immediately after endoscopy, suction water through the instrument in the usual manner to remove any loose material.
2. Remove the biopsy port as well as the suction valve (when possible). Using a cotton-tip applicator, vigorously clean the biopsy port, suction port and suction valve.
3. Clean the insertion tube of the instrument with a sponge dampened with Betadine or Hibitane (do *not* put any water-soaked material on control head. Scrub the area of the distal biopsy ports with the toothbrush.
4. Clean the control head with 4×4 in gauze pads sequentially dampened with soap, 70% alcohol and water. A toothbrush dipped in alcohol and shaken can help clean the areas difficult to reach.
5. Clean the biopsy channel by suctioning a mixture of water and disinfectant soap through the channel, then vigorously brush the entire length with the cleaning brush. Rinse again with soapy water. Use a total of 200–400 cc of water for suctioning.
6. Immerse the insertion tube in a solution of 2% activated glutaraldehyde for 5–20 min. Then, suction 1500 cc of clean tap water through the biopsy channel and thoroughly dry it. A manoeuver that greatly reduces bacterial growth (pseudomonas) during storage is the total elimination of moisture in the biopsy channel by air-drying with vacuum or forced air through the channel for 5 min as the final act of the last cleaning of the day.
7. For overnight storage, the instrument should be hung to dry.
8. The need for cleaning the air/water insufflation system has not been established. This can be accomplished by filling the reservoir bottle sequentially with soapy water, disinfectant and water and forcing them through the channel. Air-drying should then be performed.
9. Biopsy forceps are initially mechanically cleansed; then, they may be gas-sterilized and packaged. An alternative is to place them in an ultrasonic washer to loosen any particulate matter (dried blood), following which they may be disinfected and stored. The routine use of steam sterilization for biopsy forceps is possible but dries the internal wire lubrication, with resulting breakage problems. Gas sterilization may require acquisition of additional forceps because of time factors – sterilization takes 4–6 hours, followed by an aeration time of 12 hours if an aerator is used. Gas sterilization is consistent with long life of

forceps, however, colonoscopic snare devices should be routinely mechanically cleansed and disinfected.

Several uncertainties exist regarding the use of disinfecting solutions. Contact time necessary for disinfection should be prolonged if organic soiling remains in a channel after mechanical cleansing. Total and uniform absence of bacteria is not achieved, nor is it probably necessary for patient safety. Viral agents cannot be routinely tested for, but no endoscopic transmission of viral disease has ever been reported. Recommendations vary as to length of disinfection time depending on the studies performed. Skin allergies to glutaraldehyde solutions are an occasional problem.

Soaking the instrument for twenty minutes or more between patients is considered impractical by many. We have just completed a study comparing bacterial colony counts following mechanical cleansing alone or with the addition of 5-, 10- or 20-min glutaraldehyde soaks (Vennes, Gerding and Peterson, unpublished data). There was a slight difference in both parameters (negative cultures or log-units of bacterial growth) between mechanical cleansing alone and mechanical cleansing plus five minutes of glutaraldehyde soaking. There was no significant difference between 5, 10 or 20 min glutaraldehyde soaks. When 5 min of air drying (vacuum or forced air by attached tubing to the distal tip) was added to 5-min glutaraldehyde contact times, 19 of 20 cultures were negative 24–72 hours after hanging the instrument.

5.10 Summary

Major advances in design have occupied the first decade of colonoscopy. Recent changes in instrumentation are minor, with a tendency to reducing the overall diameter, and with an increase in size of the biopsy/suction channel. Endoscopic records are becoming easier to obtain with further development of photography systems, television and video-tape recorders. The possibility of cross-infection remains a concern when using the colonoscope, which performs in a bacteria-laden environment. In spite of the paucity of transmitted infections which have been reported, it is currently suggested that scrupulous mechanical cleansing and disinfection should be carried out to prevent cross-contamination.

References

Chmel, H. and Armstrong, D. (1976), Salmonella Oslo. A focal outbreak in a hospital. *Am. J. Med.*, **60**, 203.

Gulbis, A. and Lammens, P. (1980), The miniaturized colonoscopes and the patient's comfort (Abstract), *4th European Congress of Gastrointestinal Endoscopy* (June), Hamburg, Germay.

Hedrick, E. (1978), Guidelines for cleaning and disinfection of flexible fiberoptic endoscopes (FFE) used in GI endoscopy. *J. Am. Pract. Inf. Control*, **6**, 8–10.

CHAPTER SIX

The Gastrointestinal Assistant

BRIAN WRIGHT and ANNA M. RICOMA

The management of a safe, successful and efficient endoscopy unit is largely the responsibility of the chief nurse and a well-trained staff of gastrointestinal assistants and ancillary personnel all working toward the common goal of excellent and safe patient care. The endoscopy nurse plays a critical role in the total care of the patient before, during and after endoscopy (Banks, 1980). This care begins in the patient's ward, where the endoscopy assistant should ideally visit all in-patients prior to the performance of an endoscopic procedure. Direct patient contact provides reassurance to the patient and a continuity of care when the patient once again meets the assistant in the endoscopy unit. During the patient interview, the endoscopy assistant has the opportunity to explain fully the nature of the examination to the patient and to talk to the floor nursing staff concerning preparation for the procedure. For ambulatory patients, it is a great asset if a nurse from the endoscopy department is available in the out-patient clinic to explain the procedure to the patient, for this can instill confidence and give the patients moral support when they report for colonoscopy (Wright 1980).

The patient coming to endoscopy should be greeted by an atmosphere that is friendly, relaxed and efficient. This will help to alleviate some of the natural anxieties experienced by all patients upon entering a strange and seemingly hostile environment. The assistant must check that all relevant information is available (informed consent, X-ray, letters of referral, nursing check list, an example of which is shown in Fig. 6.1 and other paperwork), and that the preparation has been adequate for the procedure. The patient should be once again reassured and allowed to ask any last-minute questions that may be of concern regarding the procedure, and a repeat explanation of the examination should be offered. Specific inquiry should be directed concerning the patient's history of allergies, previous operations and reactions to drugs.

Only after all preparations have been completed should the patient enter the endoscopy room. Once the patient has assumed the desired

51

Endoscopy Unit
Gastroenterology Department

SISTER IN CHARGE

WARD . . . .

M R
MRS . . . .　has been booked for Colonoscopy on
MISS

. . . . 　at　. . . . .

NURSING CHECK LIST

I certify that the following have been carried out:　　　　　　*Please Tick*

1. One week before stop iron tablets

2. Two days before Low Residue Diet

3. Day before Fluid Diet (no milk). Senokot 4 tablets at 1800

4. Day of Colonoscopy 1 Litre 10% Mannitol to drink between 0700 - 0800
   followed by 1 Litre Water to drink

5. Patient starved from 0800 (except diabetic patients)

6. Identification label attached to patient

7. Dentures and /or Contact Lenses removed

8. Transport and Porters arranged

9. Patient dressed in Operating Gown

To accompany patient:

1. Notes with SIGNED consent form (colonoscopy and polypectomy)

2. X-rays (Barium Enema)

3. Nursing Check List

Patient should be advised not to
drive a car
return to work　　　　　　　　　　　　　　　　　} for 24 hours
operate any machinery (kitchen equipment included)
not to drink alcohol

Signature . . . .

Fig. 6.1 An example of a nursing check list which should accompany the patient.

position on the table or trolley, a safety belt should be placed around the patient, or side-rails should be raised on the side opposite the physician.

During the procedure, while the doctor is engaged in the endoscopic examination, the assistant should monitor the colour, vital signs and overall condition of the patient (Curtis, 1975). Respiratory depression is a sign of over-sedation, and observation of the breathing pattern must be made frequently during the examination. If electrocautery is to be used during the procedure, it is important to ascertain whether the patient has a cardiac pacemaker, since its function may be altered by the passage of electrical current through the patient. Electrical burns may be received by the patient if skin is touching a metal portion of the table, or if the conductive grounding plate is not properly placed.

Throughout the entire examination, the assistant must maintain a reassuring presence for the patient while simultaneously managing the technical aspects of the procedure for the endoscopist. A medical emergency may occur at any time during colonoscopy and is best handled by being completely prepared to cope with unexpected complications at all times.

Following the examination, the patient is taken to the recovery area prior to being returned to the ward or discharged home in the company of a relative or friend. The floor staff require a full report of the patient's condition, the medication used, and notes on appropriate aftercare.

6.1 Standard set-up and check list (Table 6.1)

A complete check of the room and equipment should be performed prior to commencement of any endoscopic procedure. The examination trolley or table is locked in position and covered with absorbent pads. Selection of the desired instrument is made after discussion with the endoscopist, and then attached to the light source with connections for suction and the air/water feed bottle. The instrument should be visually checked for a clear image and for proper function of suction, air and water (Salmon, 1974). The shaft of the colonoscope must be closely observed for cracks or sharp edges that could cause injury to the patient or further damage to the instrument.

Supplies to be used during the endoscopic examination should be placed on the accessory trolley (Fig. 6.2) within working distance of the physician. These include lubricant, 4 × 4 in gauze swabs or paper towels, disposable gloves, loaded camera, teaching attachment, and large pails to accommodate soiled swabs. The jaws of biopsy forceps should be checked for function and a drop of silicone fluid applied to the joint if necessary (Hollanders, 1979).

The endoscopic set-up should include several specimen jars that contain formalin, specimen carriers (lens paper, filter paper or Gelfoam), needles and blank labels. The tray for cytology studies should include a long disposable brush, slide holders, microscope slides, fixa-

Table 6.1 Endoscopy trolley

Major equipment
  Colonoscope
  Light source
  Suction apparatus
  Teaching attachment
General equipment
  Camera
  Containers for biopsy (filled with formalin)
  Needles/toothpicks for removing specimen
  Carrier for mounting specimen (filter paper or Gelfoam)
  Flushing catheter
  Force flushing tube and syringes
  50-ml syringe filled with water
  Examination gloves
  4×4 in gauze swabs
  Lubricating jelly
  Silicone fluid
  Medications
Standard accessories
  Cleaning brush
  Biopsy forceps
  Cytology equipment
    Sheathed brush
    Cytology slides
    Spray fixative
Polypectomy accessories
  Hot biopsy forceps
  Two diathermy snares
  Polyp retriever
  Diathermy equipment
    Cautery unit
    Patient grounding plate
    Foot pedal
  Carbon dioxide cylinder (optional)
Optional equipment
  Stiffening tube
  Methylene blue dye
  Local anaesthetic jelly
Extra Equipment
  Spare films
  Spare light bulbs
  Spare valves
  Back-up endoscope

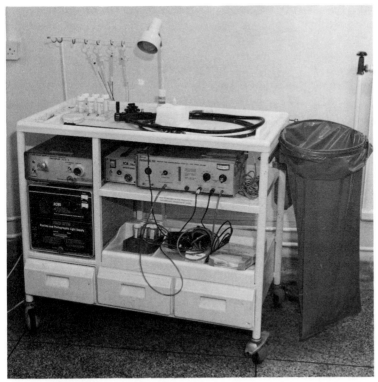

Fig. 6.2 A modified endoscopy trolley prepared for colonoscopy and polypectomy, showing a rack for biopsy forceps, etc., spotlight, waste disposal bag with a carbon dioxide cylinder located behind it.

tive spray and a vial with 1 cm^3 50% alcohol. Two 50-cc syringes and a proper adapter (14 Angiocath) should be made available for cleaning of the biopsy channel port. The medication tray must include a tourniquet, alcohol swabs, butterfly needles, adhesive tape and medication drawn up in syringes which are appropriately labelled.

An intravenous line should be prepared for possible connection to the butterfly needle, which is usually kept patent with a syringe of normal saline. A footstool should be positioned for the patient to use when getting onto the trolley.

For polypectomy, two polypectomy snares should be available. If bleeding occurs following severance of the polyp, the second snare can be immediately passed through the endoscope channel if the original snare malfunctions. A back-up snare is always appropriate should the primary equipment fail. The snare wires should be opened and closed as a functional check prior to use. The electrosurgical diathermy unit should have the power switch placed to the 'on' position and observed for proper setting. The conductive plate should be placed on the examining table, and the foot pedal positioned within the working area of the endoscopist. If carbon dioxide is to be used, the cylinder must be checked for an adequate supply of gas, and attached to the appropriate port on the endoscope, so that it can be insufflated as required. Having completed the pre-endoscopic checks, the endoscopy assistant is now ready to receive the patient.

6.2 Assistance during examination

The patient lies on the table in the supine position until the medications have been given. The patient is then turned into the left lateral recumbent position, with the buttocks at the edge of the examining table. It is in this position that the one-person technique can be best employed. The endoscopist can hold the scope in position beside the table with the right thigh while control manipulations are accomplished with both hands (see Chapter 9). The assistant stands on the opposite side of the trolley from the endoscopist and is free to give help when needed while still observing the patient. During the course of the procedure, the assistant may be required to apply abdominal compression to act as an external splint, when loop formation occurs during intubation, to give additional medication as ordered, or to reposition the patient when necessary. During the endoscopic examination, the assistant continually replenishes the supply of gauze swabs within the working area or adds lubricant to the instrument shaft at the anal canal for easier insertion as the area becomes dry rapidly. During all these manoeuvres, it is important to monitor the patient's response to the procedure, and observe any changes in vital signs or colour, and to check for abdominal distension.

More frequently, a two-person endoscopy technique is employed, with the endoscopy assistant assuming a passive role as the first assistant. Most endoscopy nurses assist during intubation by holding the colonoscope at the anus to ensure that the instrument does not slip back after each insertion. When the stiffening sleeve is used (only under fluoroscopic control), it should be placed over the colonoscope before insertion and adequately lubricated with water-soluble jelly. Once the stiffening sleeve has been carefully inserted and its position checked by the endoscopist to prevent it from moving in or out with the movements of the colonoscope, the assistant must hold it in place at the anus to prevent the possible risk of bowel perforation. Even when the endoscopist uses a one-person technique, the assistant must hold the instrument in place whenever the position of the patient is changed, while the operator uses both hands on the controls.

Occasionally, the assistant assumes a more active role in a two-person technique and assists by advancing, withdrawing or rotating the instrument at the request of the endoscopist.

Histological specimens may be obtained with the biopsy forceps. After passing the forceps through the channel, the jaws are opened upon request, a specimen is taken, and the forceps withdrawn. The assistant may use a needle or toothpick to extract the specimen from the forceps cups, being careful not to smear, crush or alter the pattern of the specimen (Dean, 1976) which should then be orientated on a small piece of filter paper or ground glass.

Whenever specimens have been taken during an examination they should be labelled promptly with the patient's name, hospital number and site of biopsy. The appropriate pathological request forms should be completed before starting the next procedure. This avoids the possibility of any confusion of specimens obtained from other patients.

If diathermy is to be used, the patient conductive plate must be positioned under the patient's thigh or between the knees, and care must be taken that the patient is not in contact with any metal parts of the table or trolley. These two points are essential to avoid a serious skin burn. During polypectomy, the assistant closes the snare loop gently but steadily until resistance is felt. If tightened too swiftly before coagulation current has been applied, the polyp stalk may be guillotined, resulting in a primary haemorrhage.

Following polypectomy, on retrieving the specimen, a sharp needle should be placed through the resected stalk to ensure proper location of the stalk site by the pathologist, since retraction of elastic tissue within the pedicle may interfere with proper orientation of histological sectioning.

It is important to keep the endoscopist informed of the power settings on the electrosurgical appliance during polypectomy procedures and whether the diathermy unit is set to cutting, coagulating or blended current.

When obtaining a cytology smear, a sleeved brush is advanced through the biopsy channel into the bowel lumen. Upon request, the assistant advances the brush forward, and the endoscopist rubs it across the lesion. The brush is then withdrawn into the sleeve to prevent loss of material from the bristles before being extracted. Smears are made directly on two to four slides and sprayed with fixative. The brush may then be immersed in a vial of alcohol for subsequent centrifugal cellular separation.

6.3 Emergency resuscitation

An alert assistant is usually the first to become aware that a patient's condition is deteriorating. The endoscopist must be informed immediately if the patient shows any sign of cardiorespiratory difficulties or collapse (Rogers, 1974). Such complications may be due to oversedation, vasovagal stimulation or hypotension. Cardiorespiratory support must be maintained while resuscitation efforts are begun. The endoscopy unit should be self-sufficient with emergency equipment including an Ambu bag, face masks, airways of various sizes, working laryngoscopes and endotracheal tubes, as well as oxygen and other back-up equipment, including drugs necessary to handle infrequent but life-threatening emergencies. All proper equipment for resuscitation must be available whether procedures are performed in a hospital environment or in a physician's private office and must be thoroughly checked weekly to ensure proper function.

6.4 Cleaning and disinfection

Before, between cases and at the end of the endoscopy test, the colonoscope shaft should be placed in a soapy solution of water, which is then aspirated through the instrument. After first removing the valve, the cleaning brush is passed through the biopsy channel and the tip of the cleaning brush is cleaned with a toothbrush before it is drawn back through the instrument the shaft of which is then soaked in activated glutaraldehyde (Cidex). The toothbrush is again used to scrub gently the distal tip. Cidex is then aspirated through the channel and the instrument shaft is left in Cidex for 10–20 min before rinsing through and wiping down with clean water. The lens of the instrument is cleaned using a specialized lens cleaner and rubbed with a 'cotton bud' or a clean piece of gauze. The control head of the instrument is swabbed with a clean piece of gauze which has been moistened but not saturated with 70% alcohol. Cotton buds may be used to clean around the drive wheels and the suction, air and water buttons. Finally after it has been rinsed with clean water, 30% alcohol is used to wipe the shaft of the instrument and also to clean the umbilicus (McCloy, 1978). Disinfection is discussed in more detail in Chapter 5. The instrument is best stored hanging vertically, to allow fluid to drain, in a purpose built cupboard.

6.5 Records

A record book of all procedures performed should be kept in the department. The findings for each patient should be entered including the instruments used, biopsies, cytology and photographs if taken, and the endoscopist performing the procedure. Drugs and dosages used should be recorded in both this book and the departmental Drug Record Book and on the Endoscopy Report. The assistant should

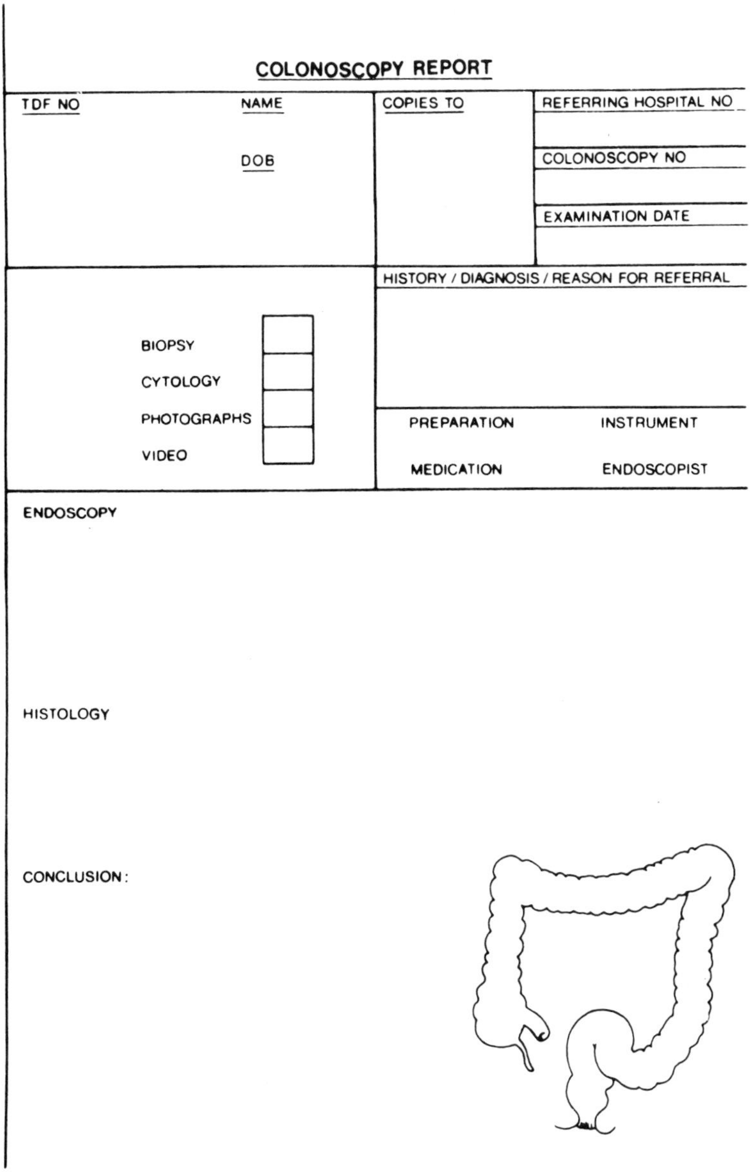

COLONOSCOPY REPORT

TDF NO

NAME

DOB

COPIES TO

REFERRING HOSPITAL NO

COLONOSCOPY NO

EXAMINATION DATE

HISTORY / DIAGNOSIS / REASON FOR REFERRAL

BIOPSY

CYTOLOGY

PHOTOGRAPHS

VIDEO

PREPARATION

INSTRUMENT

MEDICATION

ENDOSCOPIST

ENDOSCOPY

HISTOLOGY

CONCLUSION:

Fig. 6.3 An example of a specially designed colonoscopy report form.

ensure that the patient's report is written or dictated by the endoscopist, with postoperative care instructions where appropriate. A purpose-designed report form in duplicate or triplicate can be especially useful an example of which is shown in Fig. 6.3.

A patient record file can be most helpful when kept in the Department and can include a duplicate endoscopy report, together with the barium enema, cytology and histology reports, endoscopic films and other relevant gastroenterological investigations for this can save much time when preparing statistics etc. Most radiologists in turn appreciate a copy of the colonoscopy report and this helps to establish a co-operative rapport between departments.

6.6 Stores

In order to maintain a comprehensive service it is wise to ensure an adequate supply of spare biopsy forceps, cytology brushes, snares, polyp retrievers, cannulae, cleaning brushes, spare valves, extra lamps for light sources, films and videotapes etc. The nurse/assistant should check with the endoscopists who use the department as to which drugs or special accessories etc. they prefer to use and then maintain an adequate stock.

6.7 Conclusion

The endoscopy nurse/assistant, being the organizer and co-ordinator of the unit and its activities, is called upon constantly to cover several different job categories throughout the day and often fulfils many roles: nurse, technician, secretary and administrator (Cotton and Williams, 1980). Of all these, the most difficult is to maintain high standards of workmanship so that the ultimate goal – excellent patient care – is provided. The endoscopic assistant must combine professionalism with good humour and a sense of efficiency to provide the support needed for the endoscopy unit.

References

Banks, J. (1980), Colonoscopy, *Nursing*, 759–760.
Cotton, P. B. and Williams, C. B. (1980), *Practical Gastro intestinal Endoscopy*, Blackwell Scientific Publications, London.
Curtis, C. (1975), Colonoscopy: the nurses' role. *Am. J. Nurs.*, **75** (3), 430–2.
Dean, A. C. B. (1976), Colonoscopy In: *Modern Topics in Gastroenterology* (eds K. F. R. Schiller and P. R. Salmon) William Heinemann Medical, London, pp. 229–42.

Hollanders, D. (1979), *Gastrointestinal Endoscopy. An Introduction for Nurses.* Bailliere, Tindall, London, pp. 112–30.

McCloy, R. (1978), Getting the best from your endoscope, *Br. J. Clin. Equip.,* 271–9.

Rogers, B. H. G. (1974), Colonoscopy: The OR nurse's function, *AORN,* **19,** 656–70.

Salmon, P. R. (1974), *Fibreoptic Endoscopy,* Pitman Medical, London, pp. 78–101.

Wright, B. (1980), Nursing and technical aspects of a gastro-intestinal unit. *Endosc. Today,* (June), 3–4.

CHAPTER SEVEN

Radiology of the Large Bowel

DAVID E. BECKLY and GILES W. STEVENSON

With the advent of colonoscopy the clinician now has two techniques for the routine examination of the large bowel mucosa. Although almost always complementary investigations the differences between barium enema and colonoscopy depend on a number of factors including comfort, accuracy, time involved, complication rate, radiation dose and cost and indeed, local expertise may be the most important single factor. There are however several advantages of the barium enema over colonoscopy. It provides a permanent record of the large bowel for later evaluation, and the configuration of the colon and extrinsic relationships can be assessed. At colonoscopy, for example, the presence of a complete malrotation may not be appreciated. The depth of fissures and presence of fistula or paracolic abscess are more readily shown on X-ray, and in good hands the whole colon can almost always be examined. In one series only 57% of colonoscopies reached the caecum (Gelfand, Wu and Ott, 1979) and the figure of 85 to 90% quoted by experts may be quite unrepresentative of average practice. Barium enema is cheaper and may often be more comfortable and quicker. Only the most skilled endoscopists can undertake twelve colonoscopies in an afternoon, a number handled comfortably by a radiologist doing double contrast examinations in two X-ray rooms simultaneously. All these advantages however become irrelevant if the X-ray examination is unreliable.

In the upper gastrointestinal tract fibreoptic endoscopy exposed the shortcomings of the traditional barium meal and stimulated the development of double contrast techniques. In the colon the description of the double contrast enema preceded fibreoptic endoscopy by many years but the technique was slow to develop. It was first described in 1923 (Fischer, 1923), vigorously developed by Welin in the 1950s (Welin, 1967), and popularized in Britain by Allen Young from St. Mark's Hospital in the 1960s (Young, 1964). In the United States over the last few years various authors have urged the widespread adoption of double contrast techniques (Brown, 1968; Miller, 1975; Laufer, 1976; MacEwan et al., 1978). The view of one colonoscopist is given by Williams: 'On the evidence available only the most disinterested or reactionary radiologists can continue to use the standard or single contrast technique for colitis patients' (Williams and Waye, 1978). In 1968, as few as 10% of the teaching hospitals in the United States used double contrast enemas routinely (Margulis and Goldberg, 1969). By 1974 double contrast was used routinely in patients with inflammatory bowel disease by only 16% of these teaching hospitals (Thoeni and Margulis, 1978). Widely differing views are thus still held. The authors of this chapter are convinced that the double contrast enema is vastly superior to single contrast enemas in three respects: the detection of small neoplasms, demonstration of early and superficial lesions of inflammatory bowel disease and the confidence which arises from a normal examination. The routine barium enema should be a double contrast study, and a single contrast enema can be reserved for specific problems. These include a search for fistula, demonstration of the site of large bowel obstruction, and the detection and treatment of intussusception.

It is the aim of this chapter to indicate which diagnostic method, be it radiological or endoscopic, is most appropriate to the various problems encountered in everyday practice. Where radiology is the method of choice we have attempted to describe ways in which its accuracy can be maximized.

7.1 Bowel preparation

Inadequate bowel preparation is one of the major causes of error in barium enemas and in one series the second commonest cause of failed total colonoscopy (Gelfand, Wu and Ott, 1979). A clean colon is thus equally important to radiologist and colonoscopist. Responsibility for preparation should rest with the physician performing the procedure and not the physician requesting it. A physician requesting a barium enema is asking for a professional opinion on the state of the large bowel. Reports are sometimes seen which say 'no gross abnormality found in the large bowel, but the presence of faeces prevents the exclusion of polyps or early inflammatory disease'. This is a dereliction of responsibility and analogous to a physician writing in a consultation note, 'no abnormality was found on physical examination but the presence of clothes prevented the exclusion of some lesions'.

There are three different approaches to bowel cleansing, all of which can give satisfactory results.

(a) Dietary restriction, strong laxatives, oral fluids and colon washouts. This is usually a 24-hour preparation with only oral fluids permitted and use of either a contact irritant such as castor oil, or a bulk fluid producer such as magnesium citrate. Magnesium citrate and bisacodyl combined were better than castor oil (Dodds *et al.*, 1977). The disadvantage of this technique is the time required in the X-ray department, before the barium enema, while the colon is drying out after the wash-out. The problem can be solved for outpatients by asking them to administer their tap water enemas at home using a 2-l bag. The radiology department can maintain a team of part-time nursing assistants to perform colon wash-outs on the ward for in-patients (Gardiner, 1978).

(b) A more rapid method of cleansing consists of flooding the small bowel with isotonic saline (Hewitt *et al.*, 1973; Skucas, Cutliff and Fisher, 1976), or mannitol and water either orally or by a jejunal tube. A disadvantage for barium enema, however, is that the colon is frequently wet.

(c) A more prolonged oral preparation has been advocated to avoid the need for wash-outs. A typical regime consists of two days of food restriction with abundant clear oral fluids. Milder laxatives are used twice each day. The patient is instructed to drink when hungry for this sensation is abolished when the stomach is full. This regime is reported to give 92% excellent examinations and 5% acceptable (Lunderquist, 1979).

7.2 Techniques

7.2.1 *Plain abdominal X-ray*

This should always precede barium enema. It may show abnormalities which contraindicate the enema (toxic dilatation); give information which makes the enema unnecessary (active severe colitis); or alter the choice of technique (a large bowel obstruction requires a limited single contrast enema without bowel preparation to confirm obstruction and show its level). It is not customary to precede colonoscopy with another supine abdominal film but this can help in assessing bowel preparation. A tablet of barium sulphate given as an oral marker when bowel preparation starts, will allow either a supine film or brief fluoroscopy to confirm that bowel preparation is satisfactory. This is most useful when colonoscopy to the ileocaecal region is planned, since the procedure can be postponed for further preparation if barium and stool are still present in significant amounts in the right colon.

7.2.2 *Double contrast barium enema*

Commercial barium preparations are now available for double contrast examination which produce acceptable coating of the large

Organization and Techniques

bowel mucosa. Various film combinations have been recommended (Young, 1966; Miller, 1975; Peterson and Miller, 1978). They share the principle that several films of each part of the large bowel well coated with barium, and unobscured by residual barium puddles are required. For this technique the colon must be moderately distended with air and glucagon or hyoscine-N-butyl bromide (Buscopan) are often helpful after the barium has been introduced (Miller, Chernish and Brunelle, 1979). It is our practice to obtain double contrast views of the rectum and sigmoid before barium is allowed to run to the

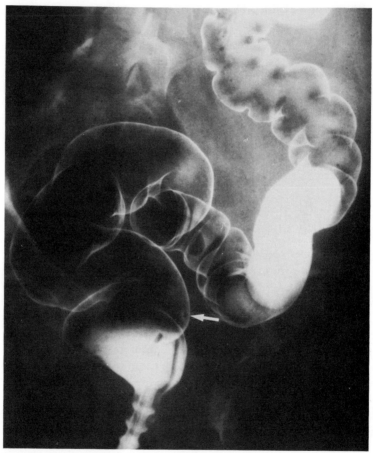

Fig. 7.1 Prone oblique film of rectum and sigmoid colon, taken after air has displaced most of the barium to the transverse colon. There may be no opportunity to obtain satisfactory rectal and sigmoid films once the caecum has been filled. Note the small anterior rectal polyp which was shown on several films.

caecum or terminal ileum (Fig. 7.1). The method is thus one of diagnosis from film rather than fluoroscopy. Traditionally the sigmoid has
been regarded as the most difficult area, and in the presence of diverticular disease, redundant loops and spasm it may occasionally not be
possible to demonstrate the sigmoid adequately even with intravenous glucagon or Buscopan. The radiologist should be honest in
recording this fact since a low level of confidence in declaring the
sigmoid normal will make the gastroenterologist reach more readily
for the colonoscope.

An advantage of the barium enema is the relative ease with which
the right colon is examined. Attention to detail must however be

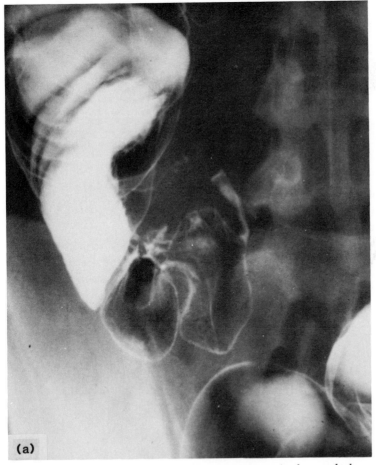

(a)

Fig. 7.2a Ileocaecal deformity. Is colonoscopy required to exclude carcinoma?

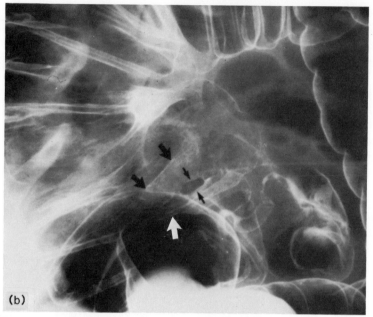

Fig. 7.2b Two minutes after (a) following injection of glucagon 0.5 mg i.v., the ileocaecal region is relaxed, normal upper and lower margins of the ileocaecal valve are sharply defined (large arrows) and the orifice of the open valve is visible (small arrows).

meticulous and common faults are inadequate air distension of the caecum (Fig. 7.2) or excessive barium within it. In Ott's series all the lesions missed radiographically were distal to the splenic flexure (Ott, Gelfand and Ramquist, 1980). In Swarbrick's series which contained many patients referred from other hospitals for colonoscopy, 90% of the missed polyps were in the sigmoid, but the radiologically missed carcinomas were scattered more evenly throughout the large bowel (Swarbrick *et al.*, 1976). The right colon can be very well demonstrated with double contrast techniques, to the extent that Williams felt able to advocate limited colonoscopy for left-sided polyps if the right colon had been well shown by the double contrast enema (Williams, *et al.*, 1974). The recognized incidence of synchronous polyps and carcinoma means that the radiologist has to take particular care to examine the proximal colon when a polypoid lesion is found on the left side. Not all colonoscopists however, share Williams reliance on barium enema and Schrock undertakes total colonoscopy routinely if barium enema shows a carcinoma, whether in the right or left colon, in order to confirm or refute the radiological diagnosis and to look

Table 7.1 Endoscopic versus radiographic detection of rectal neoplasms

	Lesion	Total	No. missed at endoscopy (%)	No. missed by Ba enema (%)
Simpkins and Young (1968)	Polyps	90	11 (12)	Not known
Laufer (1979b)	Cancer	62	9 (14)	Not known
Thoeni (1980)	All neoplasms	69	17 (25)	3 (4)

for a synchronous lesion. A synchronous lesion 5 mm or larger, missed radiographically, was found in 20% of those patients in whom the barium enema had detected a right-sided tumour. One explanation of this different approach may be that Schrock's experience is based largely on solid column barium enema whereas Williams refers specifically to double contrast examinations (Schrock, 1980a and b).

The rectum, which is in theory easily examined endoscopically, especially with the rigid proctosigmoidoscope has been a difficult area for the colonoscope. Previous studies have shown that the double contrast enema may detect lesions missed endoscopically (Table 7.1). It is possible that the practice of colonoscopic inversion will overcome this problem (see p. 145) but this remains to be shown. The majority of missed rectal lesions on barium enema are due to inattention to this area (Cooley, Agnew and Rios, 1960) and there is no place for a radiological examination that fills half the rectum with a large balloon and the other half with a solid column of dense barium.

7.2.3 *Single contrast enema*

This examination is indicated in suspected large bowel obstruction and the search for fistulae and intussusception. We prefer to use the double contrast enema on all other patients because of the higher level of confidence accompanying a report of a normal colon, and because the routine use of double contrast studies helps maintain higher radiographic standards. In the single contrast study if bowel margins cannot be seen clearly and crisply through overlapping loops, then the technique is faulty with kV too low, barium too dense or a combination of both.

7.2.4 *Instant enema*

The instant enema relies on the principle that in active ulcerative colitis the inflamed bowel expels any contents, so that the diseased distal segment is constantly 'prepared' (Young, 1963; Bartram, 1977). Barium is run into the colon until stool is reached, and the rectum is then drained. Air is introduced and double contrast films are taken. This examination shows the extent of the disease and gives an idea of the severity of disease in the colon beyond the reach of the sigmoido-scope (Fig. 7.3). Four films are sufficient including the preliminary plain film. The examination takes five minutes, and can be done on

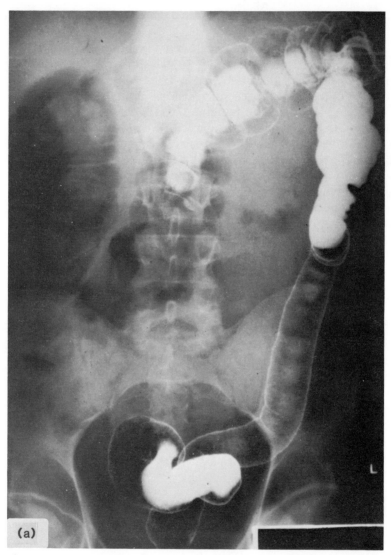

Fig. 7.3 Instant enema. At previous outpatient visits this patient had distal proctitis. At this visit, for the first time, disease extended beyond sigmoidos-

the unprepared out-patient immediately after being seen in the clinic, provided no rectal biopsy has been taken. It is of greatest use in patients with previous proctitis in whom for the first time the sigmoidoscope no longer reaches normal mucosa. It has no place as an initial examination in patients suspected of having ulcerative colitis nor as an examination for dysplasia or carcinoma in longstanding disease.

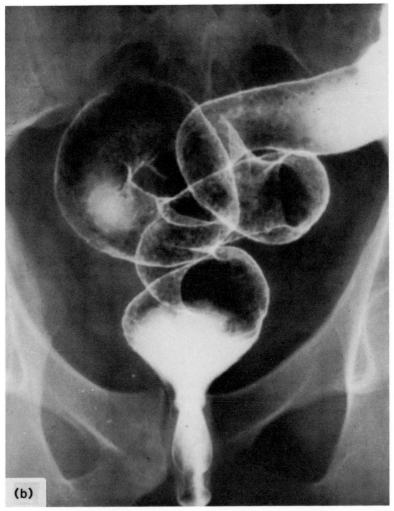

(b)

copic vision. A barium enema a few minutes later revealed normal haustra and stool in the transverse colon (a). There was active disease distal to the splenic flexure (b).

7.2.5 *Per oral pneumocolon*

Occasionally the double contrast barium enema fails on the right side of the colon. In such patients the per oral pneumocolon can be extremely useful in proving normality or giving the diagnosis (Heitzmann and Berne, 1961; Kellett, Zboralske and Margulis, 1977). Fig. 7.4 illustrates such a patient with an ileocaecal valve carcinoma, in whom colonoscopy would have been unusually arduous because part of the colon lay within the chest. The examination follows bowel preparation as for a barium enema. Barium is given orally and is

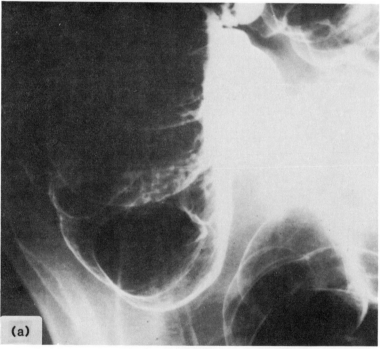

(a)

Fig. 7.4 This 81-year-old man presented with dyspnoea and had a haemo-globin of 8.0 g. He had had a 'very difficult' appendicectomy with abscess 40 years earlier. Barium meal showed a large hernia with the stomach almost entirely in the chest. At barium enema most of the transverse colon was in the chest. The 'lower pole' of the caecum appeared normal (a) but there was an unusual medial indentation (b). Neither appendiceal stump nor ileum were seen. Per oral pneumocolon (c) resolved the problem. The apparent caecal lower pole was the upper margin of a stricture (S), due to an ileocaecal valve carcinoma (large arrows). A tumour is surrounding distal ileum (small arrows) and ascending colon. The caecum is small (C). The patient survived resection of the carcinoma.

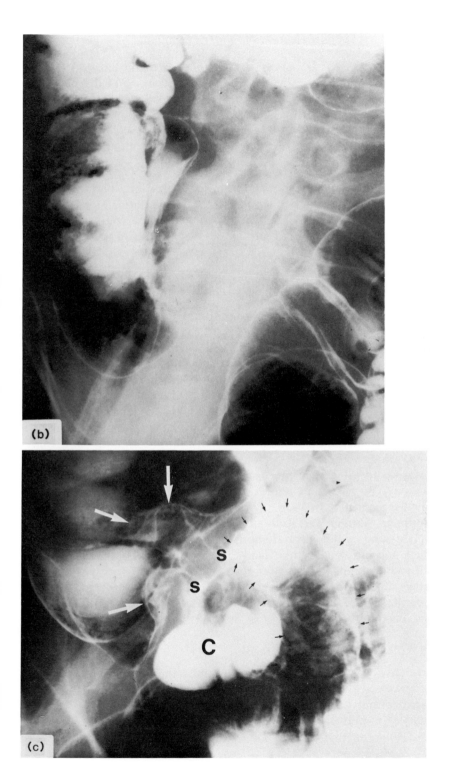

followed to the mid-transverse colon, when air is introduced rectally and antispasmodics are given to produce relaxation. Double contrast films of the right colon, ileo-caecal valve and distal ileum are then taken. Although this technique is not often needed it may sometimes be invaluable.

7.2.6 *Postoperative colon*

Following segmental, especially sigmoid, resection, barium enema, like colonoscopy, is easier to perform. High quality double contrast barium enemas can be obtained in patients with a colostomy. These are frequently patients at high risk deserving the best examination. There is a tendency on the part of patients, nurses and physicians to use less rigorous bowel preparation in colostomy patients, partly because of the problems of bag-changing and partly on the assumption that a shorter colon requires less preparation. These patients often retain stool and need vigorous somewhat unsympathetic cleansing.

In the patient with a defunctioned segment the barium can be introduced either through the rectum or through the colostomy. The former is easier but loss of air into the colostomy bag often prevents good distension. It is a little harder and messier to introduce the tube through the colostomy but better distension is obtained as the rectal sphincters are able to retain air better than the colostomy stoma.

An ileostomy can be examined by the same technique as a colostomy. Single contrast is preferable when looking for fistulae, and double contrast when mucosal detail is important. The continent ileostomy may become more popular and radiological examination may be requested because of incontinence or intubation difficulties, (Stephens, Mantell and Kelly, 1979). With early post-operative incontinence, the radiological demonstration of a normally constructed pouch and nipple valve may lead to a conservative approach and some of these patients eventually develop satisfactory function without further intervention (Stephens, Mantel and Kelly, 1979; Diner and Cockrill, 1979). The endoscopic features of the continent ileostomy have been described (Waye *et al.*, 1977) (Plates 155 and 156).

7.2.7 *Complications of barium enema*

Perforation, extravasation of barium into the vascular system and retrograde regurgitation of barium into the lungs have all been described but fortunately are rare (Seaman and Wells, 1965). Most instances of perforation near a colostomy stoma have been associated with balloon catheters, and indeed the majority of serious complications seem to be avoidable (Amberg, 1980). Minor complications such as bloating, nausea and cramps are common after barium enema but their incidence is unknown. The radiologist also needs to be familiar with the radiographic signs of complications from colonoscopy (Meyers and Ghahremani, 1977) and these are reviewed in Chapter 13.

Patients sometimes ask how much radiation they will receive from a barium enema. Reports of dosage vary considerably, but a bone marrow dose or 2 R and gonad dose (male or female) of 1 R appear to be average figures. This risk can be put in a more familiar context as it is equivalent to driving 2000 miles by car, rock-climbing for one hour, smoking 30 cigarettes, or being a man aged 60 for 12 hours (Pochin, 1978).

7.3 Inflammatory bowel disease

Bowel preparation may have to be modified in patients with active inflammatory bowel disease but in patients with clinically inactive disease full preparation should be given (Bartram, 1977; Williams and Waye, 1978).

If there is any question of toxicity, either radiographically or clinically, then barium enema is contraindicated. In general, if in doubt, do not do the enema and a patient who is too ill for bowel preparation is too ill for barium enema or colonoscopy. In those patients in whom sigmoidoscopy has established the diagnosis of ulcerative colitis, supine abdominal films may help monitor the course during the acute episodes. For practical purposes the pseudopolyposis of ulcerative colitis, cobblestoning in severe Crohn's disease, oedematous plaques of pseudomembraneous colitis and thumb-printing of ischaemic colitis are all indistinguishable on plain abdominal films (Fig. 7.5). Even amoebiasis or shigellosis may look the same. The most urgent matter is to rule out infective causes by sigmoidoscopy, microscopic examination and culture, and radiology has no role in specific diagnosis, although it may be useful in following the progress of a severe episode by plain abdominal films.

7.3.1 *Barium enema*

It is now clear that in inflammatory bowel disease barium enema should be of the double contrast type. It is no more dangerous than the single contrast enema, and is more accurate (Simpkins and Stevenson, 1972; Fraser and Findlay, 1976; Laufer, Mullens and Hamilton, 1976; Hildell, Lindstrom and Wenckert, 1979).

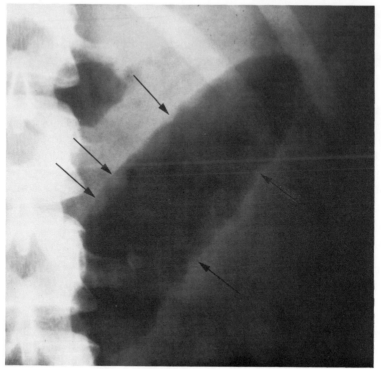

Fig. 7.5 Acute severe colitis with loss of haustra, and nodular defects (arrows). This is a non-specific appearance. In this patient it was due to pseudomembranous colitis following administration of clindamycin. This appearance contraindicates barium enema. Sigmoidoscopy was diagnostic.

7.3.2 *Ulcerative colitis*

The mildest visible mucosal change in ulcerative colitis is loss of vessel pattern. This is probably not detectable on barium enema but is readily apparent at colonoscopy. This change alone is an infrequent finding in symptomatic patients and common in quiescent disease. The degree to which barium enema underestimates the extent of disease is inversely proportional to the severity. Colonoscopy has revealed that mild right-sided changes may be present in patients in whom the more obvious disease is limited to the distal colon. The significance of this is not known. Radiological total colitis is associated with an increased incidence of carcinoma in later years but we do not know if the same applies when the ulceration is limited to the left colon but histological abnormality is more extensive.

The radiological changes in mild disease are dots, rings, nodules

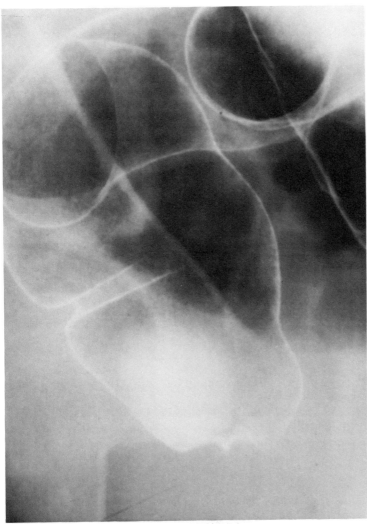

Fig. 7.6 Mild ulcerative colitis. This 'dot' pattern of extensive very superficial ulceration is unusual. More often there is associated nodularity and irregularity of the margin.

and scratches (Cole, 1978). The dots correspond to tiny superficial ulcers (Fig. 7.6) and the rings to small islands of mucosa that are oedematous and stand above the diffuse surrounding ulceration. Nodules are less common and are sometimes due to lymphoid nodular hyperplasia seen more often in mild chronic disease especially in

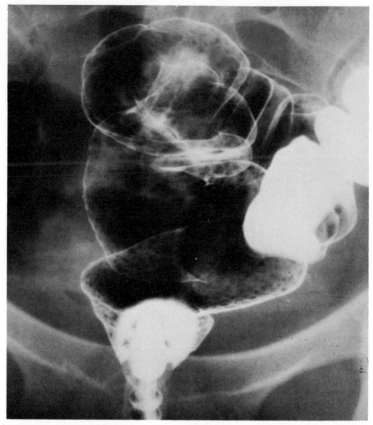

Fig. 7.7 Lymphoid nodular hyperplasia in a young adult female patient with proctitis and a biopsy consistent with ulcerative colitis.

the rectum (Fig. 7.7). Scratches are the least common finding. They run transversely and are probably related to superficial ulceration over the lymphoid nodules (Cole, 1978).

In more severe disease pseudopolyposis occurs and in fulminating disease toxic dilatation develops. A calibre greater than 5.5 cm should be a cause for concern. In long-standing ulcerative colitis shortening, loss of haustration and benign strictures may appear. Filiform polyposis occurs during recovery from severe attacks (Fig. 7.8), (Bartram and Walmsley, 1978) and large inflammatory polyps are occasionally noted (Joffe, 1977).

Double contrast barium enema probably has a 95% accuracy in detecting the visible mucosal lesions of ulcerative colitis (Simpkins and Stevenson, 1972; Laufer, Mullens and Hamilton, 1976). Not sur-

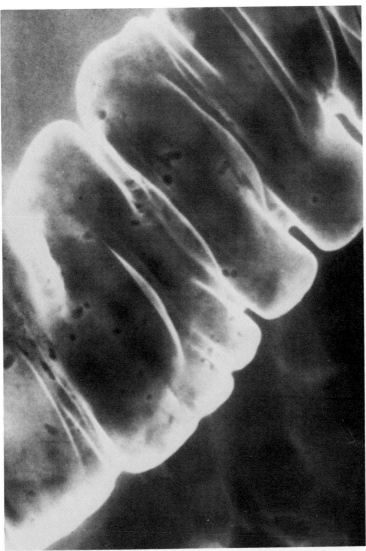

Fig. 7.8 Two years earlier there was severe pseudopolyposis in this transverse colon. The haustra have returned and the mucosa is smooth, only the small filiform and branching mucosal tags testifying to the severity of the previous attack. Biopsy showed chronic inflammatory changes still to be present, although colonoscopically the mucosa looked normal between the polyps.

prisingly, poorer accuracy is found if inactive disease is considered (Gabrielsson *et al.*, 1979). Barium enema underestimates the extent of the disease as compared to colonoscopy but colonoscopic visualization underestimates the extent as seen histologically (Dilawari *et al.*, 1973). Proctoscopy is a poor guide to the severity of proximal disease. In patients treated with rectal steroids this is readily appreciated, but in untreated patients both the enema or colonoscope may show much more severe changes in the descending colon than in the rectum. Right-sided ulcerative colitis however is unrecognized. Rarely patients will be seen in whom rectal changes are minimal in the presence of right colon ulceration, and very rarely the rectum may appear radiologically and endoscopically normal in untreated patients. In the author's experience however, rectal biopsy has always been abnormal in such patients.

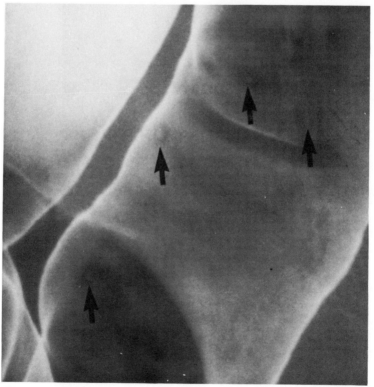

Fig. 7.9 Small aphthous ulcers in the descending colon in a 17-year-old female patient who also had Crohn's disease of the terminal ileum and duodenum. These were the only colonic manifestations.

7.3.3 *Dysplasia and carcinoma*

Long-standing ulcerative colitis is associated with an increased risk of colon cancer, especially when associated with a variety of high risk factors (see p. 328) and the same may be true in Crohn's disease to a lesser extent (p. 328). Unfortunately these tumours arise from areas of mucosal dysplasia rather than adenomas. They may be flat, penetrate early and are hard to detect radiographically. In most, but not all cases, such dysplasia is accompanied by rectal dysplasia (Lennard Jones *et al.*, 1977). It has been shown that in some cases the dysplasia is villous and macroscopically visible. It is therefore theoretically demonstrable radiographically, and this has been elegantly shown by Frank *et al.* (1978). However, the demonstration of such detail is often at or beyond the limits of radiographic resolution. Fortunately

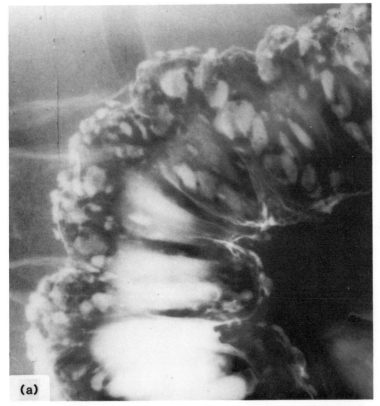

(a)

Fig. 7.10a Discrete ulcers in severe Crohn's disease with normal intervening mucosa. This patient had continuous disease from caecum to proximal sigmoid.

colonoscopy is particularly easy in these shortened colons, and as it allows multiple biopsies to be obtained it should be performed for cancer surveillance.

7.3.4 *Crohn's disease*

The early lesion is the aphthous ulcer, occurring over a lymphoid follicle. Radiographically a small central barium collection is surrounded by radiolucency (Fig. 7.9) corresponding to the small white slough and surrounding erythema visible endoscopically. Geboes and Vantrappen found aphthoid ulceration on colonoscopy in 15% of 59 patients with Crohn's colitis and preferred this method to barium enema (Geboes and Vantrappen, 1975). Radiologically it has been shown that these lesions are present in from 44 to 70% of patients

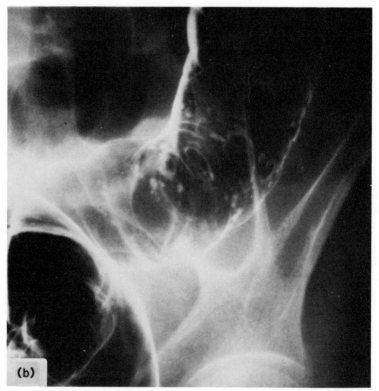

Fig. 7.10b In such a severe colonic disease, smaller aphthous ulcers may be seen at the ends of the diseased segments in 44–70% of patients.

with colonic Crohn's disease (Laufer, 1976; Kelvin *et al.*, 1978; Simpkins, 1977) often at the ends of involved segments (Fig. 7.10). A suitable barium and a clean, dry colon are necessary for these lesions to be well shown and they are not demonstrable without double contrast technique. A few patients with very early Crohn's disease or recovering from Crohn's disease, show a nodular colonic mucosa probably due to lymphoid nodular hyperplasia, and it may be that this is the earliest focal lesion in Crohn's disease. This abnormality is more readily appreciated on barium enema than at colonoscopy since there is no colour change, and these small elevations require tangential lighting to render them visible endoscopically (Fig. 7.11).

The diagnostic hallmark of Crohn's disease is the distribution. Although continuous total colitis does occur in Crohn's disease, it is more usual to have rectal-sparing, discontinuous disease and normal

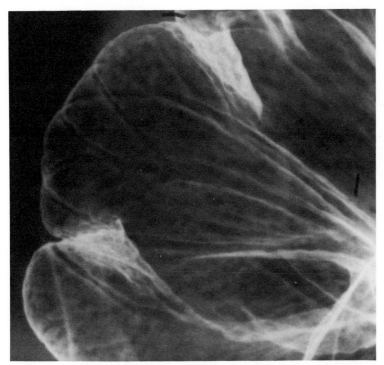

Fig. 7.11 Slight nodularity of mucosa, due to the lymphoid follicles. Characteristically some of the nodules are umbilicated. This appearance may precede Crohn's disease, but occurs in normal patients as well as a variety of diseases (Table 7.2).

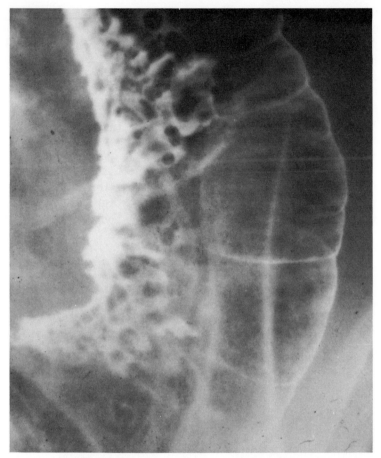

Fig. 7.12 A patch of Crohn's disease in the descending colon of a patient who had involvement of transverse colon and anal canal. This discontinuous involvement is characteristic.

mucosa between ulcers (Fig. 7.12). Anal disease is especially characteristic. Filiform polyposis and large inflammatory polyps occur, with the latter occasionally causing large obstructing masses resembling carcinoma (Joffe, 1977).

At the initial presentation of large bowel Crohn's disease, the diagnosis can be made on barium enema with a radiological accuracy of 98% (Kelvin *et al.*, 1978) and colonoscopy is usually unnecessary. In a few patients the large bowel findings are mild or non-specific (Fig. 7.13) (Hildell, Lindstrom and Wenckert, 1979). When the rectum is not involved, the small bowel normal and stool cultures negative,

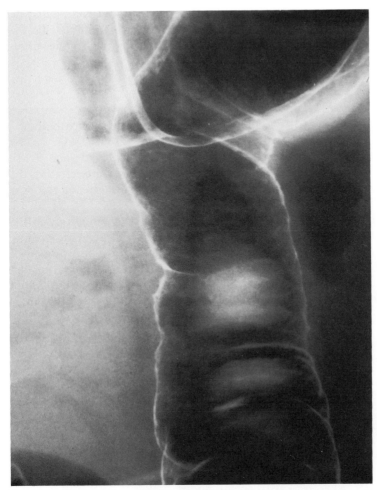

Fig. 7.13 Continuous mild disease in the descending colon in a young male patient. Colonoscopy confirmed transverse petechial haemorrhages and oedema. Biopsy was abnormal but non-specific. It was two years before the diagnosis of Crohn's disease was finally established.

there may be a diagnostic problem and in this situation colonoscopy and multiple biopsy may be very helpful. Although there is frequently delay in the diagnosis of Crohn's disease, a greater problem for the radiologist is overdiagnosis of the disease and the failure to consider conditions with which it may be confused (Chang *et al.*, 1978). Particularly troublesome are appendicitis, pelvic infection and metastatic carcinoma. The radiologist must be careful not to close the clinician's mind by giving an over-confident report of Crohn's disease when the radiographic features are simply those of non-specific full thickness involvement of bowel for which there is quite a wide differential diagnosis.

In Crohn's disease the barium enema is at its weakest in detecting early postsurgical recurrence because of retained fluid and spasm. Minimal mucosal changes may be accompanied by severe symptoms and there is no correlation between severity of X-ray or pathological change and severity of symptoms (Goldberg *et al.*, 1979). A dry colon is necessary to allow the mucosal details to be displayed (Fig. 7.14). The per oral pneumocolon may have a role here in demonstrating the anastomotic area, but this constitutes a major indication for colonoscopy in Crohn's disease.

The relative value of double contrast enema and colonoscopy in the preoperative assessment of Crohn's colitis is not clear. Furthermore the clinical importance of establishing the extent of disease remains a matter of debate. Although one report suggests that resection through diseased bowel has no influence on the recurrence rate (Pennington *et al.*, 1980; Hildell, Lindstrom and Wenckert, 1980) report that of 14 patients with preoperative Crohn's colitis (incompletely resected) 13 developed postoperative recurrence, while only three of 100 patients

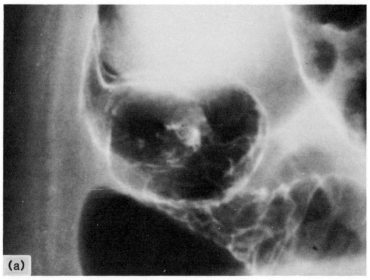

(a)

Fig. 7.14a A female patient, aged 45, with recurrent cramps and diarrhoea one year after hemicolectomy for Crohn's disease. Spasm and poor coating make this film of the anastomotic area uninterpretable.

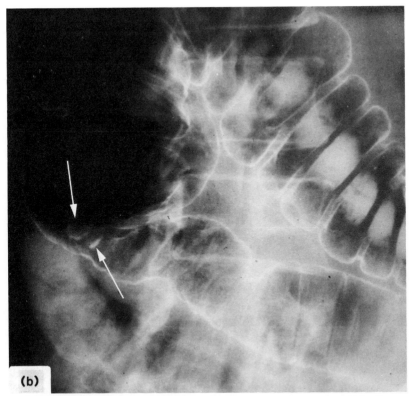

Fig. 7.14b After coating with more barium and relaxation with Buscopan 20 mg i.v., the area can be examined, and ulcers are clearly visible (arrows). Colonoscopy confirmed the presence of discrete anastomotic ulcers (c).

with resections through normal colon did so. Furthermore, of 12 patients in whom a 'normal' ileum was connected to a colonic segment that was diseased post- and usually preoperatively, ileal disease appeared postoperatively in 11. When diseased ileum was connected to normal colon in 31 patients no colitis ensued. In another study, colonic Crohn's disease was found to heal rarely (six out of 86 patients) and then only transiently, with relapse occurring within two years (five out of the six patients) (Brahme and Fork, 1975).

The reports from Hildell, Lindstrom, Wenckert, and Brahme and Fork have considerable implication for both clinician and radiologist and need to be confirmed. For the radiologist and endoscopist the demonstration of the extent of colonic Crohn's disease would become essential. For the surgeon, if the barium enema is not of sufficient quality to show the mucosa clearly then colonoscopy would be required. Double contrast enema will occasionally fail in patients with Crohn's disease in the presence of strictures, fistulae or very severe anal and perirectal disease. We have found a caudal block useful in permitting a comfortable and unhurried barium enema in one patient with extensive perianal disease.

We agree with Hildell, Lindstrom and Wenckert (1979) that when double contrast barium enema is technically satisfactory there is very little indication for colonoscopy in patients with Crohn's disease. Routine follow-up barium studies are also of little value in Crohn's disease because of the lack of correlation between symptoms and X-ray findings. This suggests that barium studies in patients with established Crohn's disease should be reserved for preoperative assessment, postoperative recurrence and severe exacerbations or change in symptoms (Goldberg *et al*, 1979).

7.3.5 *Other forms of inflammatory bowel disease and differential diagnosis*

Gross pathological appearances seen on the barium enema films are nonspecific. Although it is possible to make the correct diagnosis of ulcerative colitis and Crohn's disease in 80 to 90% of cases (Laufer and Hamilton, 1975), this is partly on grounds of distribution of pathology and associated clinical features, and partly because some of the mimicking conditions are much less common. Most of the radiological signs described as typical of either ulcerative colitis or Crohn's colitis can also occur in a variety of other forms of colitis (Fig. 7.15). Thus 'collar stud' ulcers occur in tuberculosis, salmonella, shigella, staphylococcal colitis and amoebiasis. Deep ulcers occur in ischaemic colitis, lymphogranuloma venereum, actinomycosis and Behçet's disease. Aphthous ulcers are seen in tuberculosis, yersinia enterocolitis, amoebic colitis, shigellosis and Behçet's disease as well as in Crohn's disease. In most cases careful consideration of clinical, bacteriological and histological evidence will allow the correct diagnosis to be made but this does illustrate the importance of the team approach.

In radiation colitis a history of radiation some six to twelve months earlier will usually be given. In the early stages the barium enema may be normal while colonoscopy shows changes in the appearance of the mucosa and contact bleeding. The barium enema is however useful since it is sensitive at detecting displacement of the rectum or sigmoid by recurrent or residual tumour masses. CT scanning may also have an important role in this respect.

7.3.6 *Lymphoid nodular hyperplasia*

Lymphoid nodular hyperplasia is quite often seen on double contrast

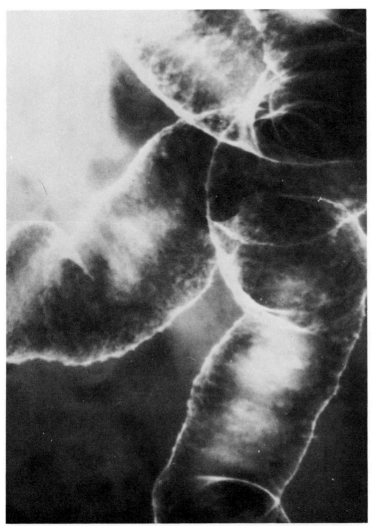

Fig. 7.15 Radiographic changes that would be consistent with ulcerative colitis in a patient with acute bloody diarrhoea. *Campylobacter* was cultured from the stool, and the patient recovered quickly with erythromycin.

barium enema. In children the lymphoid follicles will be visible in some 50% of barium enemas (Laufer and de Sa, 1978) and from the age of 10 onwards its incidence declines. Lymphoid follicles however may be large enough to be detectable in some normal adults (Kelvin *et al.*, 1979) (Fig. 7.16) and in a variety of diseases (Table 7.2)

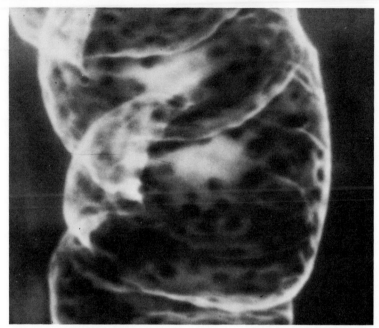

Fig. 7.16 Unusually prominent lymphoid nodular pattern in the descending colon in a 15-year-old boy with a six-week history of diarrhoea. Such marked changes are more commonly seen in hypogammaglobulinaemia but this was not the case in this patient. The infective agent was not identified.

Table 7.2 Colonic lymphoid nodular hyperplasia

Childhood
Agammaglobulinaemia ± giardiasis
Crohn's disease
Yersinia enterocolitis
Ulcerative colitis
Post-pseudomembranous colitis
Post-infective diarrhoea
Proximal to obstruction after necrotizing enterocolitis
Adjacent to carcinoma
Chronic lymphatic leukemia-lymphosarcoma
Glandular fever
Normal adults

7.4 Investigation and management of rectal bleeding: radiological aspects

This subject has been revolutionized by the application of angiography and colonoscopy. Initially angiography had a purely diagnostic role, but more recently has become useful in the management and therapy of these patients (Johnsrude and Jackson, 1978; Whitley and Hunt, 1979). It is convenient to consider acute rectal bleeding and chronic or intermittent blood loss separately.

7.4.1 *Acute massive rectal bleeding*

In many patients presenting with a brisk rectal haemorrhage the bleeding will stop spontaneously. In these cases investigation can proceed along the lines described for chronic or intermittent bleeding (*vide infra*). In some cases, however, severe bleeding persists despite conservative measures and an urgent search for the cause of the bleeding must be undertaken. Barium enema is contraindicated in these circumstances as it will delay angiography. Upper gastrointestinal haemorrhage, generalized bleeding disorders and rectal lesions must be excluded by the appropriate clinical, laboratory or endoscopic examinations. When this has been done selective superior and inferior mesenteric angiography should be performed. This is preferred to colonoscopy since small bowel lesions can also be demonstrated. If angiography is not available or is impossible then colonoscopy has been found to be a worthwhile alternative (Hunt, 1980). Emergency angiography for gastrointestinal bleeding is demanding since the patient is often very sick and the lesions being sought require impeccable technique if they are to be demonstrated successfully. Close co-operation between anaesthetist, surgeon and radiologist is essential. A wide variety of techniques for selective catheterization have been described but are beyond the scope of this chapter. Angiography will show the source of bleeding in about two-thirds of patients but must be performed during active bleeding when the site of extravasation of contrast medium can be demonstrated. Once bleeding has stopped the angiogram can only show the morphological vascular changes produced by the lesion and these may be inconspicuous (Allison, 1980) (Fig. 7.17).

Therapeutic angiography
Treatment of lower gastrointestinal bleeding by emergency colectomy carries an average mortality of 28% (Brookstein, Naderi and Walter, 1978). This has encouraged the use of non-operative methods for the control of large bowel haemorrhage. The choice lies between intra-

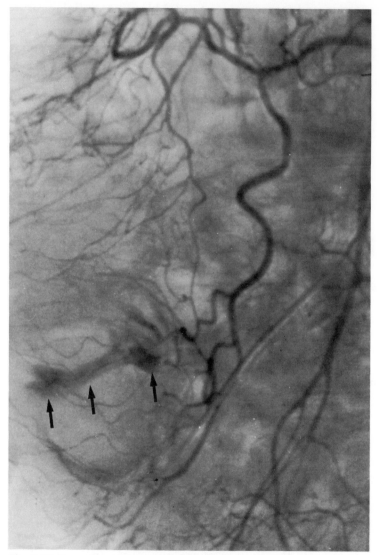

Fig. 7.17 Superior mesenteric injection in an elderly female patient with massive rectal bleeding. Contrast medium is extravasating from an angiodysplasia in the caecum. The morphological vascular changes are inconspicuous.

arterial infusion of pitressin and transcatheter embolization. Infusion of pitressin has the advantages of not requiring such subselective catheter placement and having a lower risk of bowel infarction. It has been shown to be effective in stopping bleeding from diverticula in up to 96% cases (Baum and Athanasoulis, 1974). Pitressin infusion is, however, less effective in bleeding from angiodysplasia (Rösch, Dotter and Antonovic, 1972; Giacchino *et al.*, 1979). Transcatheter embolization of the right colic artery using particles of Gelfoam or Ivalon has been successfully used in stopping bleeding from both diverticula and angiodysplasia, but even this method is not immune from episodes of rebleeding (Brookstein, Naderi and Walter, 1978). Furthermore, colonic stricture has been reported following embolization of a branch of the inferior mesenteric artery in a patient bleeding from a diverticulum in the descending colon (Mitty, Efremidis and Keller, 1979). The technical details of selective embolization are beyond the scope of this chapter but have been reviewed elsewhere (Johnsrude and Jackson, 1978; Whitley and Hunt, 1979).

Scintigraphic demonstration of acute rectal bleeding
One recent report (Alavi, 1980) shows that scintigraphy can detect the site of acute rectal bleeding. It appears to be more sensitive than arteriography, detecting bleeding at rates of 0.05–0.1 ml per minute. At present bleeding in the upper abdomen may be obscured by isotope uptake in liver and spleen. The exact role of scintigraphy is not yet clear, but its simplicity, safety and sensitivity make it an attractive technique that deserves further investigation.

7.4.2 *Chronic or intermittent rectal bleeding*

After proctosigmoidoscopy, barium enema is the examination of choice. Colonoscopy is indicated if barium enema is normal since a review of six series has indicated that colonoscopy may be expected to show the cause of bleeding in about 45% of patients, with carcinoma being found in 13% (Hunt, 1978; Tedesco *et al.*, 1978). This figure does not indicate the true potential of the barium enema since it is taken from series in which many single contrast barium enemas have been performed but it does indicate the reality of clinical practice and the great value of colonoscopy in barium enema negative rectal bleeding. Ott, Gelfand and Ramquist (1980) have examined the causes of radiological error and found that failure of technique was rare with the double contrast examination. Almost half of the mistakes were due to errors of interpretation and the remainder were perceptive errors compounded by failures of technique (Fig. 7.18). Complete invisibility of lesions on review of films is rare when double contrast techniques have been used. The implications of these observations suggest the first step after receiving a negative barium enema report in a patient with rectal bleeding should be to have the films rescrutin-

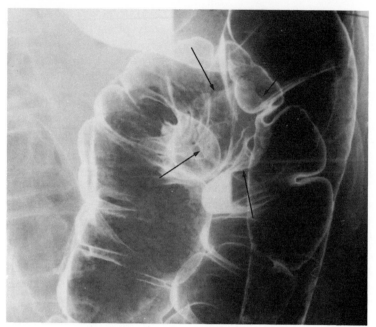

Fig. 7.18 At the apex of the sigmoid colon a polyp is present that turned out to be a carcinoma. It was not reported. The majority of such errors with double contrast examinations are perceptive, sometimes compounded by minor technical problems. In this case there is a clear double density sign. Reporting of enemas by two separate radiologists would probably eliminate many of these mistakes.

ized by a radiologist, with particular attention to the sigmoid colon where the majority of missed lesions occur (Swarbrick *et al.*, 1976; Ott, Gelfand and Ramquist, 1980). In younger patients a technetium scan should probably be considered to exclude bleeding from a Meckel's diverticulum.

If colonoscopy is negative and bleeding persists, angiography may show the cause in approximately half such patients (Sheedy, Fulton and Atwell, 1975). An angiodysplastic lesion, usually in the right colon will be the commonest finding. The radiographic signs are an early filling vein, an enlarged feeding artery and a capillary tuft. Colonoscopy is capable of detecting angiodysplasia and although its sensitivity has not been established it is probably quite high (Hunt, 1980). In patients in whom acute bleeding has stopped, and in whom angiography is therefore less useful, barium enema should be withheld in favour of colonoscopy. The cathartic effect of the blood that has been passed will have cleared the colon so that it is often well prepared and the use of barium at this stage will prevent colonoscopy and particularly angiography which might be needed should bleeding restart.

7.5 Colorectal neoplasia

The reliability of radiology for polyp and cancer detection can be looked at in various ways. Using the double contrast enema, Welin (1967) found polyps in 12.5% of patients which corresponded to the autopsy findings in patients at Malmö. The best figure reported for single contrast examinations is 7.8% (Figiel, 1973) but 1 to 3% is more usual (Seaman, 1971). Ott's review gives a range from 1 to 7.8% for single contrast examination and 9.8 to 13.1% for double contrast (Ott and Gelfand, 1978). Figiel's results do emphasize that well performed single contrast studies remain superior to poorly performed double contrast examinations.

Clark and Jones (1970) reported that 17.5% of sigmoid carcinomas were missed on barium enema and Cooley found 34 of 70 rectal carcinomas missed on the preceding barium enema (Cooley, Agnew and Rios, 1960). In contrast Williams, Hunt and Loose (1974) reported 98% of polyps greater than 1 cm in diameter were detected by double contrast enema at St. Mark's Hospital compared with 77% by single contrast; 73% of polyps under 5 mm were found on the double contrast examination. Other authors give slightly lower figures for double contrast but a reliability of from 89 to 97% is quoted (Leinicke *et al.*, 1977; Thoeni and Menuck, 1977). Thoeni reported 89.3% detection of 219 polyps of all sizes in 112 patients by double contrast enema, and 54.8% detection by single contrast. Colonoscopy detected 87.3%; 10% of the polyps were missed because the colonoscope could not reach them and 2.7% were overlooked. The average size of the polyps missed by double contrast enema was 5 mm. This careful study suggests that the increased sensitivity of colonoscopy is almost exactly offset by its inability to reach the caecum routinely.

We conclude that the reliability of colonoscopy for polyp detection is probably similar to air contrast barium enema for lesions over 1 cm, but higher than radiology for smaller polyps. Miller has collected 54 examples of polypoid lesions diagnosed radiographically and missed endoscopically, 31 by colonoscopy and 24 by proctosigmoidoscopy (Miller and Lehman, 1978). Polyps missed at colonoscopy are likely to be behind sharp folds especially at flexures (Laufer, Smith and Mullens, 1976), obscured by blood or on the right side beyond the

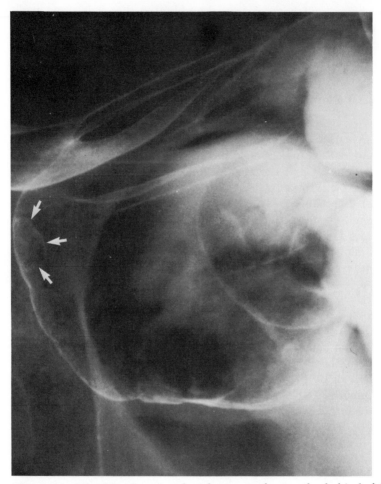

Fig. 7.19 Colonoscopic missed polyps are frequently behind folds. This 7-mm sessile polyp has been demonstrated on three barium enemas over five years, and has not grown. It could not be found on two colonoscopic examinations despite knowledge of its presence, although the ileocaecal valve and lower pole of the caecum were inspected on each occasion. The polyp lies immediately below the deep haustral fold on the lateral aspect of the caecum opposite the ileocaecal valve.

reach of a colonoscope (Fig. 7.19). Radiological misses are most likely to be in the sigmoid colon. Since perceptive errors are the major cause of missed lesions, double-reading is the single most effective remedy. The free use of hypotonic agents, adequate contrast drainage and bowel cleansing all play their part.

7.5.1 *Polyp characteristics*

The radiographic features of polyps have been well described (Simpkins and Young, 1968; Laufer, Mullens and Hamilton, 1976). Differentiation of a polyp from a diverticulum is sometimes a problem if the lesion cannot be seen in profile. When a diverticulum is seen *en face* the outer margin is sharp and inner margin less well defined, while the reverse is true of a polyp. This is due to meniscus formation by the barium layer coating the walls of the polyp or diverticulum. This sign is usually reliable, but better is the finding of a fluid level in the lesion on an erect film which never occurs with a polyp. Detection of small polyps is more difficult in the presence of diverticular disease and where the bowel is convoluted as in the sigmoid. In these circumstances a polyp is rarely seen entirely in double contrast and use must be made of other signs. Part of the polyp may appear as a filling defect within a pool of barium (Fig. 7.20). A double density is produced by the barium coated polyp as the X-rays must traverse four barium coated layers instead of two (Fig. 7.21). Occasionally line shadows produced by the polyp stalk may be the

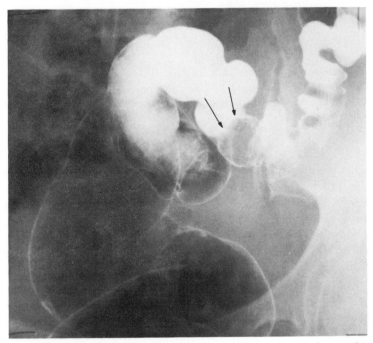

Fig. 7.20 Sigmoid polyp appearing as a partial filling defect within a pool of barium (arrows).

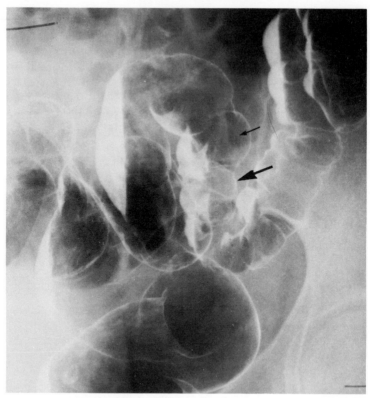

Fig. 7.21 Double density produced by the same polyp as in Fig. 7.20. Note the abrupt increase in density (large arrow) compared with the adjacent bowel (small arrow).

most obvious feature. A polyp is more likely to be malignant if it has an irregular head, indented base or lacks a pedicle. Polyps under 1 cm in size have approximately 1% chance of being malignant and those over 2 cm approximately 50% (Muto, Bussey and Morson, 1975). Although size is the single most reliable criterion (Rose *et al.*, 1980), two of Glick's 26 cases of early colon carcinoma were under 1 cm in diameter (Glick *et al.*, 1980). Thoeni also reported five cases of malignancy in polyps of 1 cm or less (Thoeni and Menuck, 1977).

Before colonoscopy was widely available polyps larger than 1.5 cm to 2 cm in diameter were operated upon, smaller ones were followed radiographically (Schrock, 1980a) and accurate measurement of polyp size was therefore thought to be important (Rose *et al.*, 1980). Colonoscopic practice varies at present, some practitioners finding it unre-

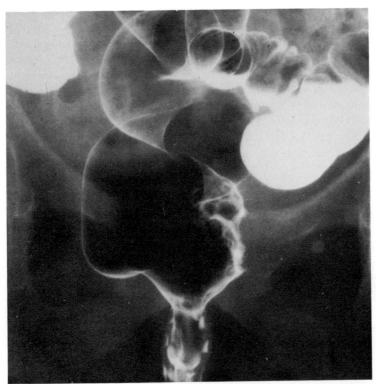

Fig. 7.22 Sessile villous adenomas may appear malignant on radiographs as in this case, with an apparently rigid infiltrated base. This was successfully treated by repeated fulguration, and all removed tissue was benign. Follow-up revealed no recurrence after two years.

warding to pursue polyps of a few millimetres diameter, others preferring to remove all polyps when first detected (Schrock, 1980a).

It is important not to make an overconfident diagnosis of carcinoma in a flat sessile villous lesion in the rectum or recto-sigmoid. These lesions may on occasion appear rigid and obviously carcinomatous and yet be benign and amenable to fulguration (Fig. 7.22).

7.5.2 *Carcinoma — usual appearance*

Most carcinomas are obvious on double contrast films but when coating is poor only the edges of the tumour may be visible. In some cases irregularity in bowel profile may be the only abnormality (Laufer, 1979a). Carcinoma coexisting with diverticular disease causes problems, both false positives and false negatives occurring with greater frequency than in normal bowel. In diverticular disease with severe spasm or obstruction it is frequently impossible to make the diagnosis radiologically and wiser not to try when the bowel mucosa cannot be clearly displayed. Colonoscopy may be invaluable in these patients, particularly when diverticular disease is complicated by stricture or associated with chronic bleeding. In a recent series 11% of 135 patients with diverticular disease and chronic bleeding were shown endoscopically to have a carcinoma unsuspected radiologically (Hunt, 1979) In the same series an additional diagnosis was made colonoscopically in 37%.

7.5.3 *Unusual appearances*

Seaman (1976) has reviewed some of the unusual radiological manifestations of colon carcinoma (Table 7.3). Two of these are likely to cause particular difficulty radiologically. Long segment carcinoma, like metastatic disease, may readily be mistaken for Crohn's disease or ischaemia. The radiologist should be alerted to the possibility of malignancy by the nodular submucosal thickening and circumferential striations mimicking cobblestoning, and yet lacking any of the specific features of Crohn's disease such as aphthous ulcers, large irregular ulcers, composite ulcers or fissures. Ulcerating colitis occurring proximal to a small obstructing carcinoma may be due to localized acute ischaemic colitis, and the changes in the ulcerating segment may be so dramatic that the small causative carcinoma is overlooked.

7.5.4 *Follow-up*

After surgical resection for colon carcinoma or after colonoscopic polypectomy the patient remains at increased risk for the develop-

Table 7.3 Unusual radiological manifestations of large bowel cancer

---
Multiplicity
Carcinoma in young people
Calcification in cancers
Perforating colon cancer
Long segment cancer
Cancer in ulcerative colitis
Ulcerating colitis proximal to an obstructing cancer
Intramural gas
Intussusception

---

ment of further tumours. Various follow-up regimes have been advocated (Strum, 1980). No one protocol is adequate for all hospitals or all patients. If the barium enemas in a hospital are poor, all the follow-up examinations should be by occult blood examination and colonoscopy. If the barium enemas are excellent, and there is no appreciable diverticular disease, all the follow-up may be by occult blood examination and barium enema. Each X-ray examination has to be assessed for technical adequacy and completeness, a rule that should also apply to colonoscopy but is impractical until television video-recording is more readily available. If the patient had a poor barium enema before resection of a partially obstructing sigmoid carcinoma, colonoscopy may be advisable three months after surgery to exclude a synchronous lesion. Palpation of the colon at surgery is of no value in excluding second tumours and cannot be relied upon. On the other hand if wide resection of a small carcinoma was preceded by a good barium enema showing the entire colonic mucosa, follow-up may be by six-monthly occult blood examinations and a barium enema at two years.

7.6 Conclusion

Barium enema remains the initial examination of choice for the large bowel and it should be of primary double contrast type. The referring physician should be able to examine the entire large bowel mucosa from the films and especially the caecum, rectum and sigmoid.

One criterion of a satisfactory standard is a polyp detection rate of 10 to 12%. This type of X-ray examination will miss about 10 to 15% of all polyps and 2 to 5% of polyps over 1 cm, mainly in the sigmoid. In patients in whom a left-sided polyp is seen, radiologists should take care to demonstrate the right colon especially clearly as this is where most of the colonoscopic misses occur. Careful demonstration of the right colon may then allow the colonoscopist to feel confident in limiting a difficult examination to the left side. This is particularly important in large teaching centres where many colonoscopies will continue to be performed by less experienced gastroenterologists in training.

In patients with inflammatory bowel disease there are three areas where barium enema may be inadequate. First is in ulcerative colitis where barium enema may not detect early carcinoma or dysplasia. The second is failure reliably to identify early postoperative recurrence in Crohn's disease which is made difficult by spasm or poor coating. The third, is the non-specificity of the radiological signs in some patients with a normal rectal mucosa. In all these instances colonoscopy will be helpful. Barium enema can detect early lesions clearly, but underestimates the extent of disease especially when it is quiescent. The clinical relevance of this underestimation is not clear. Colonoscopy may be invaluable in some patients with inflammatory bowel disease, but has little part to play in the routine management of most patients for whom sigmoidoscopy and double contrast barium enema are sufficient.

In acute rectal bleeding angiography is the primary investigation, as unlike colonoscopy it includes the small bowel in the diagnostic net. Diagnostic angiography followed by therapeutic colonoscopy may become a more common sequence of events in the future. In chronic rectal bleeding colonoscopy must always be considered when proctosigmoidoscopy and properly performed double contrast barium enema are normal.

Radiologists and colonoscopists tend to become aware of each other's deficiencies; if there is communication and dialogue this can form the framework of a team approach to the management of patients with colonic disease.

Acknowledgement

It is a pleasure to thank Dr Richard Gardiner from Chicago, Dr Igor Laufer from Philadelphia, Dr Anders Lunderquist from Lund and Dr Rudi Thoeni from San Francisco for kind permission to quote their unpublished work. We also thank Dr Fred Cole of McMaster University for Figs. 7.10, 7.11 and 7.12.

References

Allison, D. (1980), Gastrointestinal bleeding: radiological diagnosis. *Br. J. Hosp. Med.*, **23**, 358–65.

Alavi, A. (1980), Scintigraphic demonstration of acute gastrointestinal bleeding. *Gastrointest. Radiol.*, **5**, 205–208.

Amberg, J. R. (1980), Complications of colon radiography. *Gastrointest. Endosc.*, **26**(2) supplement, 15S–17S.

Bartram, C. I. (1977), Radiology in the current assessment of ulcerative colitis. *Gastrointest. Radiol.*, **1**, 383–92.

Bartram, C. I. and Walmsley, K. (1978), A radiological and pathological correlation of the mucosal changes in ulcerative colitis. *Clin. Radiol.*, **29**, 323–8.

Baum, S. and Athanasoulis, C. A. (1974), Angiographic diagnosis and control of large bowel bleeding. *Dis. Colon Rect.*, **17**, 447–53.

Bigard, M. A., Gaucher, P. and Lassalle, C. (1979), Fatal colonic explosion during colonoscopic polypectomy. *Gastroenterology*, **77**, 1307–10.

Brahme, F. and Fork, F. T. (1975) Dynamic aspects of Crohn's disease. *Radiologe*, **15**, 463–8.

Brookstein, J. J., Naderi, M. J. and Walter, J. F. (1978), Transcatheter embolization for lower gastrointestinal bleeding. *Radiology*, **127**, 345–9.

Brown, G. R. (1968), The direct air contrast examination: a rapid simplified highly diagnostic procedure. Paper presented at *Ann. Mtg Radio. Soc. N. Am.*, Chicago, December,

Chang, S., Burrel, M., Beelleza, N. and Spiro, H. (1978), Borderlands in the diagnosis of regional enteritis. *Gastrointest. Radiol.*, **3**, 67–2.

Clarke, A. and Jones, L. (1970), Diagnostic accuracy and diagnostic delay in carcinoma of the large bowel. *N.Z. Med. J.*, **71**, 341–7.

Cole, F. M. (1978), Innominate grooves of the colon: morphological characteristics and etiologic mechanisms. *Radiology*, **128**, 41–43.

Cooley, R., Agnew, C. and Rios, G. (1960), Diagnostic accuracy of the barium enema study in carcinoma of the colon and rectum. *Am. J. Roentg.*, **84**, 316–31.

Dilawari, J. B., Parkinson, C., Riddell, R. H., Loose, H. and Williams, C. (1973), Colonoscopy in the investigation of ulcerative colitis (abstract). *Gut*, **14**, 426.

Diner, W. and Cockrill, H. (1979), The continent ileostomy (Kock Pouch): roentgenologic features. *Gastrointest. Radiol.*, **4**, 65–74.

Dodds, W. J., Scanlon, G. T., Shaw, D. K., Steward, E. T., Youker, J. E. and Metter, G. E. (1977), An evaluation of colon cleansing regimens. *Am. J. Roentg.*, **128**, 57–59.

Figiel, S. (1973), Colon examination technique in detection of colon lesions. *First Standardization Conference*, 1969, Chicago. American College of Radiology, pp. 132–43.

Fischer, A. (1923), A roentgenologic method for examination of the large intestine: combination of the contrast material with insufflation with air. *Klin. Wochenschr.*, **2**, 1595.

Frank, R., Riddell, R., Feczko, P. and Levin, B. (1978), Radiological detection of colonic dysplasia (pre-carcinoma) in chronic ulcerative colitis. *Gastrointest. Radiol.*, **3**, 209–20.

Fraser, G. and Findlay, J. (1976), The double contrast enema in ulcerative and Crohn's colitis. *Clin. Radiol.*, **27**, 103–12.

Freeark, R. J. (1979), Changing perspectives in massive lower intestinal haemorrhage. *Surgery Gynec. Obstet.*, **86**, 368–76.

Gabrielsson, N., Granqvist, S., Sundelin, P. and Thorgeirsson, T. (1979), Extent of inflammatory lesions in ulcerative colitis assessed by radiology, colonoscopy and endoscopic biopsies. *Gastrointest. Radiol.*, **4**, 395–400.

Gardiner, R. (1978), Personal communication. (Presbyterian St. Luke's Hospital, Chicago).

Geboes, K. and Vantrappen, G. (1975), The value of colonoscopy in the diagnosis of Crohn's disease. *Gastrointest. Endosc.*, **22**, 18–23.

Gelfand, D., Ott, D. and Tritico, R. (1978), Cost of gastrointestinal examinations. A comparative study. *Gastrointest. Radiol.*, **3**, 135–8.

Gelfand, D., Wu, W. and Ott, D. (1979), The extent of successful colonoscopy: its implication for the radiologist. *Gastrointest. Radiol.*, **4**, 75–78.

Giacchino, J. L., Geis, W. P., Pickleman, J. R., Dado, D. V., Hadcock, W. E. and Gilbertsen, V. (1974), Proctosigmoidoscopy and polypectomy in reducing the incidence of rectal cancer. *Cancer*, **34**, 936–9.

Glick, S., Laufer, I., Kressel, H. and Thompson, J. (1980), Radiographic and clinical features of early colon cancer. *Gastrointest. Radiol.*, **5**, 83.

Goldberg, H., Carruthers, S., Nelson, J. and Singleton, J. (1979), Radiographic findings of the National Cooperative Crohn's Disease Study. *Gastroenterology*, **77**, 925–37.

Heitzmann, E. and Berne, A. (1961), Roentgen examination of the caecum and proximal ascending colon with ingested barium. *Radiology*, **76**, 415–20.

Hewitt, J., Reeve, J., Rigby, J. and Cox, A. G. (1973) Whole gut irrigation in preparation for large bowel surgery. *Lancet* **2**, 337–40.

Hildell, J., Lindstrom, C. and Wenckert, A. (1979), Radiographic appearances: Crohn's disease I. Accuracy of radiographic methods. *Acta Radiol. Diag.*, **20**, 609–25.

Hildell, J., Lindstrom, C. and Wenckert, A. (1980), Radiographic appearances in Crohn's disease III. Colonic lesions following surgery. *Acta Radiol. Diag.*, **21**, 7–78.

Hunt, R. H. (1978), Rectal bleeding. *Clin. Gastroent.*, **7**, 725–30.

Hunt, R. H. (1979), The role of colonoscopy in complicated diverticular disease. *Acta Chir. Belg.*, **6**, 349–53.

Hunt, R. H. (1980), Massive bleeding from the large bowel. *Br. Med. J.*, **280**, 1320–1.

International Commission on Radiological Protection (1977), Recommendations. ICRP Publication No. 26. *Anns ICRP*, **1**,(3).

Joffe, N. (1977), Localized giant pseudopolyposis secondary to ulcerative or granulomatous colitis. *Clin. Radiol.*, **28**, 609–16.

Johnsrude, I. S. and Jackson, D. C. (1978), The role of the radiologist in acute gastrointestinal bleeding. *Gastrointest. Radiol.*, **3**, 357–68.

Kellett, M. J., Zboralske, F. F. and Margulis, A. R. (1977), Per oral pneumocolon examination of the ileocaecal region. *Gastrointest. Radiol.*, **1**, 361–6.

Kelvin, F., Oddson, T., Rice, R., Garbutt, J. and Bradenham, B. (1978), Double contrast barium enema in ulcerative colitis and Crohn's disease. *Am. J. Roentg.*, **131**, 207–13.

Kelvin, F. *et al.* (1979), Lymphoid follicular pattern of the colon in adults. *Am. J. Roentg.*, **133**, 821–5.

Lane, N. (1977), Precursor tissue of ordinary large bowel cancer: implications for cancer prevention. In *The Gastrointestinal Tract* (eds J. H. Yardley, B. C. Morson and M. R. Able) (International Academy of Pathology Monograph No. 18) Williams and Wilkins, Baltimore, pp. 95–100.

Laufer, I. (1976), The double contrast enema: myths and misconceptions. *Gastrointest. Radiol.*, **1**, 19–31.

Laufer, I. (1979a), Principles of double contrast diagnosis. In: *Double Contrast Gastrointestinal Radiology with Endoscopic Correlation* (ed. I. Laufer), W. Saunders, Philadelphia, pp. 11–58.

Laufer, I. (1979b), Tumours of the colon. In: *Double Contrast Gastrointestinal*

Radiology with Endoscopic Correlation (ed. I. Laufer), W. Saunders, Philadelphia, p. 541.

Laufer, I. and de Sa, D. (1978), Lymphoid follicular pattern: a normal feature of the paediatric colon. *Am. J. Roentg.*, **130**, 51–55.

Laufer, I. and Hamilton, J. D. (1975), The radiologic differentiation between ulcerative colitis and granulomatous colitis by double contrast radiology. *Am. J. Gastroent.*, **66**, 259.

Laufer, I., Mullens, J. and Hamilton, J. (1976), Correlation of endoscopy and double contrast radiology in early stages of ulcerative and granulomatous colitis. *Radiology*, **118**, 1–5.

Laufer, I., Smith, N. and Mullens, J. (1976), The radiological demonstration of colorectal polyps undetected by endoscopy. *Gastroenterology*, **70**, 167–70.

Leinicke, J., Dodds, W., Hogan, W. and Stewart, E. (1977), A comparison of colonoscopy and roentgenography for detecting polypoid lesions of the colon. *Gastrointest. Radiol.*, **2**, 125–8.

Lennard Jones, J., Morson, B., Ritchie, J., Shove, D. and Williams, C. (1977), Cancer in colitis – assessment of the individual risk by clinical and histologic criteria. *Gastroenterology*, **73**, 1280–9.

Lunderquist, A. (1979), Personal communication. (University of Lund, Sweden).

MacEwan, D. W., Kavanagh, S., Chow, P. and Tishler, J. M. (1978), Manitoba barium enema efficacy study. *Radiology*, **126**, 39–44.

Margulis, A. and Goldberg, H. (1969), The current state of radiologic technique in the examination of the colon: a survey. *Radiol. Clinics N. Am.*, **7**, 27–42.

Meyers, A. M. and Ghahremani, G. G. (1977), Complications of gastrointestinal fibreoptic endoscopy. *Gastrointest. Radiol.*, **2**, 273–80.

Miller, R. E. (1975), Examination of the colon. *Curr. Prob. Radiol.*, **5**, 3–40.

Miller, R. E., Chernish, S. M. and Brunelle, R. L. (1979), Gastrointestinal radiography with Glucagon. *Gastrointest. Radiol.*, **4**, 1–10.

Miller, R. E. and Lehman, G. (1978), Polypoid colonic lesions undetected by endoscopy. *Radiology*, **129**, 295–7.

Mitty, H. A. Efremidis, S. and Keller, R. J. (1979), Colonic stricture after transcatheter embolization for diverticular bleeding. *Am. J. Roentg.*, **133**, 519–21.

Morson, B. (1974) The polyp cancer sequence in the large bowel. *Proc. R. Soc. Med.*, **67**, 451–7.

Muto, T., Bussey, H. and Morson, B. (1975), The evaluation of cancer of the colon and rectum. *Cancer*, **36**, 2251–70.

Ott, D. and Gelfand, D. (1978), Colorectal tumours: pathology and detection. *Am. J. Roentg.*, **131**, 691–5.

Ott, D., Gelfand, D. and Ramquist, N. (1980), Causes of error in gastrointestinal radiology. *Gastrointest. Radiol.*, **5**, 99–106.

Pennington, L., Hamilton, S. R., Bayless, T. M. and Cameron, J. L. (1980), Surgical management of Crohn's disease: significance of disease at margin of resection. To be published in *Ann. Surg.*, (October or November).

Peterson, G. H. and Miller, R. E. (1978), The barium enema. A reassessment looking toward perfection. *Radiology*, **128**, 315–20.

Pochin, E. E. (1978), Why be quantitative about radiation risk estimates? Lauriston S. Taylor Lecture No. 2. National Council on Radiation Protection and Measurements, Washington.

Rösch, J., Dotter, C. T. and Antonovic, R. (1972), Selective vasoconstrictor infusion in the management of arterio-capillary gastrointestinal haemorrhage. *Am. J. Roentg.*, **116**, 279–88.

Rose, C., Stevenson, G., Somers, S. and Mather, D. (1980) Radiographic measurement of colon polyp size: errors and surgical implications. To be published in *J. Can. Ass. Radiol.* (March).

Rosenstein, M. (1976), *Organ Doses in Diagnostic Radiology*. HEW Publication (FDA), 76-8030. US Department of Health, Education and Welfare, Bureau of Radiological Health, Rockville, MD.

Schrock, T. R. (1980a), Management of the discovered colon lesion. *Gastrointest. Endosc.*, **26**(2) supplement, 36S–37S.

Schrock, T. R. (1980b), Colon cancer: panel discussion. *Gastrointest. Endos.*, **26**(2) supplement, 41S–42S.

Seaman, W. B. (1971), Disease of the colon: new concepts, old problems. *Radiology*, **100**, 251–69.

Seaman, W. B. (1976), Unusual roentgen manifestations of large bowel cancer. *Sem. Roentg.*, **11**, 89–99.

Seaman, W. B. and Wells, J. (1965), Complications of the barium enema. *Gastroenterology*, **48**, 728–37.

Sheedy, P., Fulton, R. and Atwell, D. (1975), Angiographic evaluation of patients with chronic gastrointestinal bleeding. *Am. J. Roentg.*, **123**, 338–47.

Simpkins, K. C. (1977), Aphthoid ulcers in Crohn's colitis. *Clin. Radiol.*, **28**, 601–8.

Simpkins, K. C. and Stevenson, G. (1972), The modified Malmö double contrast barium enema in colitis: an assessment of its accuracy in reflecting sigmoidoscopic findings. *Br. J. Radiol.*, **45**, 486–92.

Simpkins, K. C. and Young, A. (1968), The radiology of colonic and rectal polyps. *Br. J. Surg.*, **55**, 731–5.

Skucas, J., Cutcliff, W. and Fisher, H. W. (1976), Whole-gut irrigation as a means of cleaning the colon. *Radiology*, **121**, 303–5.

Stephens, D., Mantell, B. and Kelly, K. (1979), Radiology of the continent ileostomy. *Am. J. Roentg.*, **132**, 717–21.

Strum, W. B. (1980), Surveillance of the tumour-prone colon. *Gastrointest. Endos.*, **26**(2) supplement, 38S–40S.

Swarbrick, E. T., Hunt, R. H., Fevre, D. and Williams, C. B. (1976), Colonoscopy in unexplained rectal bleeding. *Gut*, **17**, 823.

Tedesco, F. J., Waye, J. D., Raskin, J. B., Marns, S. J. and Greenwald, R. A. (1978), Colonoscopic evaluation of rectal bleeding: A study of 304 patients. *Ann. Int. Med.*, **89**, 907.

Thoeni, R. (1980), personal communication.

Thoeni, R. and Margulis, A. (1978), The state of radiographic technique in the examination of the colon: a survey. *Radiology*, **127**, 317–23.

Thoeni, R. and Menuck, L. (1977), Detection of small colon polyps. *Radiology*, **124**, 631–5.

Waye, J. D., Kneel, I., Bauer, J. and Galesnt, I. M. (1977), The continent ileostomy: diagnosis and treatment problems by means of operative fiberoptic endoscopy, *Gastrointestinal Endoscopy*, **23**, 196–98.

Welin, S. (1967), Results of the Malmö technique of colon examination. *J. Am. Med. Ass.*, **199**, 119–21.

Whitley, N. and Hunt, T. (1979), Angiography in the diagnosis and management of gastrointestinal bleeding. *Appl. Radiol.*, (Nov–Dec), 63–75.

Williams, C., Hunt, R. and Loose, H. (1974), Colonoscopy in the management of colon polyps. *Br. J. Surg.*, **61**, 673–82.

Williams, C. B. and Waye, J. D. (1978), Colonoscopy in inflammatory bowel disease. *Clinics Gastroent.*, **7**, 701–17.

Young, A. C. (1963), The instant barium enema in proctocolitis. *Proc. R. Soc. Med.*, **56**, 491–4.

Young, A. C. (1964), The Malmö enema at St. Mark's Hospital. A preliminary report. *Proc. R. Soc. Med.*, **57**, 275–8.

Young, A. C. (1966), Radiology of the colon and rectum. In: *Modern Trends in Surgery* **2**. (ed. W. T. Ervine), Butterworths, London, pp. 32–53.

CHAPTER EIGHT

Colonoscopy Intubation Techniques with Fluoroscopy

RICHARD H. HUNT

The experienced colonoscopist can reach the caecum in the majority of patients without the use of X-ray screening and soon becomes acquainted with those endoscopic landmarks which can assist in localizing the tip of the instrument (Waye, 1975). Despite reliable and effective techniques of intubation without fluoroscopy there are a number of advantages in the regular use of X-ray screening when colonoscopic procedures are being performed: it helps the endoscopist who is learning the technique to understand the effects of control movements on the tip or shaft of the instrument; the procedure is often quicker to perform; and keeping the colonoscope straight reduces stress on the instrument, making the investigation more tolerable for the patient. Fluoroscopy allows the endoscopist to confirm that total colonoscopy has been performed to the caecum which on occasion may be difficult despite a knowledge of intraluminal landmarks. X-ray screening allows the endoscopist to site lesions and biopsy locations within the colon more accurately and to search confidently those areas questioned by the barium enema examination.

It is however in those patients who have either unusual or altered anatomy of the colon that X-ray screening is most valuable. This is especially so in those patients who have a redundant colon (Fig. 8.1), those with complicated diverticular disease of the sigmoid colon, following abdominal and especially pelvic surgery, after previous infections or peritonitis and following radiotherapy for pelvic malignancy. In any of these situations adhesions between loops of colon or of colon to loops of small bowel may accentuate the angulations of the sigmoid colon and especially the sigmoid descending colon junction.

8.1 X-ray units

Colonoscopy may be performed most easily and efficiently in a purpose-built endoscopy room in which the X-ray screening facility

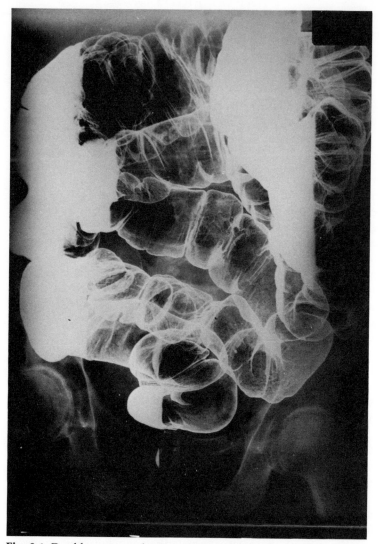

Fig. 8.1 Double contrast barium enema showing extremely redundant colon loops.

has been incorporated. An example of this can be seen in Fig. 8.2 which shows the arrangement of the endoscopy room at St. Marks Hospital for Disease of the Colon and Rectum, London. The endoscopy table has a four-way mobile top and the screening unit is suspended on a telescopic mount from the ceiling above the table so that

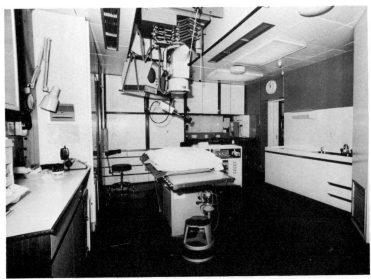

Fig. 8.2 The endoscopy suite at St. Marks Hospital, London. The table has a four-way mobile top, the X-ray unit is suspended from the ceiling and the X-ray and video monitors are also mounted above the table to leave the floor space as free as possible (by courtesy of Dr Christopher Williams).

it may be lowered when required. The X-ray screen is also conveniently suspended from the ceiling thus freeing valuable floor space.

Other purpose designed endoscopy rooms may be equipped with a cheaper but more versatile C-arm screening unit such as that shown in Fig. 4.3 (p. 32).

Most endoscopists who wish to have access to an X-ray screening facility will have an arrangement for a number of sessions in a suitable room in the X-ray Department. The largest available room should be used in order to allow adequate access for the necessary accessories for colonoscopy such as light source, trolley, suction unit, etc. and the typical arrangement in the X-ray department can be seen in Fig. 8.3.

The protective lead gowns which are often uncomfortable and heavy need not be worn until a situation requiring screening is encountered, for X-ray screening is not used continuously but only as an aid to perform a number of manoeuvres which may ease and speed intubation. With increased experience the mean time of screening drops from 2 min to a mean of less than 1 min per patient (Hunt, 1978).

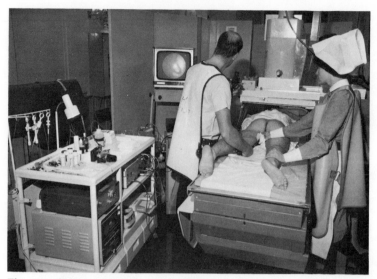

Fig. 8.3 Colonoscopy may be performed relatively easily in a conventional X-ray department. The assistant can prevent the colonoscope from slipping back at the anus when standing opposite the endoscopist but still has access to the accessory trolley.

Modern X-ray units may be fitted with an intermittent exposure facility and video disc recorder which can reduce significantly the radiation exposure to patients, staff and colonoscopes. This equipment is known as the X-ray dose reduction system.

8.2 Anatomy of the colon

The colonoscopist must know the basic features of colonic anatomy to understand the difficulties which may be encountered during insertion of the instrument.

The rectum is bound to the posterior abdominal wall as are both the descending and ascending colon. The sigmoid colon and transverse colon therefore move freely between these fixed points and it is in these regions that the colonoscopist encounters most of the problems of intubation.

The large bowel is about 150 cm in length. The anal canal is approximately 4 cm long and its abrupt posterior angle is maintained by the sling of puborectalis muscle formed from the levator ani muscle. The lower part of the rectum is dilated into the rectal ampulla at the level of the third sacral vertebra. The valves of Houston are encountered in the upper rectum and they are seen as mucosal projections – two on the left and one on the right side.

The sigmoid colon is suspended from the pelvic wall on a double fold of mesentery which is V-shaped and attached between the point where the left external iliac artery bifurcates, and the third sacral vertebra in the mid-line. The sigmoid colon may rest on the bladder in the male or the bladder, uterus and ovary in the female. Lying between the fixed points of the rectum and descending colon, the sigmoid colon, which is about 40 cm in length, may loop in a variety of ways on its mesentery of variable length and can be stretched at colonoscopy high into the abdomen.

The sigmoid colon may make a sharp angulation with the descending colon, which is about 25 cm in length and lies in the left paracolic gutter. The colon is at its highest point at the splenic flexure in contrast to the lower, more dilated hepatic flexure and the high acute angulation of the splenic flexure is normally mobile and suspended on the mesentery of the transverse colon. The true anatomical splenic flexure lies over the posteroinferior tip of the spleen and may often be seen as an angulation of the descending colon on the barium enema films (Fig. 8.4).

Both the descending colon and the ascending colon lie posteriorly while the transverse colon passes from the posterior aspect anteriorly across the abdomen and posteriorly again. Whalen (1976) has pointed out that when viewed laterally the depth of the colon from anterior to posterior aspect is much greater than normally appreciated. The anterior position of the transverse colon can be seen in Fig. 8.5 which shows lateral screening with the colonoscope inserted to the ascending colon.

The transverse colon is about 50 cm in length and suspended entirely on the transverse mesocolon which, as already mentioned, usually suspends the splenic flexure and occasionally the hepatic flexure also. When the transverse colon is suspended on a long mesocolon it may be stretched by the colonoscope deep into the pelvis in a V-shaped configuration.

The transverse colon meets the ascending colon at the hepatic flexure. The ascending colon lies anterior to the right kidney and is about 15 cm in length with the lower portion lying in the right paracolic gutter below the right kidney.

The caecum occupies the right iliac fossa. The terminal ileum normally enters posteromedially at the ileocaecal valve which characteris-

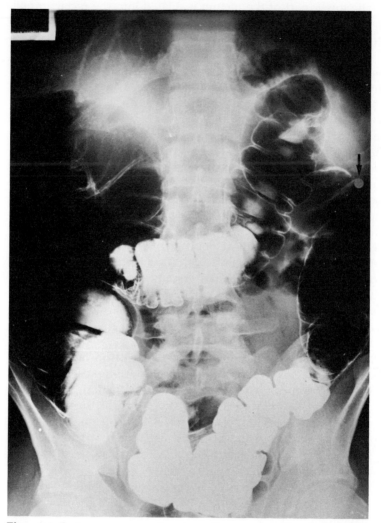

Fig. 8.4 Barium enema showing the true anatomical splenic flexure (arrowed).

tically appears as a horizontal slit-like aperture. Also on the posteromedial wall a few centimetres below the ileocaecal valve lies the orifice of the appendix, situated at the meeting point of the triradiate folds of the caecal pole.

Although the colon is about 150 cm in length, when the colonoscope is inserted, without loops, the caecum normally lies at about 70 cm, the hepatic flexure at about 60 cm, the splenic flexure at about

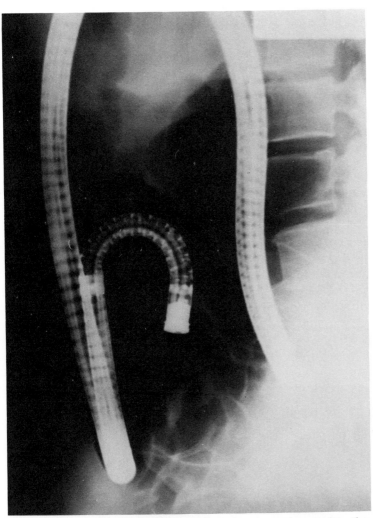

Fig. 8.5 Lateral screening showing the colonoscope inserted to the ascending colon. The transverse colon lies anterior and can easily be manipulated by abdominal pressure from the hand.

50 cm and the descending colon sigmoid colon junction at about 35 cm from the anal margin.

Many of these observations on the anatomy of the colon have been beautifully demonstrated by Whalen and Riemenschneider (1967) and help to explain why difficulties may be encountered during intubation of the colonoscope especially in the sigmoid colon, at the sigmoid colon/descending colon junction but also at the splenic and hepatic flexures and in the transverse colon.

8.2.1 *Unusual colonic anatomy*

When using fluoroscopy the experienced endoscopist will sometimes encounter unusual and unexpected configurations of the colonoscope which do not fit with concepts of the normal anatomy.

An example of this can be seen in Fig. 8.6. The X-ray shows a reversed splenic flexure and a descending colon which lies in the centre of the abdomen on a mesentery rather than in the left paracolic gutter as expected.

Other variations which may be encountered include a caecum in the right hypochondrium, or in the mid-abdomen in the pelvis rather than in the right iliac fossa.

Surgeons are usually aware of the considerable variation of colonic anatomy between patients and a persistent descending mesocolon has been found in 36% and ascending mesocolon in 10% of subjects (Cotton and Williams, 1980).

Excessive looping may occur in patients with a long transverse mesocolon as can be seen with the gamma loop shown in Fig. 8.7.

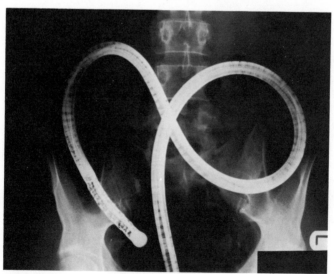

Fig. 8.6 The descending colon is on a mesentery in continuity with the sigmoid colon. This anatomic configuration reverses the splenic flexure.

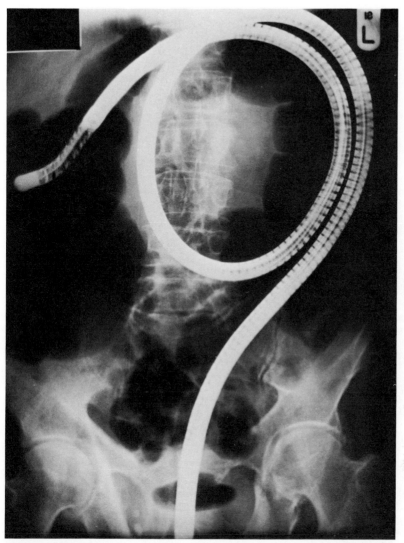

Fig. 8.7 A gamma loop may sometimes form in the mid-transverse colon. This configuration prevents much of the propulsive force given to the shaft from reaching the colonoscope tip.

Both this and the unusual appearance seen when there is a persistent descending mesocolon (Fig. 8.6) can usually be reduced to represent the expected question mark shape (Fig. 8.8) when the colonoscope is inserted to the caecum.

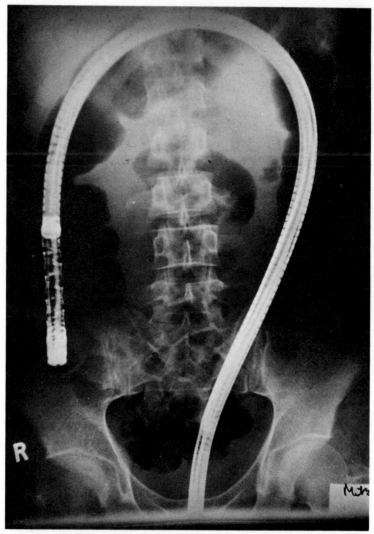

Fig. 8.8 The ideal 'question mark' configuration for the colonoscope when inserted to the caecum.

8.3 The technique of colonoscopy using fluoroscopy

Early reports of colonoscopic intubation suggested that the best technique of insertion was to pass the colonoscope into the colon and allow the mucosa to 'slide by', especially around sharply angulated bends where the limited tip flexion of earlier instruments did not permit visualization of the lumen. If the mucosa blanched or insertion was difficult the instrument was then withdrawn a little. In general this was not a successful technique. Although the caecum could often be reached successfully, patients were frequently subjected to severe discomfort due to the formation of many large loops. Loops stretch

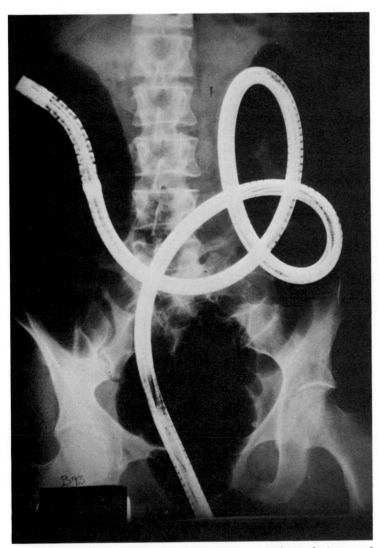

Fig. 8.9 Numerous loops produced during early techniques of 'slide-by' insertion. The drive wires become so stretched that the colonoscope tip cannot be moved.

the control wires and place the instrument under considerable stress (Fig. 8.9) which can be the frequent cause of damage and expensive repair bills.

The development of colonoscopes with a tip capable of deflection through 230° and wider angles of view means that it is now possible to visualize the lumen of the colon during most of the insertion. These advances coupled with a better understanding of the anatomy of the colon have considerably affected the endoscopist's approach to technique.

The handling of the colonoscope remains the same whether or not fluoroscopy is used to assist in intubation. The head of the instrument is held in the left hand and the 'up-down' control is manipulated by the thumb and forefinger of the left hand. The 'right-left' control is usually kept locked and manipulated when required by the right hand which otherwise controls the manipulation of the shaft of the instrument, which can then be torqued, advanced or withdrawn simultaneously with hooking the tip, using the left hand on the up-down control. A nursing assistant can, if necessary, prevent the shaft of the colonoscope from slipping back by holding the colonoscope at the anus (Fig. 8.3) whenever the endoscopist's right hand is off the shaft of the instrument. Most endoscopists do not employ their assistant to advance the scope, however, preferring to retain their own sensitive control over intubation.

The patient lies in the left lateral position and following a careful rectal examination, which helps to relax the anal sphincter, the well lubricated colonoscope is inserted through the anus along the forefinger of the right hand. Residual fluid in the rectum is usually aspirated and the lens flushed before insertion of the instrument begins. If the lens is coated with lubricant jelly or faeces the instrument should be withdrawn at this stage and the lens cleaned before reinsertion. Intubation requires careful steering up the lumen of the colon without the insufflation of too much air which may increase the angulations of the bowel especially at the sigmoid/descending colon junction.

X-ray screening is not necessary for the endoscopist to know that a loop is forming. If the tip of the colonoscope is not advancing within the lumen in a one-to-one relationship with the shaft of the instrument entering the anus, then one or more loops are forming. If, in this situation, advance of the tip has not been achieved after withdrawal, reorientation and reinsertion, fluoroscopy can be most helpful and time-saving.

It is normally necessary to change the position of the patient in order to use X-ray screening most effectively, although some endoscopists are able to interpret the position of the colonoscope when screening in the left lateral position (Fig. 8.5). Most of those who use fluoroscopy place their patient in the supine position but it is my own practice to place the patient in the prone position (Fig. 8.3) although this does take additional time. This position has a number of advantages; it provides natural abdominal compression which is often helpful to intubation but does still not hinder access for an assistant to add manual abdominal compression should it be necessary; patients are generally more comfortable lying prone, are less embarrassed in this position and the endoscopist has better access to the colonoscope with more control over manipulations of the shaft at the anus.

Alternatively, the patient may remain in the left lateral position when the experienced endoscopist can interpret lateral screening. This position is also comfortable for most patients except those with arthritis; it is not embarrassing and gives good access for insertion of the colonoscope, abdominal compression by the assistant and for nursing observations.

8.4 The sigmoid colon

The most common loops which may form in the sigmoid region are the natural alpha loop (Fig. 8.10) which can be helpful allowing an easy passage to the descending colon and splenic flexure. It is usually readily resolved by withdrawal of the colonoscope while applying clockwise rotation to the shaft (Fig. 8.12d and e). X-ray screening is rarely necessary to perform this procedure. The second most common loop in the sigmoid region is the N-shaped configuration which may be less easy to negotiate (Fig. 8.11). There is also a variety of more complex and less well recognized configurations which may occur in the sigmoid region. In some cases these may be caused by poor intubation techniques, especially from inserting too much colonoscope at the anus with little or no advance of the tip thus allowing loops to form. Sigmoid loops can often be prevented by frequent withdrawal of the instrument. Stretching makes natural angulations of the colon more acute and tends to decrease the diameter of the bowel lumen. This distorts the natural landmarks which assist intubation; for example, the sigmoid folds may be less obvious and the helpful signs of circular muscular folds and arcuate highlights (Plate 5) disappear: consequently, the lumen is less easily seen and followed. Another common error is to insufflate too much air within the sigmoid region which also makes the natural angulations of the colon more acute and the lumen less easy to see. This is especially true at the sigmoid/des-

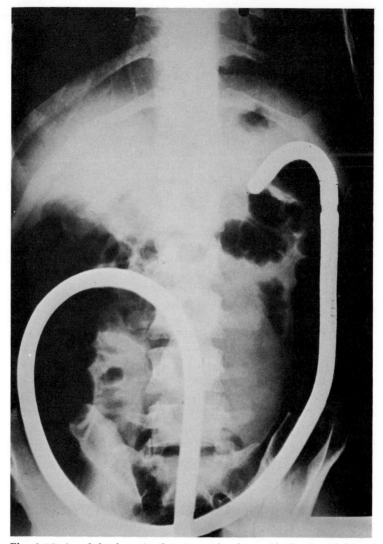

Fig. 8.10 An alpha loop in the sigmoid colon with the tip of the colonoscope at the splenic flexure.

cending colon junction, which is the most common site of difficulty. Loops which have been distended by over inflation with air are difficult to reduce by mechanical manipulation.

Occasionally, double loops may occur in the sigmoid region and these may present a problem if they keep recurring. It may not be possible to resolve either one or both the loops until the tip of the

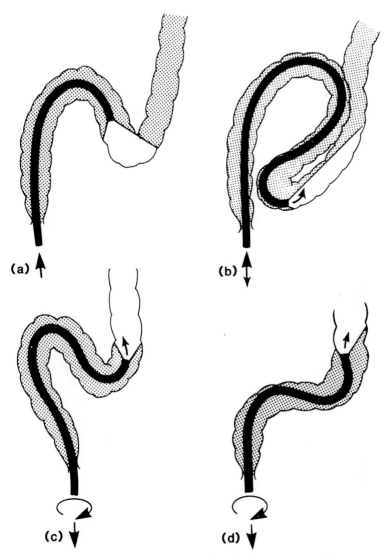

Fig. 8.11 The 'N'-shaped configuration of the colonoscope which may occur at the sigmoid colon/descending colon junction. Advancement by wriggling and jiggling (b) into the lower descending colon is followed by withdrawal with clockwise torque (c) and then straightening of the instrument to achieve a paradoxical advance up the descending colon.

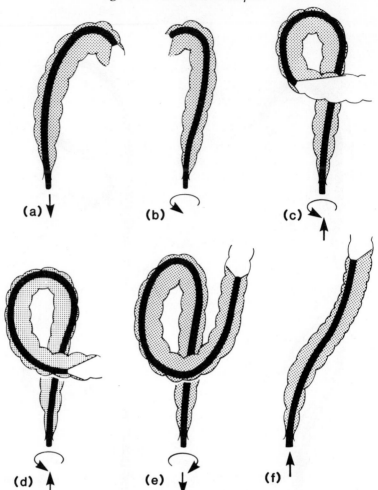

(a) (b) (c)

(d) (e) (f)

Fig. 8.12 The alpha loop may be created by withdrawal of the instrument tip to the apex of the sigmoid (a). Anticlockwise rotation through 180° (b) is followed by advance monitoring torque (c and d). Once the colonoscope tip is inserted well into the descending colon the instrument is straightened by clockwise rotation and simultaneous withdrawal (e) before further advancement (f).

colonoscope has advanced to the splenic flexure. Screening is usually necessary to resolve looping of this nature and may indicate the need to 'push through' the loops for the tip to attain and then maintain, a purchase at the splenic flexure. Hooking the tip at the splenic flexure will prevent the tip slipping back into the descending colon or even the upper sigmoid colon.

It is wise to use X-ray screening when pushing through a loop to avoid damage to the bowel wall. Serosal lacerations may occur during some procedures (Livstone and Kerstein, 1976; Sjogren *et al.*, 1978) and by monitoring with fluoroscopy stretching of loops may be kept to a minimum. The mildly sedated patient will complain of pain as the mesentery becomes seriously stretched. Resolution of a double loop usually requires clockwise rotation on withdrawal followed by anticlockwise rotation as the withdrawal is continued. Resolution of such loops is always best performed under both visual and X-ray control to prevent damage to the sigmoid mesentery.

In practice it is those patients who have moderate to severe sigmoid diverticular disease that pose most problems in the sigmoid region probably as a consequence of pericolic inflammation which has resulted in fixation of the sigmoid colon. The lumen may also be difficult to find and associated poor bowel preparation may be an added problem which obscures the view.

Intubation difficulties may also commonly be encountered in patients who have had abdominal or especially pelvic surgery and women patients following a previous hysterectomy constitute a particular problem in this group. Previous radiotherapy for pelvic malignancy may make the situation even more difficult, when fixation of the colon may be almost complete. Such patients may be submitted for colonoscopy because of bleeding when the differential diagnosis includes radiation colitis or possible recurrence of the pelvic malignancy with local invasion of the colon. A successful examination is essential but is not always possible although helpful information may still be obtained. In patients with this kind of problem an N-shaped configuration (Fig. 8.11) may be commonly encountered. This has been described as S-shaped by Matsunaga and Tajima (1970) who described difficulty in entering the descending colon when this configuration is encountered. Deyhle (1972b) suggested a technique for intubating such a sigmoid colon. By coaxing the tip under X-ray control around the sigmoid colon/descending colon junction with short movements of insertion and withdrawal to lie 5 or 10 cm into the descending colon (Fig. 8.11b). Then by applying clockwise torque to the colonoscope at the anus with the tip of the instrument angled up and pressed against the colonic wall, the shaft could be withdrawn (Fig. 8.11c) again under X-ray control thus 'straightening' the sigmoid colon and achieving a paradoxical advance of the tip of the colonoscope up the descending colon (Fig. 8.11d). It is important to look through the instrument and visualize the lumen while the loop is being reduced by withdrawal in order to steer up the descending colon during the final act of straightening the sigmoid.

The junction of the sigmoid colon and the descending colon is likely to be the first point of difficulty for the experienced endoscopist and the position of the patient may be changed at this point in order to use X-ray screening. This act of repositioning the patient onto the front (or back) may in itself make passage of the colonoscope easier (Overholt 1975) and screening will not always be required.

Some authors have in the past suggested that when the sigmoid colon/descending colon junction cannot be easily passed, the endoscopist should attempt to create an alpha loop (Williams and Teague, 1973; Williams, 1974; Wolff and Shinya, 1974; Sakai, 1974). This manoeuvre is seldom employed now that individual expertise has increased and modern instruments are capable of such extreme tip deflections.

However, an alpha loop may still, on occasion, be useful and is therefore described: it is wise to use X-ray screening to control the manoeuvre. The colonoscope is withdrawn so that the tip of the instrument lies about halfway around the sigmoid loop (Fig. 8.12) which is usually reached at 35 ± 5 cm during intubation. The shaft of the instrument is torqued anticlockwise through 180° (Fig. 8.12a and b) and the instrument is advanced as the anticlockwise torque is maintained. This allows the tip of the colonoscope to slide around the 'outside' wall of the alpha loop to enter the descending colon (Fig. 8.12d and e). The tip should be advanced to the splenic flexure before the loop is resolved. The endoscopist should be viewing this blind 'slide-by' manoeuvre while intermittently screening. Straightening of the colonoscope is achieved by simultaneous 180° clockwise rotation and withdrawal (Fig. 8.12e and f). The colonoscope can then be advanced directly to the splenic flexure.

Severe fixation of the sigmoid colon may result in a 'spiral' configuration when the shaft is viewed fluoroscopically (Fig. 8.13). The fixation usually results from severe pelvic inflammation, previous surgery or radiation and poses a special problem for the colonoscopist since a fixed loop makes it difficult to transfer the force of insertion to the tip of the instrument. When fixation occurs together with acute angulation of the sigmoid/descending colon junction intubation may be particularly difficult and constant advance and withdrawal to straighten the angle of the junction is necessary in the attempt to enter the descending colon.

8.4.1 *Reformation of sigmoid loops*

After straightening any configuration of sigmoid loops, further advance will often lead to reformation of a loop which need not necessarily comply with that which was first encountered. The modern

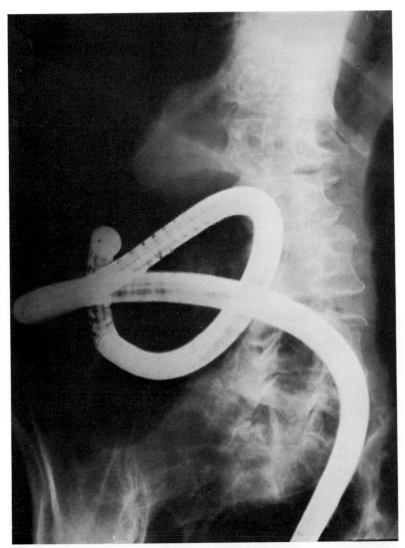

Fig. 8.13 The spiral configuration often seen in a fixed sigmoid colon. the instrument tip is almost at the sigmoid descending colon junction. Advance is usually achieved by a little withdrawal and wriggling and jiggling but the instrument often slips back.

colonoscope makes it easier to maintain a 'straight' sigmoid colon by virtue of the torque stability of the shaft as exemplified by the four-stage stiffening inherent in the construction of the ACMI long colonoscope. Despite these advantages and greatly improved techniques, sigmoid loops may still reform and in some cases constitute a problem. Attempts to stiffen the colonoscope by the use of internal wires or external sigmoid splints have thus been described (Deyhle, 1972a, 1972b) and widely used (Nagy, 1973; Sakai, 1974; Williams and Teague, 1973; Shinya and Wolff, 1976).

8.4.2 *The sigmoid splint/stiffening sleeve*

A sigmoid stiffening device was first advocated for use by Deyhle (1972b) and those currently available consists of a 45 cm tube of plastic material strengthened by a wire spiral (Fig. 8.14a). There is a washer at the proximal end to prevent leakage of air and fluid from the colon.

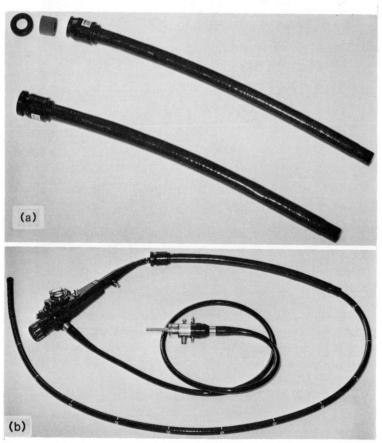

Fig. 8.14 (a) A colonoscope stiffening sleeve (Olympus) showing the seal and the assembled tube. (b) The stiffening sleeve placed over the colonoscope before endoscopy.

When use of the sigmoid sleeve is anticipated, fluoroscopy is mandatory. The sleeve is placed over the colonoscope before intubation is started (Fig. 8.14b). It is usually necessary to unscrew the tip of the instrument before passing the sleeve over the shaft. The tip should then be replaced and the sleeve passed as far as it will go towards the control head of the instrument; lubrication with silicone or water soluble jelly is helpful. The sleeve then remains in this position until required. It is difficult to use the stiffening sleeve with shorter colonoscopes because not enough shaft is left free for manipulation and insertion, with the sleeve in place on the proximal end of the instrument.

Intubation of the sigmoid colon is performed as usual. Any sigmoid loops encountered are straightened as described and once the colonoscope is in the upper descending colon or at the splenic flexure the sleeve may be inserted safely.

The anus is liberally lubricated with a water soluble lubricant jelly and the stiffening sleeve carefully advanced through the anus over the shaft of the 'straightened' colonoscope. Clearly the instrument is not entirely straight for there is a gentle S-shape in both the AP and lateral planes. Gentle traction on the colonoscope is maintained as the sleeve is advanced in order to keep it 'straightened' and gentle rotation of the sleeve permits a more controlled and gentle insertion. The insertion procedure is carefully monitored by X-ray screening, and is necessary in only one plane. Fluoroscopy is essential to ensure that the colonoscope has remained 'straight', that the tip has not slipped back from the splenic flexure and to confirm that the sleeve is correctly sited (Fig. 8.15). Once in position, the assistant must hold the head of the sleeve firmly in place at the anus allowing the colonoscope to slide freely in or out. The sleeve is not normally taken out until the caecum has been reached and the colonoscope has been withdrawn to the region of the hepatic flexure.

The sigmoid stiffening sleeve should never be used without the facility for X-ray screening. Even with this precaution perforation may occur and damage may be caused to the shaft of the colonoscope, although this device is less likely to damage the instrument than the use of stiffening wires previously described (Deyhle, 1972a). Severe diverticular disease and pelvic adhesions may make the use of the stiffening sleeve difficult or even impossible.

The stiffening sleeve will prevent reformation of sigmoid loops which are often associated with pain and may slow insertion of the colonoscope beyond the splenic flexure. Well planned and careful use of the sigmoid sleeve in patients with a long and redundant sigmoid colon may make total colonoscopy a less painful and more rapid procedure.

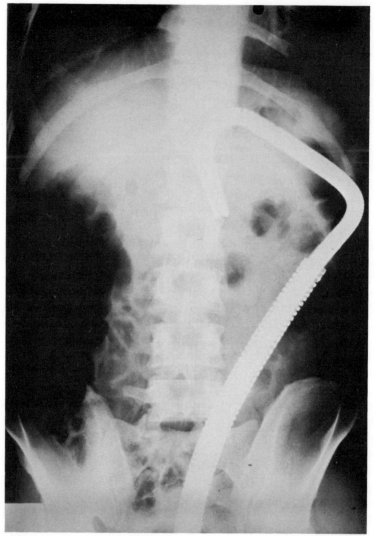

Fig. 8.15 The colonoscope inserted to the distal transverse colon with the stiffening sleeve in place.

8.5 The splenic flexure

X-ray screening may not be necessary during passage up the descending colon (Plate 4) unless this part of the colon has an aberrant mesentery. A 'gate-like' fold is frequently seen (Plate 8) just below the splenic flexure, which is recognized by the blue venous colouration of the spleen seen through the colon wall (Plate 7). The colonoscope is advanced into the flexure, where the acute angulation between descending and transverse colon often causes difficulty in obtaining a view of the lumen. This problem has been partially solved with advances in technological design and with greater instrument tip deflection. Careful steering to the left permits the characteristic triangular format of the transverse colon to be seen (Plates 9 and 10). Angulation to the left, clockwise rotation on the shaft and withdrawal of the colonoscope (Fig. 8.16) brings down the high but mobile splenic flexure which is possible because it is usually suspended on the mesentery of the distal transverse colon. It may be helpful to monitor this manoeuvre by X-ray screening. The acute angulation of the tip of the colonoscope is reduced (thumb back on the up-down control) as the colonoscope is advanced into the distal transverse colon (Fig. 8.16 d–f). Clockwise torque helps to advance the tip of the colonoscope anteriorly as the transverse colon leaves the left paracolic gutter and simultaneously helps to maintain the previously 'straightened' configuration of the sigmoid region.

Passage into the transverse colon is accomplished by a combination of the manoeuvres which have been described. Continuous gentle insertion and withdrawal of the shaft of the colonoscope is used while pulling the flexure down with each withdrawal; and then by reducing tip flexion with each reinsertion (Fig. 8.16). These manoeuvres are all performed with clockwise torque applied to the shaft. Although this technique clearly does not work in every patient it is the most reliable approach in the majority of cases. When a patient has a high and relatively fixed splenic flexure (Fig. 8.17), it may be necessary to 'push through the loop'. This procedure is always best performed under X-ray screening when the size of the loop may be observed. Such a manoeuvre is not without hazard if a large loop is formed when it carries the risk of a linear tear at the flexure or possible damage to the spleen (Telmos and Mittal, 1977; Ellis, Harrison and Williams, 1979).

Variations of anatomy at the splenic flexure do cause confusion. Passage is always more difficult with a high fixed splenic flexure (Fig. 8.17). The most difficult configuration however is the reversed splenic flexure (Fig. 8.6) which may make intubation of the right colon more difficult. Although this appears rather like the alpha loop in the sigmoid colon it cannot always be reduced in the same way because of the anatomical attachments. The use of X-ray to help passage of the colonoscope in this kind of problem is most helpful, because it allows the endoscopist to ascertain when the colonoscope tip has been hooked around the hepatic flexure before withdrawal which may then succeed in reducing the reversed splenic flexure.

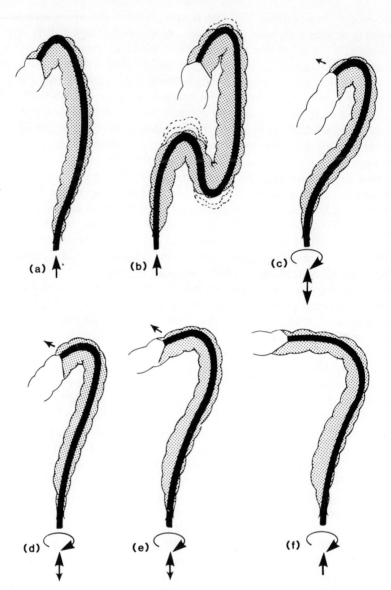

Fig. 8.16 Negotiation of the splenic flexure. Insertion of the colonoscope with the tip at the splenic flexure may stretch both the flexure or the sigmoid colon (b). To negotiate the flexure the instrument is withdrawn with clockwise torque and reintroduced (c). Further advance is achieved by bringing the acutely angulated flexure downwards with each withdrawal and reducing flexion on the tip with each reinsertion (d and e). Clockwise torque is maintained with each advance to prevent recurrence of loops in the sigmoid.

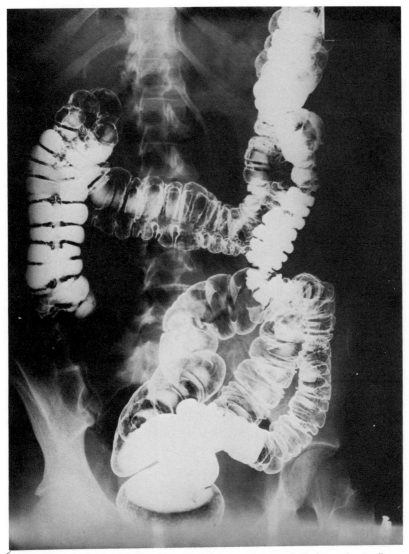

Fig. 8.17 Intubation difficulties may be encountered if the splenic flexure is very high and acute as seen in this barium enema.

8.6 The transverse colon

Insertion of the colonoscope through the transverse colon seldom presents any difficulty. Progress should be made steadily with repeated insufflation of small amounts of air to distend the bowel. Repeated withdrawal of the instrument helps to provide continuous visualiza-

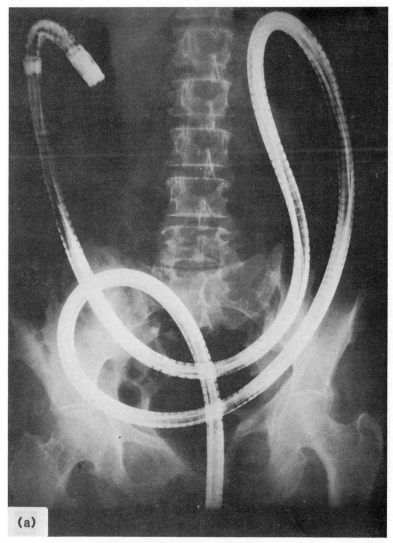

Fig. 8.18a Deep looping of the transverse colon into the pelvis is common as in this case. An alpha loop has recurred in the sigmoid region. The tip is hooked at the hepatic flexure.

tion of the lumen which may be lost from view if too enthusiastic or rapid an advance is made. Initially the lumen lies slightly to the left until the lumbar spine is crossed when both application of right control and upward angulation is usually required. A variety of loops may occur in the transverse colon; those in Figs. 8.18 and 8.19 are the most commonly encountered.

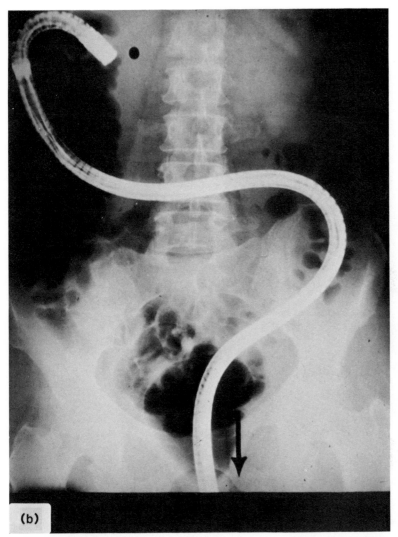

(b)

Fig. 8.18b Withdrawal and clockwise torque resolves both loops. The clockwise rotation on the shaft should be maintained during reinsertion.

In the case of a configuration such as Fig. 8.18 advance is usually achieved by hooking up the tip against a fold in the colon wall (Fig. 8.20a) and withdrawing the shaft thus shortening the transverse colon. A paradoxical advance of the tip towards the hepatic flexure may often then occur when the tip is straightened and the shaft reinserted (Fig. 8.20b). Alternatively, two, three or more repetitions of the same manoeuvre may be required – insertion; hook up; with-

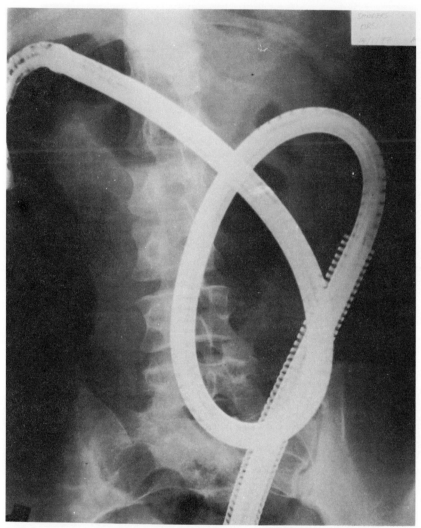

Fig. 8.19 A gamma loop occurring in the distal transverse colon. The stiffening device has been inserted because of troublesome recurrent looping in the sigmoid colon. The caecum can now, however, be reached easily.

draw; reinsert – a little advance being made on each occasion. X-ray can be helpful here to speed progress by intermittent monitoring of these movements.

The use of abdominal compression by the nurse assistant will often prevent reformation of this transverse loop. The assistant's

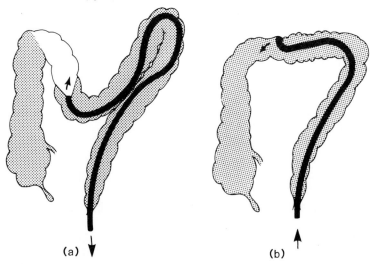

(a)   (b)

Fig. 8.20 Looping in the mid-transverse colon when the tip has not reached the hepatic flexure may be resolved by hooking the tip against the bowel wall and withdrawing (a). On straightening the tip a paradoxical advance towards the hepatic flexure occurs (b). Advance may be continued by repetitive motions of (a) and (b).

hand is passed under the prone patient and compression is applied upwards with the palm of the hand just above the umbilicus and directed posterosuperiorly. X-ray screening should not be applied while the assistant's hand is in place but may be used both before and after the manoeuvre. The technique of placing the patient prone on the screening table helps abdominal compression and if a nurse/assistant is not readily available a pillow under the abdomen can help to compress the area from the umbilicus to the pubic symphysis.

Despite these manoeuvres a dependent transverse colon may still present difficulties and advance may only be achieved by pushing through the loop.

8.7 The proximal transverse colon and hepatic flexure

Passage along the proximal transverse colon is closely related to those manoeuvres which are required to round the hepatic flexure and enter the upper ascending colon: these two regions should therefore be considered together.

As the hepatic flexure is approached the tip of the colonoscope is usually angled upwards (thumb forward on the up-down control wheel). A small amount of right angulation and clockwise torque is applied since the proximal transverse colon lies somewhat posterior.

The hepatic flexure is much wider than the splenic flexure and has prominent arcuate folds which do not fully encircle the lumen. The blue venous colour of the liver (more prominent than the spleen) can be seen through the colonic wall where the right lobe of the liver causes a flattened impression on the superior aspect of the flexure (Plate 11).

Passage around the hepatic flexure is achieved by approaching from below and steering to the right (posteriorly) carefully avoiding the prominent arcuate folds. Then by angling the tip downwards (with the thumb fully back on the up-down control) the ascending colon can usually be visualized. When this is not possible acute left angulation of the full downward deflected tip will often bring the ascending colon into view. In addition, clockwise torque is frequently helpful at this point. Once the ascending colon has been seen, advance of the colonoscope to the caecum is usually achieved by hooking the tip into a fold and withdrawing the shaft at the anus while simultaneously applying clockwise torque (Fig. 8.21). As the tip of the instrument paradoxically enters the ascending colon, advance to the caecum can be aided by using suction to remove air from the right colon. In the ascending colon there is often a gravy-like fluid (Plate 13); the prominent muscular folds do not completely encircle the lumen (Plate 12) and the colon here readily dilates with air. The pole of the caecum, the caecal sling fold, appendix orifice and ileocaecal valve can usually be identified. Loops may occur at the hepatic flexure which

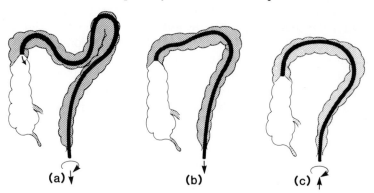

(a)   (b)   (c)

Fig. 8.21 At the hepatic flexure, careful steering to avoid the prominent folds will usually allow the ascending colon to be seen (a). Withdrawal to reduce the transverse loops produces a paradoxical advance (b). The aspiration of air, gentle insertion and clockwise torque, advances the tip down the ascending colon.

may make these ideal manoeuvres less successful, especially when there is a reversed hepatic flexure (Fig. 8.22).

When the configuration in Fig. 8.23a is seen it is often possible to change the configuration by applying left angulation and clockwise torque followed by withdrawal. If this succeeds as shown in Fig. 8.23b then advance of the tip can continue as already described (Fig. 8.23).

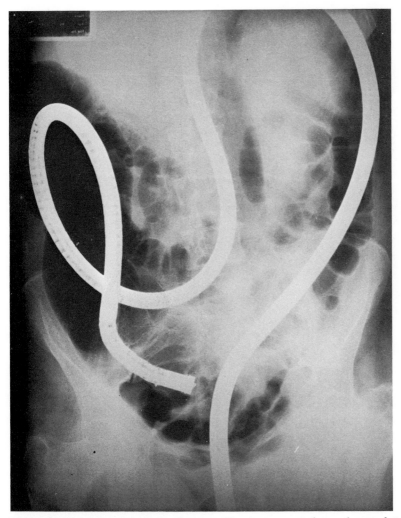

Fig. 8.22 A reversed hepatic flexure. The instrument has advanced to the caecum by 'pushing through the loop' at the hepatic flexure.

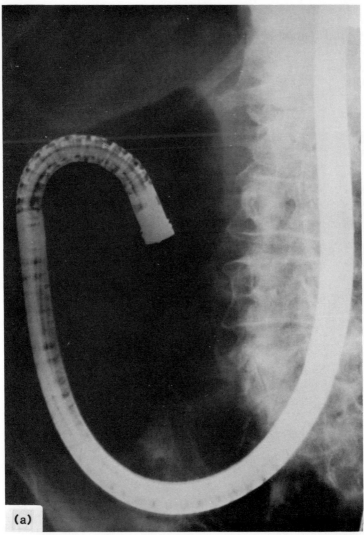

Fig. 8.23a A reversed hepatic flexure with the tip of the instrument in the ascending colon.

However this manoeuvre is not always successful and attempts to withdraw the colonoscope result in the tip of the instrument slipping back around the outside of the loop, losing both the depth of insertion gained and the purchase of the colonoscope tip around the hepatic flexure. After changing the patient's position back to the left lateral or supine position withdrawal of the instrument tip to the mid trans-

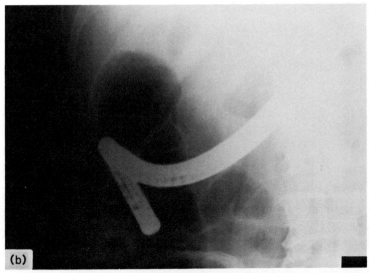

(b)

Fig. 8.23b Withdrawal of the instrument with clockwise torque reduces the loop.

verse colon followed by reinsertion of the colonoscope may help to resolve the problem. Failing that, it is normally preferable to push through the loop to advance the tip of the colonoscope far enough into the ascending colon or even the caecum (Fig. 8.22) for withdrawal and clockwise torque to again be attempted. If the tip has advanced well into the ascending colon this withdrawal manoeuvre will often work. Should this fail then advance into the caecum may only be achieved by pushing through the loop when abdominal compression on the transverse colon can again be helpful or X-ray control can be used. A further attempt to resolve any loops should be made before inspection of the caecum is carried out (Fig. 8.8). This is because control of the tip of the instrument and consequently angulation are compromised when the drive wires are stretched by looping of the colonoscope shaft; this is one of the main reasons for attempting to keep the instrument as 'straight' as possible.

One of the more difficult and unusual anatomical variations encountered by the colonoscopist in this region of the colon is what is known as the right colon loop (Rhodes, Zvargulis, Moffat and Hartong, 1978). This configuration may easily mislead the endoscopist who does not have fluoroscopy available and even with screening a false sense of security may sometimes be engendered. Insertion of the colonoscope to the proximal transverse colon is achieved and this

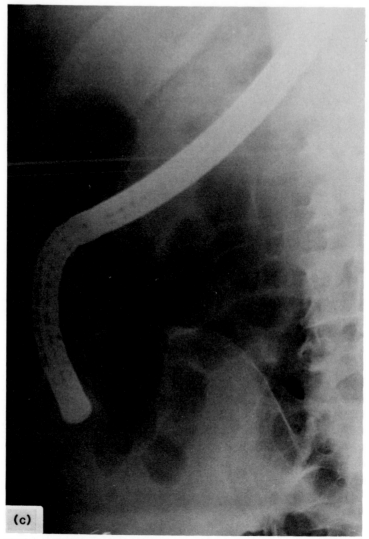

Fig. 8.23c The tip of the instrument then paradoxically advances down the ascending colon to the pole of the caecum.

point then lies in the right lower quadrant of the abdomen. The depth of insertion on the colonoscope will show between 60 and 70 cm; transillumination may be seen in the right iliac fossa and palpation at this point may be seen to indent the colon wall. Due to stretching of the 'superior' wall of the transverse colon no further lumen may be observed. The appendiceal orifice and ileocaecal valve will not be visible here. X-ray screening may suggest that insertion to the caecum has occurred via a low hepatic flexure. However a careful look at the 'pneumogram' will show that the hepatic flexure has not been passed and that the ascending colon has not been intubated. The colonoscope should be withdrawn and the tip angled upwards to take the tension off the stretched colonic wall; a careful search can then be made for the lumen of the proximal transverse colon which has probably been occluded by stretching, a prominent fold or muscle spasm.

The manoeuvres which have been described in the proximal transverse colon, at the hepatic flexure and in the right colon are all made easier if the sigmoid colon remains straightened. This may be achieved by keeping clockwise torque applied to the colonoscope in the case of both Olympus or Fuji instruments. The increased proximal stiffness of the four staged shaft ACMI colonoscope makes this technique less necessary. Alternatively the use of the sigmoid stiffening device may be favoured and this will often allow rapid intubation of the transverse and right colon, with less discomfort for the patient.

8.8 The ascending colon, caecum and terminal ileum

The ascending colon is usually short and dilated with prominent arcuate folds which do not fully encircle the lumen (Plate 12), but on occasion may be found to be deceptively long. Advance down this part of the colon is achieved by withdrawal of the shaft of the instrument accompanied by suction to deflate the caecum, collapsing it towards the tip of the colonoscope. Application of abdominal pressure above the umbilicus to reduce any looping of the transverse colon will help to advance the tip of the instrument to the caecum. X-ray screening is seldom of help in the right colon except to document total colonoscopy (Fig. 8.8). Which can also be confirmed by the easily identifiable landmarks such as the ileocaecal valve (Plate 14). The valve usually lies well above the pole of the caecum to the left or inferiorly in the field of view but may occasionally be on the right. The orifice of the appendix may be seen (Plate 15) as well as the characteristic caecal sling fold. Transillumination of light from the tip of the instrument may be in the right iliac fossa (Plate 20) and finger palpation just distal to this will indent the caecal wall (Plate 19). If there are no loops in the colonoscope and the tip is in the caecum, approximately 70 cm of instrument will be inserted.

It is essential to make a careful search of the caecum which may be difficult if the instrument has not been straightened by resolving all existing loops. Blind spots can certainly occur in this part of the colon and an attempt should be made to invert the tip of the colonoscope. After straightening the colonoscope the tip should be advanced to the pole of the caecum and angled fully up with maximum left control applied. Careful advance with intermittent and gentle withdrawal will usually allow the endoscopist to visualize the inferior aspect of the ileocaecal valve and surrounding arcuate folds (Plate 17). Any residual fluid in the caecum should be aspirated to permit a careful search especially for vascular abnormalities (see Chapter 14).

It is important to have good visualization of the caecum in order to enter the ileocaecal valve and terminal ileum (Nagasako and Takemoto, 1973; Gaisford, 1974). The superior aspect of the valve is normally identified as a flattening of the arcuate fold but may also be seen to take a labial form (Plate 18). The tip of the colonoscope is advanced past the valve and angled acutely upwards and towards it. The colonoscope is then gently withdrawn and when the tip of the colonoscope lifts the superior lip of the valve the angulation is reduced and the tip straightened to advance into the terminal ileum (Plate 25). Direct intubation by advancing the instrument down the ascending colon under visual control is rarely achieved. Radiology is seldom helpful for intubation of the terminal ileum but may assist the trainee endoscopist to understand how to perform the manoeuvre which has been described.

8.9 Withdrawal and examination of the colon

Examination of the colon should be made on both insertion and withdrawal of the colonoscope, for small lesions may otherwise be missed. However, the most searching examination is made during withdrawal. After the caecum (and perhaps terminal ileum) has been examined withdrawal of the colonoscope is controlled by the thumb and fingers of the right hand on the shaft of the instrument held 15–20 cm from the anus. The thumb and forefinger of the left hand are used to rotate the up-down control wheel as described during intubation. Full visualization of the lumen can be obtained by a combination of the up-down control and rotation of the shaft of the colonoscope thus quickly sweeping through the whole visual field. If the instrument suddenly slips back past a prominent fold, the right hand can rapidly reinsert the colonoscope. A careful search should be made behind prominent muscular folds and occasionally an antispasmodic drug may be given such as hyoscine-*N*-butyl bromide (Buscopan) 20–40 mg i.v. to reduce spasm and motility.

X-ray screening is seldom of value during this stage of the examination except to identify the anatomical site of biopsies when these are taken (especially in chronic total ulcerative colitis), when searching for a lesion which has been suspected on the barium enema films or for locating smooth long strictures. Several passes of the colonoscope can then be made through that region of the colon which is under suspicion.

Examination of the lumen may be more difficult at the flexures and at the sigmoid colon/descending colon junction. A better view may occasionally be obtained by changing the position of the patient. Insufflation of air is helpful in the sigmoid region although this part of the colon is always difficult to examine if there is extensive diverticular disease.

Once the rectum has been reached the colonoscope should be inverted to visualize the 'blind zone' which lies just within the rectum (Plate 1) (Huber and Weiss, 1977). The colonoscope is advanced towards the rectosigmoid junction and angled acutely upwards with maximum left angulation applied and then gently withdrawn and rotated to visualize the internal margin of the anus (Plate 2).

After straightening the instrument residual air should be aspirated from the rectum before withdrawal in order to make the patient more comfortable.

8.10 Conclusion

Colonoscopy is now clearly established and the demand for both diagnostic and therapeutic procedures is growing rapidly together with the increasing awareness of the clinical potential of this procedure. Although intubation may be safely and confidently accomplished without the assistance of X-ray facilities, access to screening may be a valuable asset especially to those endoscopists who are providing a referral service and who need to be sure that they can accomplish total colonoscopy whatever the configuration of the patient's colon.

Acknowledgement

I should like to thank Mr Colin Light and Mr Bob Wright of the Department of Clinical Illustration and Mr Ted Over and Mr Steve Hardman of the Department of Clinical Photography for their help in the preparation of this chapter.

References

Cotton, P. B. and Williams, C. B. (1980), Anatomical variations in colonoscopy, In: *Practical Gastrointestinal Endoscopy*, Blackwell Scientific Publications, Oxford, pp. 99–101.

Deyhle, P. (1972a), Flexible steel wire for maintenance of the straightening of the sigmoid and transverse colon during colonoscopy. *Endoscopy*, **4**, 36–37.

Deyhle, P. (1972b), A new technique for the fibrendoscopic passage through the S-type loop of the sigmoid colon. *Endoscopy*, **4**, 102–4.

Ellis, W. R., Harrison, J. M. and Williams, R. S. (1979), Rupture of spleen at colonoscopy. *Br. Med. J.*, **1**, 307–8.

Gaisford, W. D. (1974), Fibrendoscopy of the caecum and terminal ileium. *Gastrointest. Endosc.*, **21**, 13–19.

Huber, A. and Weiss, W. (1977), Coloscopic inversion. *Endoscopy*, **9**, 42–43.

Hunt, R. H. (1978), *Colonoscopy – Technique and Clinical Practice*. Thesis for Gilbert Blane Medal, Royal College of Surgeons, London.

Livstone, E. M. and Kerstein, M. D. (1976), Serosal tears following colonoscopy. *Archs Surg.*, **111**, 88.

Matsunaga, F. and Tajima, T. (1970), *An Outline of Colonofibreoscopy*, First Department of Internal Medicine, Hirosake University, Japan.

Nagasako, K. and Takemoto, T. (1973), Endoscopy of the ileocaecal area. *Gastroenterology*, **65**, 403–11.

Nagy, G. S. (1973), Fibrecolonoscopy, *Med. J. Aust.*, **1**, 378–82.

Overholt, B. (1975), Colonoscopy – a review. *Gastroenterology*, **68**, 1308–20.

Rhodes, J. B., Zvargulis, J., Moffat, R. and Hartong, W. (1978), Right colon loop: A potential pitfall for total colonoscopy. *Endoscopy*, **10**, 295–7.

Sakai, Y. (1974), Further progress in colonoscopy. *Gastrointest. Endosc.*, **20**, 143–7.

Shinya, H. and Wolff, W. (1976), Flexible colonoscopy. *Cancer*, **37**, 462–70.

Sjogren, F. W., Johnson, L. F., Butler, M. L., Heit, M. A., Gremilton, D. E. and Cammerer, R. C. (1978), Serosal ulceration: a complication of intraoperative colonoscopy explained by transmural pressure gradients. *Gastrointest. Endosc.*, **24**, 239–42.

Telmos, A. J. and Mittal, V. K. (1977), Splenic rupture following colonoscopy; letter to Editor, *J. Am. Med. Ass.*, **237**, 2318.

Whalen, J. P. (1976), *Radiology of the Abdomen; Anatomic Basis*, Lea & Febiger, Philadelphia, pp. 79–93.

Whalen, J. P. and Riemenschneider, P. A. (1967), An analysis of the normal anatomic relationships of the colon as applied to roentgenographic observations. *Am. J. Roentg. Rad. Ther. Nucl. Med.*, **99**, 55–61.

Waye, J. D. (1975), Colonoscopy; a clinical view. *Mt. Sinai J. Med.*, **42**, 1–34.

Williams, C. B. (1974), *Colonoscopy According to St. Marks*, ACMI Instruction Manual.

Williams, C. B. and Teague, R. H. (1973), Colonoscopy – progress report. *Gut*, **14**, 990–1003.

Wolff, W. I. and Shinya, H. (1974), Modern endoscopy of the alimentary tract, In: *Current Problems in Surgery*. Year Book Medical Publishers, Chicago.

CHAPTER NINE

Colonoscopy Intubation Techniques without Fluoroscopy

JEROME D. WAYE

Many techniques have been developed over the past decade to achieve colonoscopic intubation (Provenzale, Camerada and Revignas, 1966; Williams and Muto, 1972; Waye, 1972, 1977; Marks, 1974; Provenzale and Revignas, 1969; Shinya and Wolff, 1976; Overholt, 1975). Currently, there are one-person techniques and two-person techniques, either of which can be used with or without fluoroscopy; there are methods using internal and external stiffeners (Gabrielsson, Grandqvist and Ohlsen, 1972; Deyhle, 1972a and b; Nagy, 1973; Sakai, 1972; 1974; Wolff and Shinya, 1974.), and different techniques are utilized with different instruments (American Society for Gastrointestinal Endoscopy, 1975). Some colonoscopists prefer their patients to be in the left lateral position, and others with the patient supine, and a few even start with the patient in the right lateral position. It should be stated at the outset of this chapter that any technique is acceptable that permits the examiner to perform a total colonoscopy in a high percentage of cases, with safety and patient comfort carefully considered. The length of time for the performance of a total colonoscopy is variable and always decreases with increasing experience. In the performance of colonoscopy, 'experience' refers to a vast body of knowledge concerning the actual performance of the procedure, which can only be learned by sharpening the endoscopist's capacity for observation through the flexible fiberoptic endoscope. Much of the initial experience should be learned in an endoscopic training programme, where a preceptor demonstrates techniques and points out landmarks, and then by an endoscopic teacher watching, the students perform many procedures via a lecture-scope on a one-to-one basis. Training should be given under tutelage, so that the student will learn how hard to push, when to pull back the instrument and when to torque the instrument to the right or left; and will learn many of the nuances of colonoscopy, such as interpreting light reflections from the colonic wall.

Practically speaking, there are only a limited number of options

147

available to the endoscopist during the performance of colonoscopy. The instrument can be: pushed inward, pulled outward, torqued (twisted) to the right or left; air may be insufflated or evacuated; the instrument tip may be deflected up or down, or a combination of right or left; the patient's position may be changed, or external compression may be placed on the patient's abdomen. Speed during colonoscopy is gained by choosing the fewest options sequentially to enable the instrument to be passed farther into the colon. This ability can be partially taught but, for the most part, must be learned over a span of time (experience).

This chapter will detail my personal experience with colonoscopy. The techniques of non-fluoroscopic colonoscopy have been developed over the past ten years, and it has been determined that a one-person colonoscopic technique is more efficient than a two-person procedure (Overholt, 1975; Waye, 1974). Fluoroscopy is usually unnecessary for the performance of total colonoscopy, for there are now many other indications for the colonoscopist that a loop is forming, and the location of the loop is not of great import, since all loops may be removed by withdrawing the instrument (Nagasako and Takemoto, 1972). In the absence of fluoroscopy, the location of the tip of the instrument can be ascertained by paying strict attention to intracolonic landmarks; each area of the colon has its own characteristic configuration and appearance.

The hand that holds the shaft of the colonoscope is the important one (Waye, 1977). The colonoscope should be guided by the operator's hand on the shaft of the instrument. The hand that holds the shaft allows the colonoscopist to torque or twist the instrument to the right or to the left, to advance it or withdraw it, to jiggle it and to feel resistance to forward motion at the end of the instrument. Holding the shaft with the right hand permits perfect coordination between rotatory movements of the colonoscope and guidance of the up/down control with the left hand. If two operators are performing colonoscopy, one holds the head of the instrument and 'steers' the dial controls, while the other handles the instrument itself. Even with two trained operators, there must be constant communication as to the location of the lumen and the direction of steerage, so that their motions will not be counterproductive. However, when a relatively untrained assistant handles the instrument and 'pushes and pulls', most of the skill of performing colonoscopy is lost, and the procedure becomes prolonged and tedious.

In the performance of a one-person technique, the shaft of the colonoscope is held in the right hand, while the head of the instrument is held in the operator's left hand. The left thumb reaches under the head to manipulate the large 'up/down' dial (Waye, 1980). Simultaneously, the left index finger is in position to depress the air/water/suction buttons. Although the easiest and most comfortable position is to hold the head of the instrument in the left hand so that the weight of the instrument rests on the thumb and the thenar eminence, this does not allow the thumb to move the up/down dial freely. The colonoscope head should be held high up in the hand toward the metacarpophalangeal joints, to allow the thumb to rotate the large dial freely. To accomplish this, the thenar eminence should not be in contact with the instrument, but the weight of the head is supported with the distal three fingers squeezing the instrument. This is an awkward position for the beginner but, like the grip in tennis, must be learned. The left thumb should not be utilized to rotate the right/left dial, which is in the outermost position. When changes in the right/left direction are desired, the right/left dial should be turned with the right hand, which travels from the shaft of the instrument to that dial frequently during the course of colonoscopy.

The major function of the right hand is to manipulate the shaft of the instrument, torquing to the right or left, and advancing or withdrawing; however, it is frequently moved between the instrument shaft and the dial control knob.

9.1 Position of the patient

Most endoscopists prefer to begin the examination with the patient in the left lateral position. When colonoscoping with a one-person technique, the patient's buttocks and anus should be at the very edge of the examining table near the endoscopist. The knees should be drawn up so that the thighs are at right angles to the back. The endoscopist stands on the left side of the table immediately to the back of the patient, at a position just caudal to the rectum. The examiner faces the head of the table with the right thigh next to the edge of the endoscopy table. The most comfortable level for the examining table is at the endoscopist's mid to upper thigh, with the patient in the left lateral position. The endoscope can be easily manipulated, holding it near the rectum with the same grip as that used when holding a screwdriver.

When the patient is prone or supine, the examiner must either reach toward the middle of the table or underneath the patient's leg to manipulate the shaft of the instrument. The proper positioning of the patient during colonoscopy is of great importance for the one-person technique.

The position of the light source should be almost directly behind the examiner, so that the umbilicus can cross over in front of the examiner from the left. This positioning of the equipment eliminates confusion between the shaft of the instrument held in the right hand, and the umbilicus of the colonoscope.

9.2 Position of the assistant

Although the technique of colonoscopy is referred to as 'one-person' or 'two-person', these terms refer to the actual performance of endoscopy. An assistant is an essential member of the endoscopic team and performs many functions. During one-person colonoscopy, the position of the gastrointestinal assistant should be on the opposite side of the table, across from the examiner. The light source is located behind the examiner and the assistant has a tray on wheels which can be drawn up close to the examining table near to the patient's knees. On this tray are biopsy specimen bottles containing fixative, biopsy forceps, snares, extra medications, etc. The assistant can observe the patient, pass intruments as required, and apply pressure to the abdomen without interfering with the movement of the examiner.

9.3 Position of observers

Students or other physicians desiring to observe colonoscopy may watch through the teaching 'lecture-scope'. When that has been attached to the colonoscope, the easiest position for the observer is to stand on the left side of the table (the same side as the examiner) at about the level of the patient's shoulders. If video equipment is available, the screen is best positioned near the head of the examining table, and observers may watch the screen and the endoscopic manipulations from the foot of the table.

9.4 Technique of performing one-person colonoscopy

Once the instrument is inserted into the rectum, endoscopists are concerned that release of the grip on the shaft may allow the endoscope to fall out of the colon. This can be prevented by one of three methods:

9.4.1 *Using an assistant*

The endoscopic assistant (nurse/technician) may hold the instrument close to the rectum at all times, so that it will be secure. This technique is acceptable but may be cumbersome for the assistant, who frequently has many other functions to perform during the examination.

9.4.2 *Coil scope on table*

The instrument may be coiled on the examining table. Since torque is a very important part of performing colonoscopy, it will readily become apparent that a loop of instrument coiled upon the examining table tends to resist torquing manoeuvres, especially clockwise torque. However, if the instrument is inserted into the rectum and is permitted to hang down toward the floor, the shaft may be easily rotated 360° with the right hand. In contrast to this is the 15–20° torque, which can be accomplished by twisting the scope once it has been draped onto the examining table.

9.4.3 *Holding the shaft*

The weight of the shaft alone tends to drag it out of the rectum when the scope hangs down beside the examining table. Since the weight is not great, the scope may be held in position by gently pressing the right lateral thigh against the colonoscope shaft as it drapes over the edge of the examining table, holding the instrument there as it hangs down toward the floor. Whenever a 'shaft manoeuvre' (advance, withdrawal or torque) is desired, the examiner grasps the instrument with the right hand and simultaneously releases pressure with the thigh holding the instrument. Once the shaft manoeuvre is completed, the right thigh again gently holds the instrument against the side of the table. The technique is easily learned and applied and permits shaft manoeuvres to be accomplished without difficulty. With very little practice, the position of the instrument may be maintained with the right thigh, as the right hand leaves the shaft of the instrument to turn the right/left control wheel. This technique avoids the necessity for an assistant to hold the instrument and prevents the shaft from slipping out of the rectum.

Colonoscopy is more easily accomplished when the distance between the rectum and the 'holding position' by the right lateral thigh is as short as possible. This distance is usually about 20 cm when the instrument is straight between the rectum and the edge of the table. If the patient's position is not maintained with the rectum just at the edge of the table, the distance from the rectum to the 'holding position' is greater, and the instrument then has a tendency to coil and slip out of the rectum. Using the technique of holding the instrument at the edge of the table with the right lateral thigh, the length of the instrument loses its significance, and it could be 160 cm long, 200 cm, or 250 cm long. The important length, therefore, is *not* the amount that hangs down toward the floor, but the length traversed by the instrument from the rectum to the edge of the table where it is held by the lateral thigh. A long instrument is then converted to an instrument that is functionally only 20 cm long (the distance between the rectum and the edge of the table). Any length instrument can be used in this fashion, and even the novice colonoscopist need not start with a short instrument, since this technique turns any length scope into a functionally short instrument. The examiner should try to keep as little slack in the exposed portion of the instrument as possible. If a large loop forms between the rectum and the holding position at the edge of the table, the elasticity of the instrument may cause it to slide out of the colon for several centimetres, even while it is being held by the thigh.

9.5 Medication for endoscopy

The patient should be sedated but not unconscious. General anaesthesia should not be used (Teague, Salmon and Read, 1973; Colcher, 1974; Waye, 1975, 1977). Excellent control of discomfort induced by passage of the colonoscope may be obtained by meperidine/pethidine, 50 mg iv., and diazepam, approximately 10 mg i.v. (to be titrated according to the patient's age, weight and general condition) just before the examination commences. If a patient complains of discomfort, further aliquots of meperidine/pethidine may be given i.v. in 25 mg increments.

9.6 Instrument characteristics

9.6.1 *'Floppiness'*

With the tip of the instrument bent 90° upward, it may be directed to the right by either turning the right/left dial (away from the examiner), or by torquing the shaft of the instrument a quarter-turn in a clockwise direction. This concept is an important one in performing colonoscopy, i.e. if one desires to turn right, there are two different methods of achieving that goal. To ensure that the tip of the instrument actually turns right as the instrument shaft is rotated (torqued), the instrument must be torque-stable at its tip. This means that the instrument must remain fairly rigid in its tip portion, so that, as the instrument is torqued 90° clockwise, such as in turning around a fold, the tip will bend in the direction of torque and push away folds that are encountered. If the instrument tip is 'floppy', when clockwise rotation is imparted to the shaft, the tip may not rotate to the right but instead may be pushed toward the midline of the lumen by the colon wall. This 'floppiness' is an undesirable characteristic of some instruments, and, if the scope tends to be straightened out by pressure against the folds or colon wall with torque, a great deal of the rotational directional capability of the instrument is lost. Rotation of a straight instrument within the colon is of little benefit, since the corkscrew action of torquing a bent instrument is lost. To keep the tip of the instrument in the direction which one desires, and to decrease 'floppiness' of the tip, the right/left dial should be locked during the entire colonoscopic examination, from the moment the instrument is inserted in the rectum until it is withdrawn. The setting of the locking mechanism does not mean that the tip of the instrument is fixed in one direction, for the right hand is continually 'flying' back and forth from the shaft of the instrument to the right/left knob to redirect tip orientation within the bowel.

9.6.2 *Stiffness*

Many instruments are available, with a varying degree of 'stiffness' of the instrument shaft. The larger-diameter instruments, especially those with two channels, are somewhat less flexible than the single-channel instruments. Pain that occurs during colonoscopy is usually due to traction on the root of the mesocolon, caused by the formation of a large loop within the abdominal cavity (Fig. 9.1). As a loop enlarges, the mesenteric attachments become taut and then cause pain when excessively stretched. An ideal instrument, therefore, would be one that is stiff enough to be advanced through the colon and yet flexible enough to comply to the curves of the large bowel and not cause excessive stretching of the mesocolon. If an instrument had the proper characteristics of stiffness to prevent excessive bending, and yet would conform to the anatomical configuration of the bowel and not overstretch the elasticity of the mesocolon, introduction would cause very little patient discomfort. Such an ideal instrument is not available. However, the greater flexibility of the single-channel instruments allows the colonoscope to conform to the bowel configuration and gives a tendency for the tip of the instrument to advance, even when a loop is formed. The stiffer instruments tend to make the bowel, and therefore the mesocolon, conform to the shape of the instrument. When a loop is formed with the stiffer instrument, and the operator continues to insert more of the shaft into the rectum, a larger loop forms and causes traction on the root of the

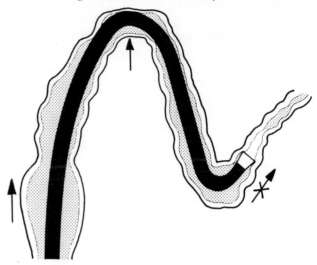

Fig. 9.1 Painful sigmoid loop. Frequently, the tip of the instrument cannot be passed beyond the sigmoid-descending colon junction due to angulation (previous pelvic surgery, diverticular disease, anatomic variation). Further advancement of the instrument into the rectum only causes a large sigmoid loop to form. The traction on the root of the mesocolon by a large loop is responsible for pain.

mesentery with resulting pain. When using the larger-calibre instruments, it is very important to pull back the instrument continually to straighten out the loops. In this fashion, the instrument can be advanced slowly, with slight clockwise torque to keep the instrument as straight as possible (Fig. 9.2). If a loop tends to reform, the instrument should again be withdrawn and reintroduced with clockwise torque.

9.6.3 *Tip deflection*

The tip of modern colonoscopes can be deflected in a circle by manipulation of the two dials at the instrument head. However, when the instrument has been introduced into the colon, and multiple bends made along the course of the instrument, the tip frequently does not respond with the same degree of deflection as when the instrument is straightened outside the patient. Looping of the instrument causes stretching of the deflection control wires, with limitation of further deflection.

Tip deflection characteristics are markedly changed once the end of

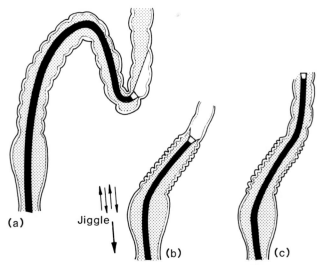

(a)   Jiggle   (b)   (c)

Fig. 9.2 Advancement beyond the sigmoid-descending colon junction. (a) When the instrument cannot be passed beyond the sigmoid-descending colon junction, the tip should be bent upward toward the descending colon, which hooks the instrument. (b) The instrument should be withdrawn with a jiggling to-and-fro motion at the rectum to pleat the bowel onto the instrument. (c) With the sigmoid-descending colon straightened by accordian pleating, the instrument may then be advanced in a straight fashion up to the descending colon. Clockwise torque on the instrument helps to maintain straightness.

the instrument comes in contact with the colonic mucosa. Ideally, the distal 6–8 cm of instrument tip will travel to an arc of 270–360° when the up/down control dial is manipulated. However, whenever the end of the instrument touches the wall of the colon (even quite gently), the tip no longer can be deflected. Contact of the tip on any surface changes the deflection characteristics of the instrument, so that, instead of the tip moving, the bending 'joint' located 5–7 cm from the tip will move up and down. This is 'wasted motion' for the endoscopist, and knowledge of this change in deflection characteristics should always prompt the examiner to pull back the instrument frequently during the course of the examination. When the tip of the instrument is touching a mucosal surface, the only method to restore tip deflection capability is to withdraw the instrument from mucosal contact. This inherent characteristic of flexible endoscopes may be demonstrated by lightly holding the tip against an outstretched palm of an assistant while turning the dial controls. Withdrawal from contact by 1 mm will restore the full deflection capability.

9.6.4 *Maintaining shaft straightness*

Once the instrument has been withdrawn and straightened, rein-
troduction of the shaft may once again cause a loop to form. Reformation of a loop may be partially prevented by slight clockwise torque
on the shaft of the instrument as it is being inserted. This clockwise
torque of the shaft of the instrument tends to keep the insertion tube
stiffened and tends to prevent bowing and bending of the instrument. This characteristic is inherent in the manufacture of the flexible
fibreoptic colonoscope, since two separate inner sheaths are present.
One inner sheath is a complete woven covering of steel filamentous
strands, and the other is a circular, spiral flat wire coil. A slight
clockwise torque tends to 'tighten' the characteristics of the spiral
coiled steel protecting sheath, thus reducing the tendency for loop
formation.

9.7 Passage of the colonoscope

Following rectal examination with a well-lubricated gloved finger, the
instrument should be held in the right hand approximately 6 cm from
the tip. The control head of the instrument is held in the left hand in
the proper position, with the main body of the control panel held
high up toward the metacarpophalangeal joints. Only the distal
3–4 cm of instrument tip need be lubricated. This can easily be
accomplished by squeezing lubricant directly onto the instrument
shaft, or by placing lubricant onto a gauze pad and rotating the tip of
the instrument through the lubricant. The instrument may be
inserted directly in the rectum, for there is no need for an introducer
or to pass the scope through a 'split sigmoidoscope'. As the instrument is placed into the rectum with the patient in the left lateral position, the shaft is hung down beside the examining table and held
with the right thigh. With the light source positioned behind the
examiner, the umbilicus should cross over the examiner's left side to
prevent confusion between the shaft of the instrument and the
umbilicus of the connecting portion when both are hanging toward
the right side of the examiner.

Upon entering the rectum, a 'red-out' invariably occurs. The air
button should be depressed immediately upon entering the rectum,
and the right hand returned from the shaft of the instrument to the
right/left dial, while the left thumb controls the up/down dial. A
rapid rotation of the dials in a manner to perform a rapid 360° scan
should be accomplished. If the red-out persists even with the introduction of air, the tip is in surface contact and not moving. The right
hand should be returned to the shaft, and it should be withdrawn

with gentle clockwise rotation. During withdrawal, the left thumb should move the up/down dial in the up direction, so that, as the instrument is rotated, the tip will be simultaneously angulated. As noted previously, if the colonoscope tip is not deflected with the up/down or right/left dials, the examiner is only rotating a straight instrument which will be of little benefit. Even though the instrument has only been inserted 3–4 cm into the rectum, it is important to pull the shaft back slightly to eliminate tip contact with the mucosa, or the tip deflection characteristics will change, as noted above.

With air insufflation, the rectum will become distended, and the examiner will immediately see a prominent fold. The lumen is always situated behind a prominent fold of the colon. To intubate the lumen, the instrument should be advanced (using the right hand) slightly beyond that fold. Once the endoscopist estimates that the tip has been advanced beyond the fold (only by a few millimetres), the tip should be deflected toward the direction of maximal concavity of that fold, i.e. if a fold is seen on the left of the visual field, the instrument should be advanced slightly beyond it. Then, the tip of the instrument should be advanced directly to the left using the left/right control knob. If the fold is not directly left but is toward the left upper portion of the field, a combination of movements of both control knobs should be made to bend the tip in the direction of the fold (up and left). Almost immediately, another fold will be seen on the opposite wall of the colon, and a similar but opposite manoeuvre should be performed. The right hand should be returned to the shaft of the instrument and the instrument advanced toward the direction of the next fold. Once that fold has been reached, the instrument should be advanced slightly more and the right hand returned to the dial controls, and the controls manipulated toward the concavity of the next fold. If the estimation of the endoscopist was wrong, and the instrument tip had not advanced beyond the fold, manipulation of the dials will cause the instrument tip to be deflected before the fold, and the fold will be seen as the tip turns distal to it. Should that happen, the dials should be rotated back to their initial position, and, following further insufflation of air, the instrument should be introduced further beyond the fold and tip deflection again performed with the dial controls.

The recent generation of instruments permits the examiner to continue to see the lumen throughout most of the colonoscopic examination. However, the earlier generation of instruments and those instruments which are larger in calibre may require a considerable torquing manoeuvre in order to intubate the sigmoid colon easily. At approximately 17–20 cm from the anus, the examiner will see a fold whose major concavity is to the left. When that fold has been passed, tip deflection to the left may not demonstrate the colon lumen. This may be due to bowel angulation greater than the deflection capability of the colonoscope. The right/left dial should be locked with the tip in the direction of the concavity of the fold just passed (in this instance, to the left). The shaft of the instrument should then be rotated with the right hand in an anticlockwise direction as the thumb of the left hand slowly manipulates the up/down wheel in an up direction. This will usually spiral the tip of the instrument in a circular fashion and permit easy intubation of the sigmoid colon. As the instrument is being torqued anticlockwise with the right hand, the right hand also gradually advances the instrument during the rotation. This is not a difficult manoeuvre to perform but points out the necessity for excellent co-ordination between shaft manoeuvres and manipulations of the dial controls. The right hand is responsible for rotating the shaft anticlockwise and advancing the instrument, while the left hand holds the control head and manipulates the tip in an up direction. The tip of the instrument at this point is usually aimed at the descending colon near the junction of the sigmoid descending colon. If a large loop had been formed with this man-oeuvre, slight withdrawal of the instrument shaft may be of benefit to straighten the instrument. In order to prevent withdrawal from merely causing removal of the instrument in the same fashion in which it was introduced, small increments of withdrawal may be per-formed with slight clockwise torque applied to the instrument, which serves to straighten it as well as to reduce the anticlockwise loop previously introduced.

9.7.1 *Knowing when the shaft is straight*

The endoscopist must always look through the eyepiece of the instrument during the entire duration of the endoscopic examination. While looking through the ocular, the examiner can, with experience, estimate the distance that the tip of the instrument advances along the bowel lumen as the right hand simultaneously introduces the shaft into the rectum. If there is a one-to-one correlation between the amount of mucosa traversed and the amount of instrument intro-duced into the rectum, the instrument, for all intents and purposes, is straight. If, however, the right hand introduces several centimetres of instrument shaft into the rectum, and the eye can only appreciate a small forward movement of the tip, or none at all, the instrument is not straight. Any disparity between the amount of scope introduced and the advancement of tip indicates that a loop is forming. This observation does not require fluoroscopic confirmation. The importance is for the examiner to be aware of how much instrument is being inserted into the rectum. If manipulation of the shaft is taken over by a second party, the endoscopist loses this ability to perceive how much instrument is being advanced versus the linear amount of mucosa traversed.

Another method of determining if the instrument shaft is straight is to jiggle the instrument at the rectum. If little tip motion occurs as the instrument is being jiggled in 5–7 cm repetitive advance/withdrawal motions at the rectum, the instrument can be assumed not to be straight, and a loop is present.

9.7.2 *Loop formation* (Table 9.1)

If fluoroscopy is utilized, there is no problem with telling whether a loop has formed upon introduction of the instrument. Without the use of fluoroscopy, it rapidly becomes evident that the location of a loop makes little difference to the passage of the colonoscope, since all loops may be removed by withdrawal of the colonoscope shaft. In the absence of fluoroscopy, one can use three separate endoscopic observations to assist in determining whether a loop is present within the colon.

(a) *Lack of one-to-one advancement of the instrument*
While looking through the eyepiece, if the examiner estimates that the tip of the instrument moves across the mucosal surface a smaller distance than the amount introduced into the rectum, a loop is forming with the colon.

(b) *Lack of 'jiggle' response*
As the examiner observes the lumen through the eyepiece, rapid to-and-fro movements of the instrument at the rectum should cause the tip to undergo excursions of similar magnitude. If the magnitude

Table 9.1 Loop formation

A loop is forming when:
1. Endoscopist estimates a less than one-to-one advancement of the tip
2. Endoscopist sees retrograde motion
3. During jiggle manoeuvre, the tip does not move in 1-to-1 relation with motion at rectum

---

of the intraluminal excursions is less than those performed at the rectum, a loop is present.

(c) *Paradoxical motion* (Fig. 9.3)

If a loop has formed within the colon, and the examiner continues to advance the instrument, the tip may actually be observed (by the endoscopist watching through the eyepiece) to move in a retrograde fashion backward out of the colon. This 'paradoxical' motion of retrograde movement of the tip of the instrument despite advancement of instrument into the rectum is absolute evidence that a loop is forming. This does not usually occur with small loops but is invariably seen with large loops. The reason for paradoxical motion is that only a portion of the colonoscope which goes into forming a large loop is obtained from the amount of instrument inserted into the rectum, and a further component of this large loop is 'borrowed' from

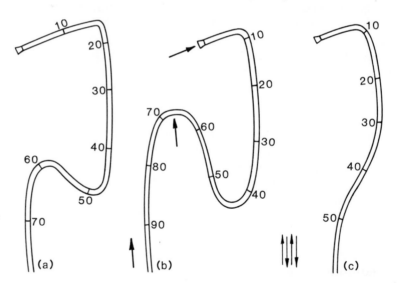

Fig. 9.3 Paradoxical motion. (a) The instrument has been advanced with a loop in the sigmoid colon (this loop may be anywhere in the colon). (b) Further introduction of the shaft into the rectum causes a large loop to form, a portion of which is created from the amount of instrument placed into the rectum, but another portion from the length of scope already lying within the colon. This causes the tip to move in a retrograde fashion through the colon, although further instrument is advanced into the rectum. This always indicates the formation of a loop. (c) Several attempts should be made at jiggling and withdrawal of any loop, so that propulsive forces may be directed through a straight instrument to the tip, rather than resulting in the formation of a large loop.

the length of instrument already in the bowel. When a loop forms in the colon, further colonoscope is pushed into the colon by the examiner. A large loop may be associated with withdrawal of the tip from its position in the colon in spite of further advancement of the instrument shaft into the rectum. Whenever a loop such as this forms, withdrawal of the instrument, usually with a slight clockwise torque, will cause reduction of the loop, and the tip of the instrument (as observed through the eyepiece) may spring forward several centimetres.

9.7.3 *Use of loops during colonoscopy*

Ideally, it should be possible to pleat the entire colon over the instrument by to-and-fro jiggling motions of the shaft durings its passage (Fig. 9.2). In this fashion, by advancing the instrument 5–10 cm and then withdrawal of 3–7 cm in fairly rapid jiggling motions, the bowel will become foreshortened over a (fairly) straight colonoscope, and the tip of the instrument will slowly progress around the entire colon. However, this is not always possible. Occasionally, no matter what the endoscopist tries, a loop will continue to form within the bowel. If this tendency persists, and the instrument cannot be advanced in a straight fashion, the examiner may elect to make a larger loop and 'push through' the loop. This technique necessarily causes stretching of the mesocolon and invariably causes discomfort for the patient. When 'pushing through the loop', the colonoscope should be advanced in a jiggling fashion with small increments of advance followed by small increments of withdrawal (Fig. 9.4). This jiggling to and fro usually causes the tip of the instrument to advance farther and farther up into the colon until a bend is reached, at which point the tip of the instrument may be deflected beyond that bend, and the loop straightened by withdrawal of several centimetres (perhaps 10–30 or even 40 cm) of instrument.

The technique of 'pushing through the loop' should be performed gently, and it is invariably successful with the more flexible single-channel instruments. The double-channel instruments, on the other hand, are stiffer and may not have a tendency to advance once a certain limit of stretch of the mesocolon has been achieved. They may instead tend to increase the loop in an ever-expanding fashion, causing increasing patient discomfort with the possibility of a perforation. Needless to say, an important technical difference in the passage of the stiffer instruments compared to the more flexible ones is that attempts should be made at every stage of insertion to keep the instrument as straight as possible by continually withdrawing the

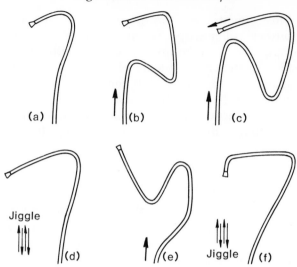

Fig. 9.4 Use of loops in intubation. (a) The instrument has been straightened at the splenic flexure by withdrawal. (b) An attempt to pass into the transverse colon produces a sigmoid loop, with some slight advancement of the tip. (c) Attempts at straightening are unsuccessful, and the instrument cannot be further advanced. Therefore, a larger loop is made in the sigmoid colon, with slight advancement of the tip. (d) Once the tip has been advanced, the instrument is withdrawn and restraightened. (e) Further advancement may cause another loop to form, either in the sigmoid or in the transverse colon. The instrument may once again have to be pushed through this loop in order to reach the hepatic flexure. (f) When the instrument has reached the desired location, pulling back on the shaft will once again straighten out all the loops, no matter where they are located.

instrument a few centimetres after it has been introduced. The technique of passage of the two types of instruments is different because the characteristics of the instruments themselves differ. The stiffer scopes tend to resist loop formation more than the flexible ones and will, therefore, tend to remain straighter. Attempts at straightening, once achieved, will be more easily maintained with the stiffer instruments than with single-channel scopes, and there should be less need to 'push through the loop'.

The endoscopist may find that several instances of 'pushing through the loop' will be necessary during the course of a colonoscopy. One may have to perform this manoeuvre in the sigmoid colon and then straighten out by withdrawing a considerable length of instrument. As the colonoscope is being jiggled and withdrawn, the instrument may be assumed to be straight when the observer notices a one-to-one movement ratio of the shaft of the tip. The instrument is then reintroduced with a slight (usually clockwise) torque on the shaft. When the tip reaches the area of the splenic flexure, the same sigmoid loop may be formed, requiring another attempt to 'push through the loop'. This same circumstance may occur near the hepatic flexure of the colon. Since a sizable loop may induce patient discomfort, it is important to attempt to straighten out the loop as soon as possible.

9.7.4 *Always know the location of the lumen*

Whether fluoroscopy is used or not, advancement of the colonoscope should not be performed unless the endoscopist knows the exact location of the lumen. When colonoscopy was in its infancy, and the instruments were not capable of the present degree of tip deflection, examiners frequently had to rely on blind 'slide-by' manoeuvres during intubation. The technique of 'blind slide-by' is totally unacceptable today but was used when the lumen could not be seen in any position of tip deflection. The method required the examiner to advance the shaft of the instrument into the rectum in the hope that the tip would advance along the luminal mucosal surface, rather than perforate and become extraluminal. There are now a number of techniques which help the colonoscopist always to know the location of the lumen. They should be observed during every endoscopic procedure.

(a) *Lumen is behind a fold*
The tip of the instrument should be advanced up to the fold, slightly beyond it, and then the instrument tip should be redirected toward the concavity of that fold. If lumen still cannot be visualized, the right/left knob should be rotated, and then the shaft of the instrument torqued toward the direction of the lumen. If lumen still cannot be seen, the instrument tip should be withdrawn until a luminal view is obtained.

(b) *Highlights*
Light is reflected from the mucosal surface back to the eye of the examiner. Just beneath the mucosal surface is the circular muscle layer of the colon. Since this is arranged in a circumferential fashion completely around the bowel lumen, light is often reflected in an arcuate fashion from the ridges caused by the circular muscle layer (Plate 5). Usually, multiple parallel arcs of light are seen reflected from successive circular muscle bundles. Even if the examiner can

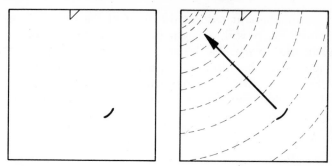

Fig. 9.5 Highlights. The figure on the left indicates a small arcuate reflection of light which should form the basis of the construction of a circle in the mind of the colonoscopist (right). The lumen lies toward the centre of a circle constructed, using the small arc of reflected light as a portion of its circumference.

only identify a small arc of reflected light, an imaginary circle should be drawn in the mind's eye using the arcuate reflection to define one arc of the circumference of a circle (Fig. 9.5). The centre of the imaginary circle then indicates the location of the lumen. The tip should be directed toward the centre of this circle and the instrument advanced with a jiggling motion (Overholt, Collman and Laing, 1971; Waye, 1977). As this is accomplished, the lumen should come into view. In this fashion, 'blind slide-by' is circumvented. Since the tip of the instrument is pointed toward the lumen, the smooth bending portion of the instrument, rather than the blunter tip, skids along the bowel wall (Fig. 9.6). Arcuate reflections from the bowel wall are useful even when a specific arc-like segment of light reflection is not identifiable. With increasing experience, 2–3 point reflections can be recognized as forming a portion of an arc, and these will be as helpful to the examiner as a single arcuate highlight. Reflections observed during jiggling movements of the intrument are also of great benefit, since the jiggle manoeuvre may cause points of reflected light to be scattered over a wider area, making the perception of highlights in an arcuate pattern easier than if one just looks through the instrument while the tip is stationary.

(c) *Ridges*
In areas of muscular hypertrophy, such as those encountered in patients with diverticular disease, thick ridges may be seen (Plate 6). These thickened muscle bundles are arranged in a circumferential pattern, and observation of the ridges may be used in a similar fashion as reflected light, with the tip of the instrument pointed toward the

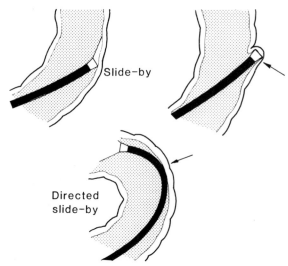

Fig. 9.6 Slide-by. The top two frames demonstrate the technique of blind slide-by, in which the blunt tip of the instrument is pushed against the colonic wall, with the hope of advancing farther into the colon, without seeing the lumen. This is dangerous, as perforation may result. The bottom portion demonstrates 'directed slide-by', during which the tip of the instrument is deflected towards the lumen, as identified by highlights. With this technique, the blunt bending portion of the endoscope skids along the bowel wall as the tip is directed toward the lumen.

centre of an imaginary circle, with the ridge as one portion of its circumference.

(d) *Endoscopy memory*
The endoscopist should always remember where the lumen was. As one identifies the lumen in the distance, and then advances the instrument, the tip does not always advance in a straight line toward the lumen previously identified. The instrument may veer off to the right or left, and if the examiner does not take care to remember in which direction the lumen was previously seen, several minutes may be spent looking in the area to which the instrument was advanced without finding it.

When the instrument has straightened out a curve in the bowel and is being withdrawn, the tendency for the bowel is to restore its normal folds and anatomical curvatures. An example follows: if the bowel has a normal curve like the letter 'C', and this has been straightened out to an 'I' configuration, as the instrument is withdrawn the tendency is for the bowel to begin reforming the 'C' loop.

When the instrument has reached the bottom of the 'C' loop, the initial bowel contour will have been restored. Sometimes, that restoration of original curvature is quite rapid, and, when the instrument is withdrawn only 1–2 cm, the endoscopist can no longer find the location of the lumen. During instrument withdrawal, as colon loops reform, the following sequence occurs: the smooth curvature of the 'C' may suddenly protrude from the right of the examiner's field and push the lumen to the left, and the endoscopist will have the instrument at the bottom portion of the 'C' within a split second. The inexperienced examiner usually turns the instrument to the right to find the lumen, which may have disappeared quickly. In actuality, however, the lumen is off to the left around the bend of the 'C'. As previously mentioned, it is most important for the endoscopist to observe the lumen continuously during colonoscopy. Once this concept is accepted, colonoscopy becomes considerably easier.

9.7.5 *Hooking the colonoscope*

Hooking manoeuvres are used to straighten the colonoscope and are frequently performed during endoscopy. With the tip flexed around a fold, the instrument may be withdrawn without fear of losing the position of the colonoscope. Hooking is also used when forward progress is impeded.

Once the tip is advanced beyond a bend and hooked on a fold, the instrument may be withdrawn and straightened. When the instrument is hooked around a fold in this fashion, part of the lumen may be seen beyond it, although there may not be a tubular view of the lumen ahead. Hooking cannot be accomplished by bending the instrument acutely across the lumen of the bowel.

9.7.6 *The splenic flexure*

As the instrument is advanced up to the area of the splenic flexure, a variable portion of the instrument will have been inserted into the patient's rectum. With a gentle loop in the sigmoid colon, the splenic flexure is usually reached at approximately 70 cm of instrument inserted into the rectum. However, the actual distance of shaft insertion may vary from 50–120 cm. In approximately half of all colonoscopies, a rounded bluish impression of the spleen may be seen lying against the colonic wall (Plate 7). The splenic flexure itself may appear to have a fold covering the entrance into the transverse colon. This has been described as the 'gate-like fold' of the splenic flexure (Plate 8) and may be completely closed or 'fish-mouthed' in configuration.

The endoscopist should always be able to identify the location of lumen, and the transverse colon is usually found by making an acute downward and left rotation of the tip controls, with clockwise torque of the instrument. In order to advance the instrument into the transverse colon, straightening by withdrawal of the instrument from the rectum is almost invariably necessary (Fig. 9.7). With the tip of the instrument bent acutely toward the distal transverse colon, introducing further instrument into the rectum may cause the bent tip of the colonoscope to act like the crook of a cane, and the entire tip and bending portion of the colonoscope may advance up toward the diaphragm when more scope is advanced into the rectum. This will cause paradoxical motion, with the tip of the instrument moving farther away from entry into the transverse colon. By withdrawal of the instrument, the flexed tip (deflected always to keep the location of lumen in view) may actually enter the transverse colon. Withdrawal brings the tip of the instrument down from its position near the diaphragm (Fig. 9.7), and the amount of deflection may require adjustment as the angle changes from acute to obtuse. Entry into the distal transverse colon may become relatively easy. Unfortunately, when the shaft is inserted into the rectum to advance the tip into the transverse colon the same problem of paradoxical motion may occur

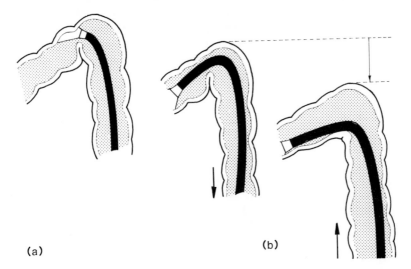

(a)   (b)

Fig. 9.7 The splenic flexure. (a) As the tip reaches the splenic flexure, it must be deflected downward and to the left. (b) Once the transverse colon is identified, the instrument should be withdrawn from the rectum to decrease the acute angle at the splenic flexure. As the instrument is withdrawn (by jiggling), the left thumb on the dial decreases the amount of tip deflection, so that the instrument enters the transverse colon with a less acute angle.

again when the deflected portion of the instrument advances toward the diaphragm. Three different manoeuvres may be of benefit in this situation:

1. Have an assistant press on the left lower quadrant of the abdomen (with the patient in the left lateral position). This may act as an external splint to the sigmoid colon, so that further coiling of the instrument does not occur, and most of the force placed on the instrument will be transmitted directly to the tip. This may straighten the sigmoid but could result in retrograde movement of the instrument, as previously described.

2. The assistant may place one hand on the patient's left upper quadrant and the other underneath the rib cage and left flank to prevent cephalad motion of the instrument, so that, as the instrument is advanced in the rectum, it will be deflected on the hands of the assistant and directed into the transverse colon.

3. One may 'push through the loop' and, although retrograde motion occurs in the beginning, further jiggling motion of the instrument with gradual slow advancement of the instrument with each jiggling motion may advance the tip into the transverse colon. Simultaneous pressure by an assistant in the left lower quadrant may prevent sigmoid looping. Once the flexure has been negotiated, the instrument is easily passed into the transverse colon after being straightened by withdrawal.

9.7.7 *The transverse colon*

The transverse colon is triangular in appearance (Plates 9 and 10) and is easily recognized by the endoscopist. Once the instrument passes into the transverse colon, the major direction of the instrument is downward toward the pelvis. A sudden angulation usually occurs in the direction of the transverse colon, which signifies that the tip of the instrument has reached the midportion of the transverse colon, forming an acute 'V' in the pelvis. Once that point is reached, the transverse colon ascends up toward the right upper quadrant. In error, many endoscopists believe they are at the hepatic flexure once this bend is reached (Rhodes *et al.*, 1978). Usually, however, a considerable portion of proximal transverse colon must yet be traversed before reaching the hepatic flexure. The endoscopist who reaches the angulated transverse colon may continue to advance the instrument in the rectum and 'push through the loop', gradually advancing the

instrument toward the hepatic flexure. Frequently, this is not possible, and the instrument should be withdrawn. With the tip of the
instrument hooked around the angle of the transverse colon ('V'),
withdrawal of the instrument from the rectum will raise the transverse colon up toward the diaphragm and cause it to straighten. This
manoeuvre itself (just pulling back the instrument with a slight clockwise torque) may cause the colonoscope to spring forward through
the transverse colon up toward the hepatic flexure. If that is not
easily accomplished, the assistant may compress the mid-abdominal area
to elevate and, therefore, straighten the transverse colon, causing the
instrument to pass more easily across the abdomen.

9.7.8 *The hepatic flexure*

The hepatic flexure is usually recognized by the sharp bluish edge of
liver shining through the colonic wall (Plate 11). Multiple convolu-
tions of the bowel may have to be negotiated in order to reach the
hepatic flexure. Although most physicians think of the hepatic flexure
as being a point area, it is several centimetres long in its anteropos-
terior direction (beginning just under the right costal margin and ending in the right flank). Because of its length, it is frequently difficult to
push the instrument around the hepatic flexure, since loops tend to
form in the transverse colon or the sigmoid colon. It makes little difference where looping occurs, and the following technique has been
devised to pass the instrument around the hepatic flexure: With the
patient in the left lateral position, the instrument is pointed upward
when in the transverse colon (toward the patient's right upper quadrant). The last fold of the hepatic flexure just before the colon turns
posteriorly is a bend to the right (posterior with the patient in this
position). Frequently, the lumen of this posteriorly directed portion of
the hepatic flexure cannot be seen even with the tip bent to the right.
The shaft should then be withdrawn from the rectum with a clockwise torque. The right control should be locked right, and air withdrawn with the left index finger as the instrument is torqued and
withdrawn by the right hand. This causes the instrument tip to rotate
(by torque) and proceed posteriorly as the loops are being removed
from the sigmoid and/or transverse colon. When the colonoscope is
at the junction of the posterior hepatic flexure area and the ascending
colon, it can frequently be advanced through most of the ascending
colon by further withdrawal (reversal of paradoxical motion). Once
the air is withdrawn from the right colon, shortening it by deflation,
a small advance of the instrument in the rectum propels the tip down
toward the caecum. If this does occur, further attempts at 'pushing

through the loop' and pressure in the mid-abdomen by an assistant may help to advance the instrument. The caecum can be recognized by the characteristic pool of ileal contents (Plate 13), by the presence of a short incomplete fold at the very tip of the caecum (which I have named the 'caecal sling fold', representing an indentation caused by the taenea coli as it passes around the caput coli), by the orifice of the appendix, and by visualizing the superior lip of the ileocaecal valve (Nagasako and Takemoto, 1973; Gaisford, 1974).

9.8 General colonoscopic tips (Table 9.2)

1. There are only a finite number of manoeuvres that can be performed with the colonoscope:

    (a) The instrument may be pushed into the rectum or withdrawn.
    (b) It may be torqued to the right or to the left.
    (c) The tip may be turned up or down, right or left.
    (d) Air may be insufflated or withdrawn.
    (e) The instrument may be lubricated.
    (f) The abdomen may be compressed to 'splint' a large loop from forming.
    (g) The patient's position may be changed (Overholt, 1975).

Table 9.2 Colonoscopic technique

1. Examiner should not sit down
2. Keep patient's rectum near edge of table
3. Do not drape instrument on table
4. To prevent scope from falling out of rectum, hold it against edge of table with your right lateral thigh

Rapid colonoscopy is performed by quickly running through the sequences available and deciding whether progress is or is not being made and moving on to another manoeuvre.

Table 9.3 Manoeuvres if scope does not advance

1. Lubricate scope at anus
2. Withdraw air
3. Jiggle
4. Straighten scope by withdrawing
5. In TVC apply pressure to abdomen
6. Push through the loop (gently)

2. A few manoeuvres may be performed if the instrument does not advance (Table 9.3):

(a) Apply lubrication to the instrument just at the anal orifice. Since the dry rectum may hold the sheath of the instrument very tightly, torquing the instrument while it is being rigidly held by a dry anus may result in inability to torque the instrument tip, and pushing the instrument in and out may also be difficult. In addition to this difficulty, the polyethylene sheath may be shorn off at the level of the rectum from the sheer stress of attempting to torque the sheath with the right hand while it is being tightly held by the rectum.

(b) Air should be withdrawn to deflate the bowel.

(c) Jiggling motions should be performed frequently with rapid to-and-fro excursions of the instrument at the rectum. These excursions should be in 5–10 cm increments. This manoeuvre alone may allow the instrument tip to creep forward across the mucosa and advance into an area previously inaccessible.

(d) Loops may be taken out of the instrument by withdrawal of the scope. Withdrawal is usually performed with a slight clockwise rotation and in a jiggling fashion to pleat the bowel, so that whatever pathway was traversed in forming a loop is not simply retraced by straight withdrawal.

(e) If straightening the instrument does not help, another man-oeuvre is to 'push through the loop' by advancing the instrument in a jiggling motion, but each insertion is a few centimetres more than the amount of instrument withdrawn during the jiggle technique. The jiggling should be performed gently to prevent perforation of the bowel and to allow bowel compliance with each greater amount of stretch induced by the short jiggling excursions.

(f) An additional manoeuvre may be to have the assistant apply pressure on various portions of the abdomen to splint the instrument and prevent large loops from forming.

3. During intubation of the colon, the following points should be observed (Table 9.4):

(a) The right/left control knob should be locked to stiffen the tip, although it is frequently moved during the examination.

(b) Movement of the right/left knob should be performed to direct the tip toward the lumen, and the lock may be left on during the entire procedure.

Table 9.4 Colonoscopy intubation

1. Lock L/R control knob to stiffen tip
2. Steer right or left toward lumen p.r.n. (over-ride lock)
3. Torque shaft
4. Jiggle often
5. Pull back often to straighten scope
6. Let scope hang down beside table

(c) The shaft of the instrument should be torqued to the right or to the left, depending on the direction of the folds in the colon.

(d) The scope should be jiggled often, both during intubation and during extubation; loops in the instrument should be straightened out by pulling the instrument back frequently, and usually with a slight clockwise torque on the shaft of the instrument.

(e) The instrument should hang down beside the table, rather than be draped on the table, since that makes torquing manoeuvres easier.

(f) The examiner should not sit down, since by so doing the instrument cannot be held in position with the right lateral thigh against the edge of the table; as soon as the examiner sits down, someone else must be available to hold the instrument so that it does not slip out of the rectum.

(g) It is important to keep the patient's rectum near the edge of the table so that the amount of instrument between the anus and the holding position at the edge of the table is as short as possible. If the patient is positioned at the centre of the table, there is a long distance between the rectum and the holding position at the edge of the table, and the instrument may begin to recoil spontaneously from the rectum rather than to be held in place by the holding position of the right lateral thigh.

Table 9.5 Colonoscopy extubation

1. Lock R/L control knob
2. Direct tip toward lumen through lock
3. Use torque more than control knobs
4. Jiggle to uncoil bowel slowly
5. Scope may lie on table

4. During removal of the instrument, once it has been advanced to the colon (Table 9.5):

(a) The right/left control knob should remain locked.
(b) Most of the observation of the bowel wall is performed with the right hand torquing the shaft of the instrument clockwise and counterclockwise, alternatively; there is more facility by handling the instrument with torque rather than by using the control knobs (Fig. 9.8).
(c) Keeping the hand on the shaft of the instrument also helps to guide withdrawal slowly so that, if the bowel begins to uncoil from its pleated position on the scope, the instrument can be rapidly advanced through the bowel to capture the uncoiled loops quickly.
(d) During extubation, the instrument may lie on the table, since the torquing manoeuvres are gentle and do not require large movements of the instrument.

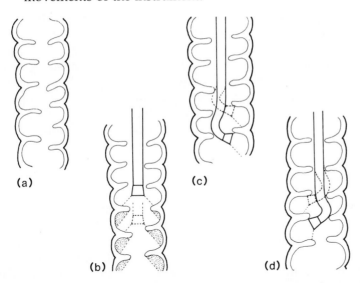

Fig. 9.8 Extubation technique. (a) The normal colon has multiple angulations and folds, especially in the sigmoid region. (b) Once the endoscope has been placed through the colon, it is accordian-pleated on the endoscope. Withdrawal of the straight instrument, no matter how wide the angle of view at the tip, will leave 'blind spots' behind the colonic folds. (c) With the tip angled upward, using the left thumb on the up/down dial, and the right/left locked to ensure tip stiffness, the instrument may be torqued to the left and to the right (d) to sweep the tip behind each of the folds during instrument withdrawal. This torquing manoeuvre allows complete visualization behind each of the colon folds.

Table 9.6 Special manoeuvres

Torque:	Tends to keep shaft from flexing
Jiggle:	Rapid 10–15 cm to-and-fro motions of shaft straightens scope, allows bowel to pleat onto scope
Lock R/L control:	Allows scope to push folds aside if not locked, tip tends to straighten
Air withdrawal:	Tends to decrease acute bowel angulations
Mid-abdominal pressure:	Lifts up and straightens transverse colon

By following these integrated but simple manoeuvres (Table 9.6), one should be able to perform colonoscopy easily, quickly and efficiently with the greatest comfort for the patient.

9.9 Colonoscopic anatomy and landmarks

Large bluish-green vessels can be seen in the rectum which extend proximally for about 15 cm. Above this level, the fine branching reticular patterns of arterial blood vessels can be identified throughout the remainder of the colon (Plate 3). The descending colon is characterized by its tubular configuration (Plate 4), but it rarely, on intubation, is straight. It is usually quite tortuous, with multiple folds and bends. The spleen may be seen in the area of the splenic flexure in about 50% of cases (Plate 7); this is better seen on intubation than extubation. The transverse colon is easily identified by its triangular configurations (Plates 9 and 10), and the bluish coloration of the liver can be seen at the hepatic flexure (Plate 11). The liver produces a sharp edge to the viewer, caused by the rolling away of the colon from the liver (Fig. 9.9). The ascending colon is composed of folds which are arcuate and involve 50–70% of the bowel wall, without being completely circumferential (Plate 12). The ileocaecal valve is pointed toward the base of the caecum (Plate 17), and its orifice is usually not identifiable during colonoscopy. The location of the ileocaecal valve can usually be seen as an indentation of a colonic valve (Plates 14 and 16), approximately 4 cm above the appendiceal orifice or the blind end of the caecum. Both lips of the ileocaecal valve are rarely identified, since only the proximal overhanging lip protrudes into the lumen.

The length of instrument inserted into the rectum usually bears little relation to the area of colon intubated. When the tip is in the caecum, and the scope is straightened to a smooth contour resembling a question mark, the scope length may be 70 cm. On the other

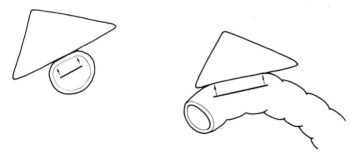

Fig. 9.9 The hepatic flexure. The liver (△) rests against one edge of the colonic wall, indenting it. As the colon rolls away from contact with the liver, a sharp edge of blue liver coloration is created. The shape of the hepatic blue coloration depends on anatomic factors of the liver and the colon, as well as the altered configuration of the colon containing the instrument.

hand, during intubation, the splenic flexure may be reached when 120 cm of scope have been introduced into the rectum. On withdrawal, however, with the scope straight, the splenic flexure is usually identified at approximately 40–50 cm from the anus. Numbers mean little to the referring physician, who questions that the endoscopist finds a lesion at the 20 cm level that could not be seen during rigid sigmoidoscopy when it is actually located in the mid-sigmoid colon. The pleating of the colon upon the flexible instruments construes the meaning of a specific centimetre level when compared with the rigid instrument.

The location of the tip of the colonoscope can be ascertained in a number of ways. One is to pay attention to the intraluminal landmarks described above. The second is to use transillumination (Table 9.7). Transillumination is best seen in the caecum, and, if the tip of the instrument is in the caecum, transillumination should be seen just above the right inguinal ligament (Plate 20). If transillumination is

Table 9.7 Transillumination

Most helpful in caecum
Rarely seen in left colon
Occasionally seen in TVC
Frequently in hepatic flexure (RUQ)
Almost always in caecum
   Look for light just above inguinal fold

---

seen somewhere near the area of McBurney's point, it is impossible to tell whether the colonoscope tip is in the transverse colon and pushed down toward the right lower quadrant, or is in the area of the ileocaecal valve. Since the transverse colon is anterior, the light may be seen in the anterior abdomen when the instrument is in the transverse colon, especially near the area of the hepatic flexure (Whalen and Riemenscheider, 1967). The light can usually not be seen when the instrument is in the sigmoid colon unless a large loop is formed, and transillumination may then be visible near the umbilicus. A third way to ascertain the location of the tip is to ballotte the anterior wall rapidly with one finger while observing the lumen through the instrument (Plates 18 and 19). The point of maximal movement of the bowel wall is always immediately over the site of ballottement, so that maximal movement when the ballotting finger is in the right upper quadrant usually means that the tip is at the hepatic flexure. The position of the tip can almost invariably be localized within 5 cm of its actual position.

When not using fluoroscopy, the examiner should be absolutely certain that the tip of the instrument is located precisely. Non-fluoroscoping colonoscopists must make every effort to know the exact location of the instrument tip at all times during the procedure, for it is easy to convince oneself that the caecum has been entered when, in reality, the endoscopy is only one-quarter or one-half completed.

The three general rules that will result in successful colonoscopy are:

1. *Pull back the instrument often.* This straightens out loops, makes further advancing easier, and takes the tip of the instrument off the mucosal surface, restoring the capability of tip deflection.
2. *Always know where the lumen is located.* This can be done by a variety of techniques, such as pulling back to look for the fold in the bowel behind which the lumen is situated, or observing the 'highlights' of light reflected from the circular muscle layers of the bowel.
3. *The hand that is on the shaft of the instrument is the hand that actually performs colonoscopy.* Most colonoscopic manoeuvres should be performed with some amount of clockwise torque, except in the sigmoid colon during initial intubation, where most of the torque is anticlockwise in rotation.

References

Am. Soc. Gastrointest. Endosc. (1975), Guidelines for standards of training and practice. *Gastrointest. Endosc.*, **22**, 46–47.

Colcher, H. (1974), Prevention and treatment of complications of diagnostic colonoscopy and polypectomy. Lecture to Am. Soc. Gastrointest. Endosc., San Francisco.

Deyhle, P. (1972a), Flexible steel wire for maintenance of the straightening of the sigmoid and transverse colon during colonoscopy. *Endoscopy*, **4**, 36–37.

Deyhle, P. (1972b), A new technique for the fibrendoscopic passage through the S-type loop of the sigmoid colon. *Endoscopy*, **4**, 102–4.

Gabrielsson, N., Grandqvist, S. and Ohlsen, H. (1972), Colonoscopy with the aid of a stiff wire to stiffen the fiberscope. *Endoscopy*, **4**, 224–6.

Gaisford, W. D. (1974), Fibrendoscopy of the cecum and terminal ileum, *Gastrointest. Endosc.*, **21**, 13–19.

Marks, G. (1974), Flexible fiberoptic colonoscopy. *J. Am. Med. Ass.*, **228**, 1411–13.

Nagasako, K. and Takemoto, T. (1972), Fibercolonoscopy without the help of fluoroscopy. *Endoscopy*, **4**, 208–12.

Nagasako, K. and Takemoto, T. (1973), Endoscopy of the ileocecal area, *Gastroenterology*, **65**, 403–11.

Nagy, G. S. (1973), Fibrecolonoscopy, *Med. J. Aust.*, **1**, 378–82.

Overholt, B. F. (1975), Colonoscopy: a review, *Gastroenterology*, **68**, 1308–20.

Overholt, B. F., Collman, R. and Laing, W. G. (1971), Fibersigmoidoscopy – clinical value. *Gastroenterology*, **60**, 826–31.

Provanzale, L., Camerada, P. and Revignas, A. (1966), La colonoscopia totale transanale mediante: Una metodica originale. *Radd. Med. Sarda*, **69**. 149–60.

Provenzale, L. and Revignas, A. (1969), An original method for guided intubation of the colon. **16**, 11–17.

Rhodes, J. B., Zvargulis, J., Moffat, R. and Hartong, W. (1978), Right colon loop: A potential pitfall for total colonoscopy. *Endoscopy*, **10**, 295–7.

Sakai, Y. (1972), The technic of colonofiberscopy. *Dis. Colon & Rectum*, **15**, 403–12.

Sakai, Y. (1974), Further progress in colonoscopy. *Gastrointest. Endosc.*, **20**, 143–7.

Shinya, H. and Wolff, W. I. (1976), Flexible colonoscopy. *Cancer*, **37**, (Suppl. Jan), 462–70.

Teague, R. H., Salmon, P. R. and Read, A. E. (1973), Fiberoscopic examination of the colon: a review of 255 cases. *Gut*, **14**, 139–42.

Whalen, J. P. and Riemenschneider, P. A. (1967), An analysis of the normal anatomic relationships of the colon as applied to roentgenographic observations. *Am. J. Roentg. Radat. Ther. Nucl. Med.*, **99**, 55–61.

Waye, J. D. (1972), Colonoscopy. *Surg. Clinics N. Amer.*, **52**, 1013–24.

Waye, J. D. (1974), *Colonoscopy* (monograph and slides), MEDCOM, New York.

Waye, J. D. (1975), Colonoscopy: a clinical view. *Mt Sinai J. Med.*, **42**, 1–34.

Waye, J. D. (1977), Colonoscopy. Guidelines and technique for diagnosis and therapy. In: *Progress in Gastroenterology*. (ed. G. B. J. Glass), Grune and Stratton, New York, pp. 991–1013.

Waye, J. D. (1980), *Technique of Colonoscopy* (monograph and slides, MEDC, Inc., New Jersey.

Williams, C. B. and Muto, T. (1972), Examination of the whole colon with the fiberoptic colonoscope. *Br. Med. J.*, **3**, 278–81.

Wolff, W. I. and Shinya, H. (1974), Modern endoscopy of the alimentary tract. In: *Current Problems in Surgery*. Year Book Medical Publishers, Chicago.

CHAPTER TEN

Flexible Sigmoidoscopy

STEPHEN E. HEDBERG

10.1 Indications

The introduction of the flexible fibreoptic sigmoidoscope has caused some consternation among those who remember the early 50-cm 'colonoscopes' as a brief phase in the rapid development of total colonoscopy (Overholt, 1969; Salmon et al., 1971). In this light, flexible sigmoidoscopy appears to some a backward step in the management of colonic disease, but this impression arises because they are attempting to equate flexible sigmoidoscopy with colonoscopy, instead of focusing upon the advantages of flexible over rigid sigmoidoscopy, and its ease of use as an office procedure (Holt and Wherry, 1980).

Determination of the value of flexible sigmoidoscopy comes at a time when the efficacy, safety, and cost of every conceivable drug, test, procedure, screen and intervention are coming under scrutiny. It is unfortunate, therefore, to discover that our baseline – rigid sigmoidoscopy – has itself never been critically evaluated in ways that permit meaningful comparisons with flexible sigmoidoscopy. Thus, we now discover as we attempt to relate cost–benefit ratios of the two procedures that the terms of the equation have never been precisely defined. The cost of instruments and procedures are readily available, but the benefits are clear: cancer detection, especially the early cancers that would not otherwise have been found until too advanced; polyps found and destroyed that would otherwise in time have become cancer; lesions detected that would not have been by barium enema or stool examination for occult blood; and colostomies avoided. The cancer deaths prevented, and these other benefits are complexly interrelated, and their precise value in each case is in turn dependent upon the indication for which the procedure is performed. Examinations made for bleeding will be fewer and give a higher yield than screening examinations; costs will therefore be lower and benefits greater. But such patients might benefit even more from total colonoscopy, and some would argue that the finding of a neoplasm on flexible sigmoidoscopy or rigid sigmoidoscopy is a strong indication for total colonoscopy, whereas a negative

179

examination in a patient with bleeding would also require colonoscopy.

When rigid sigmoidoscopy is carried out for screening in cancer detection and prevention, it has been shown that the cost per cancer death prevented is low if the population is over 40 or 45 years of age (Gilbertsen, 1974). In this group of asymptomatic patients, flexible sigmoidoscopy can detect twice as many lesions as rigid sigmoidoscopy, so that if costs can be kept down to approximately twice that of rigid sigmoidoscopy, the cost–benefit ratio of the two procedures would appear to be equivalent, with a greater absolute yield for flexible sigmoidoscopy, *in screening*. It is not likely that the advantages of flexible sigmoidoscopy would pertain in groups under 40 years, where the yield would be so low as to raise markedly the cost of each lesion detected (Lipschutz *et al.*, 1980).

Thus, critical evaluation and discussion of all the available data have persuaded the Standards of Training and Practice Committee of the American Society for Gastrointestinal Endoscopy to recommend that the indications for flexible sigmoidoscopy should be considered identical to those of rigid sigmoidoscopy and that the greater yield of flexible sigmoidoscopy does not obviate the need for total colonoscopy in patients with neoplastic lesions, chronic ulcerative colitis, change in bowel habit, anaemia, intestinal blood loss, or any abnormality suspected on barium enema. As the experienced colonoscopist knows well, the mid-to-upper sigmoid may lie deeper than the tip of a 60 cm fibrescope, so that without fluoroscopic control it may be erroneous to exonerate this area if suspicious on barium enema, even when the fibreoptic sigmoidoscope may have been fully inserted.

10.2 Instrumentation

Technically any fibrescope longer than the rectum and shorter than a colonoscope (100 cm) may be designated as a sigmoidoscope. Fibrescopes with an insertion tube length of 55 to 65 cm are available from the major manufacturers of gastrointestinal endoscopes. Shorter instruments have been tested with satisfactory results, but their distribution has been relatively limited. Fibresigmoidoscopes are rugged in comparison to colonoscopes, but their design is similar, so that the initial cost, cost and frequency of repairs, cost of cleaning and maintenance are very much higher than that of rigid sigmoidoscopes, many of which are now disposable. Necessary accessories include sources of light, air/CO_2, wash water, and suction; these units are compatible with colonoscopes from the same manufacturer, but not with rigid sigmoidoscopes. Accessory instruments for passage through the working channel of the fibrescope are identical in construction to those for colonoscopes, but may be shorter, with a consequent decrease in mechanical problems attributable to angulation and friction. Polypectomy snares and electrosurgical units are mechanically compatible with fibresigmoidoscopes, but the use of sparking devices in the bowel after the limited preparation (to be described) for flexible sigmoidoscopy does introduce an unacceptable explosion hazard, and cannot be recommended.

10.3 Preparation

Preparation of the patient for flexible sigmoidoscopy should begin with an explanation of the indication for the procedure and a general description of the instrument and its use. The risk of perforation (about 1 in 10 000) should be mentioned and dismissed. The relative advantages and disadvantages of rigid sigmoidoscopy, barium enema, and total colonoscopy should be outlined so that the patient may give his informed consent. If there is time, a printed explanation is very useful because it allows the patient an opportunity to study it in his own time and then ask any questions; the printed version also establishes beyond doubt that the patient has received the full information.

Preparation of the bowel is almost always adequate for rigid sigmoidoscopy after one prepackaged saline phosphate solution (Fleet) enema. It is preferable to administer two enemas before flexible sigmoidoscopy because fibresigmoidoscopy requires a cleaner bowel, and because the intention of flexible sigmoidoscopy is to intubate higher up the colon.

Premedication is not generally indicated any more than for rigid sigmoidoscopy, but the occasional extremely apprehensive patient may be advised to take a tranquilizer, such as diazepam, 5 or 10 mg, orally an hour before the procedure.

Intravenous medication, electrocardiographic monitoring, or pulse and blood pressure monitoring should not be necessary for the safe and comfortable conduct of flexible sigmoidoscopy. If a need for any of these is anticipated, it is likely that an alternative procedure should be elected instead of flexible sigmoidoscopy.

10.4 Instruction and training

It is generally agreed by experienced endoscopists, who are aware of the pitfalls, that fibreoptic sigmoidoscopy should not be attempted by untrained persons. Observation of a few cases followed by performance under supervision of twenty cases should suffice to lower the complication rate to an acceptable level (Katon, 1978). There is no doubt, however, that the very high yields of flexible sigmoidoscopy in relation to rigid sigmoidoscopy that have been reported, are attributable in some degree to the extensive colonoscopic experience of the authors, and that equivalent experience with flexible sigmoidoscopy will be needed before these results can be matched by a non-endoscopist. A very real concern here is that the person whose repertoire is limited to flexible sigmoidoscopy may, for whatever reason, be less attentive to recommending colonoscopy when it is in fact indicated, especially when the indication for further endoscopy is a lesion, such as a polyp, that may have been removed by flexible sigmoidoscopy. For this reason it is important that the training of the fibresigmoidoscopist should include sufficient didactic material relating to the proper use of flexible sigmoidoscopy in relation to other investigations. The experience with rigid sigmoidoscopy and barium enema, however, which are still heavily relied upon despite their relatively low yield in comparison to total colonoscopy, causes great concern that flexible sigmoidoscopy and barium enema will be similarly misused.

Whatever the training, the broader background of the individuals performing flexible sigmoidoscopy is of some importance. At present it is assumed that skilled endoscopists would have the highest yield with flexible sigmoidoscopy and the lowest complication rate. Available data are insufficient to determine the extent to which paramedical persons, non-endoscopists, physicians, or persons with other credentials would experience different yield and complication rates.

10.5 Technique

The right or better the left lateral position is comfortable for both patient and examiner. The knee-chest position, with or without the assistance of a proctoscopy table, is relatively uncomfortable and offers no advantage.

The anus and perianal skin are well lubricated with the gloved index finger. A thorough digital examination should be repeated at this time. The tip of the fibrescope is then placed in the intergluteal fold and pressed against the palmar surface of the inserted finger. The thumb of the examining hand pushes the tip of the scope into the anus as the finger is removed.

The lens is washed to remove lubricant and a little air is introduced in order to permit viewing and orientation. Retained liquid should be aspirated, carefully avoiding any residual solid faeces, which will block the suction channel, obscure the view, and nescessitate removal and manual cleaning of the tip.

Overinflation of the bowel is unpleasant for the patient and lengthens the bowel as it distends. This is not so much of a disadvantage in flexible sigmoidoscopy as in colonoscopy, but the preferable technique is still to advance the fibrescope with minimal insufflation of gas. The lumen of the bowel should be kept in view to the greatest extent possible, and when not completely in view its direction should always be known with certainty. 'Slide-by' (introduction without luminal view) is to be avoided if possible, but may be safely used if only gentle pressure is applied, and no discomfort results. Much better results will be obtained, however, with less discomfort and danger, if a combination of torquing, hooking, pulling, and jiggling motions is used to pleat the sigmoid loops over as short a length of the instrument as possible. If this can be done, the 60-cm fibresigmoidoscope can be advanced to the splenic flexure or beyond. If the sigmoid cannot be pleated onto 30 or 40 cm of instrument then advancing the fibrescope will extend the sigmoid loop, which can often accommodate the full length of the insertion tube with ease if not comfort. The so-called 'alpha loop' thus created is much more difficult to resolve than with a full length colonoscope where the necessary clockwise torquing is made easier by the shaft of the instrument remaining outside the patient. With the flexible sigmoidoscope, torquing must be done by rotating the entire control head. Further, a successful 'alpha manoeuvre' often requires hooking the tip around the splenic flexure, which is not possible with the shorter instrument in a looped configuration. Thus the operator who has not had colonoscopic training is more likely to form a loop than an experienced colonoscopist, and lacking experience and mechanical skills will be less able to resolve the loop.

Once the fullest possible insertion is achieved, the bowel is inflated with gas to flatten haustrations and other mucosal folds. Overfilling with air is painful and dangerous and is not always relieved sufficiently by evacuation around the fibrescope. With complete but not tense or uncomfortable distension, the instrument is slowly withdrawn, torquing it and deflecting the tip so as to see behind every fold (Coller, 1980).

Biopsy, brushing, or washing of lesions or suspicious areas should be done as the instrument passes any sites in question in order to avoid a second intubation. Photographic documentation of any changes provides a reference point against which to compare the findings on follow-up examinations. Though polypectomy is not recommended under the conditions of preparation described, it could be considered if carbon dioxide is used as the insufflation gas, in which case there would be virtually no hazard of explosion. Biopsy without total excision of polyps carries a 20% risk of a false negative report if the lesion is malignant. Coller, Corman and Veidenheimer (1976) and others have published data supporting the notion that any patient found to have a neoplastic polyp should have total colonoscopy, so that the question of polypectomy via the flexible sigmoidoscope would not then be raised and would be performed during total colonoscopy.

10.6 Results

Several studies have prospectively compared the results of rigid sigmoidoscopy and flexible sigmoidoscopy as performed by experienced endoscopists. Studies of flexible sigmoidoscopy done by non-endoscopists and non-physicians are underway but data are presently unavailable.

The reported series comparing rigid sigmoidoscopy and flexible sigmoidoscopy in the detection of polyps and cancers are summarized in Table 10.1.

The effective insertion length is the length of colon examined by either rigid sigmoidoscopy or flexible sigmoidoscopy. The length of colon examined is only roughly approximated by measuring the length of the instrument inserted. With both instruments the bowel will tend to be stretched by the neophyte, but gathered and pleated by the expert, who on average is usually also able to insert more sigmoidoscope. Reported series indicate that average insertion is 18–20 cm for rigid sigmoidoscopy as compared to 44–55 cm for flex-

Table 10.1 Detection of polyps and cancer

Author	No. patients	Polyps		Carcinoma	
		Number FS/RS	Ratio FS:RS	Number FS/RS	Ratio FS:RS
Deyhle, 1977	450	78/39	2.0:1	15/6	2.5:1
Katon, 1978	120	33/7	4.5:1	3/1	3.0:1
McCallum *et al.*, 1977	342	37/6	6.0:1	4/2	2.0:1
Marks *et al.*, 1979	1012	200/92	2.2:1	22/11	2.0:1
Protell *et al.*, 1978	610	47/24	2.0:1	8/4	2.0:1
Winawer *et al.*, 1979	108	35/3	12.0:1	5/1	5.0:1
Winnan *et al.*, 1980	341	36/6	6.0:1	4/1	4.0:1
Totals	2983	466/177		46/20	
Averages			2.6:1		2.3:1

ible sigmoidoscopy (Winawer *et al.*, 1979; Marks *et al*, 1979; Winnan *et al*, 1980).

It is generally reported that flexible sigmoidoscopy takes about twice as long as rigid sigmoidoscopy, but patient preference is about equal, or a little greater for flexible sigmoidoscopy (Winawer *et al.*, 1979; McCallum *et al.*, 1977; Katon, 1978; Protell, 1978).

Katon (1978) collected data for rigid sigmoidoscopy and flexible sigmoidoscopy, finding one perforation per 10 000 examinations for both procedures. The mortality rate for rigid sigmoidoscopy was 1/71 000. No deaths were reported for flexible sigmoidoscopy, but the total was less than 10 000 cases so that no real conclusions can be drawn.

With these reports and findings generally accepted, there nevertheless remains doubt amongst authorities concerning the proper utilization of flexible sigmoidoscopy. Tedesco (1979b) warns that whatever the value of flexible sigmoidoscopy for screening, if colonic disease is suspected, then evaluation with the colonoscope must be preferred over flexible sigmoidoscopy. He doubts that flexible sigmoidoscopy really adds anything to our ability to diagnose colonic disease. Marks *et al.* (1979), on the other hand, advocate flexible sigmoidoscopy not to exclude other diagnostic investigations, but only as a quicker and more convenient screening procedure. Their use of flexible sigmoidoscopy in symptomatic patients where colonoscopy was already indicated, whatever the flexible sigmoidoscopy or X-ray findings might be, may constitute unnecessary duplication. In fact, in only 203 of the 1012 cases was the indication for the examination of 'routine screening': 647 patients were seen for diagnosis of symptoms, polyp surveillance or cancer follow-up, which are widely considered to be indications for total colonoscopy. No cancers were found in the screening group, and only 26 polyps, so that the vast majority of the polyps detected were actually in patients who might have had total colonoscopy. Winnan *et al.* (1980) and others declared that flexible sigmoidoscopy was valuable in the detection of colorectal lesions and in interval screening examinations for cancer and premalignant lesions in symptomatic and asymptomatic persons, but they pointed out that many patients with symptoms or signs of colorectal disease undergo double contrast X-rays, total colonoscopy, or both, so that the important future role of flexible sigmoidoscopy may be as a routine interval examination for the asymptomatic patient.

Katon and Melnyk (1979) reviewed one year's experience with 265 patients undergoing flexible sigmoidoscopy. They found the procedure most helpful when performed for the following indications: 1. differential diagnosis and follow-up of inflammatory bowel disease;

2. hematochezia; 3. abnormal barium enema; 4. polypectomy; 5. diar-rhoea with normal barium enema; and 6. guaiac (Haemoccult)-positive stools. In reviewing this study, Tedesco (1979a) points out that these are all indications for total colonoscopy, and that the important question is not whether many lesions can be detected by flexible sig-moidoscopy, but whether a less than adequate examination will be accepted to reduce cost and effort.

Winawer *et al.* (1979) compared flexible sigmoidoscopy and double contrast barium enema against colonoscopy in 45 Haemoccult positive patients. Eight cancers were found by each method, but colonoscopy detected 18% more polyps. These findings are at variance with other reports that show an increasing incidence of carcinoma in the higher portions of the colon (Cady *et al.*, 1974; Snyder *et al.*, 1977; Rhodes *et al.*, 1977) and much lower diagnostic accuracy of barium enema than was apparently available to Winawer's patients (Tedesco, 1979a). Winawer concludes that the combination of flexible sigmoidoscopy and barium enema may not be as good as total colonoscopy, but in certain clinical situations it may be adequate, especially where superior radiology is available.

It is impossible to say at this time whether flexible sigmoidoscopy is destined to have a major impact on the detection and management of colorectal cancer. Physician and patient acceptance should be grea-ter than for rigid sigmoidoscopy, which has not achieved its potential. With Gilbertsen's data (Gilbertsen, 1974, 1980; Gilbertsen *et al.*, 1979) becoming more widely known, the potential of rigid sig-moidoscopy in the secondary prevention of cancer (by destroying premalignant polyps) is being appreciated just at the time that the next generation of physicians appears ready to abandon rigid sig-moidoscopy entirely. It is exciting to extrapolate Gilbertsen's 1974 results to flexible sigmoidoscopy and total colonoscopy, but we have no data to confirm our hope that colorectal cancer can be prevented wherever the fibrescope can reach.

In terms of detection of polyps and cancer we are on firmer ground. There is no question of the fact that, if charges and fees are roughly comparable, flexible sigmoidoscopy will detect more polyps and cancers per unit cost than will rigid sigmoidoscopy; and total colonoscopy will detect more lesions than any other method, but probably not more per unit cost. It also has to be proved that cancers detected by initial screening, by whatever method (Rhodes *et al.*, 1977), are actually cured more often than cancers presenting clinically. Cancers found by screening are more often of Dukes' stage A or B (Gilbertsen *et al.*, 1979) and less often C or D, but it seems likely that some of the early stage lesions found by screening will prove to be highly malignant, poor prognosis lesions that happened to be diagnosed earlier. Preliminary data indicate, however, that most lesions detected by screening behave as one would hope, according to Dukes' stage (Gilbertsen, 1980). If this proves true, then the benefit of colorectal endoscopy will have been clearly established as a factor of the depth of insertion – the greater the insertion, the greater the benefit in cancer deaths prevented.

The cost per death prevented will then be more easy to determine. At that point, the philosophers (or, more likely, the administrators) will take over to tell us what will be a reasonable expenditure to prevent death from colorectal cancer. Once that figure is known, the decision to screen by colonoscopy, rigid sigmoidoscopy, flexible sigmoidoscopy, rectal examination by a paramedic, occult blood testing, double contrast barium enema, or digital self-examination will become more or less clear. As for fibreoptic sigmoidoscopy, the final analysis of cost-effectiveness will have to account for the ineluctable fact that every patient saved from cancer must then survive to endure expensive follow-up and other screening tests, and finally to die of one or more diseases that may be even more costly.

References

Cady, B., Persson, A. V., Monson, D. O. and Maunz, D. L. (1974), Changing patterns of colorectal carcinoma. *Cancer*, **33**, 422–6.

Coller, J. A., Corman, M. L. and Veidenheimer, M. C. (1976), Colonic polypoid disease: need for total colonoscopy. *Am. J. Surg.*, **131**, 490.

Coller, J. A. (1980), Techniques of flexible fibreoptic sigmoidoscopy. *Surg. Clinics North Amer.*, **60**, 465–79.

Deyhle, P. (1977), Fiberoptic colonoscopy. In: *Gastroenterology*, (ed. H. L. Bockus) W. B. Saunders, Philadelphia, London, **3**, pp. 843–52.

Gilbertsen, V. A. (1974), Proctosigmoidoscopy and polypectomy in reducing the incidence of rectal cancer. *Cancer*, **34**, 936–9.

Gilbersten, V. A. (1980), Personal communication.

Gilbertsen, V. A., Williams, S. E., Schuman, L. and McHugh, R. (1979), Colonoscopy in the detection of carcinoma of the intestine. *Surgery, Gynec. Obstet.* **149**, 877–8.

Holt, R. W. and Wherry, D. C. (1980), Flexible fibreoptic sigmoidoscopy in a surgeon's office. *Amer. J. Surg.*, **139**, 708–12.

Katon, R. M. (1978), Sigmoidoscopy (rigid and flexible). In: *Screening and Early Detection of Colorectal Cancer.* (ed. D. R. Brodie), US Dept. Health, Education and Welfare, National Institute Health, pp. 115–23.

Katon, R. M. and Melnyk, C. S. (1979), The pansigmoidoscope: one year's experience in a gastrointestinal diagnostic unit. *J. Clin. Gastroent.*, 41–45.

Lipschutz, G. R., Katon, R. M., McCool, M. F., Mayer, B., Smith, F. W., Duff, E. I. and Melnyk, C. S. (1980), Flexible sigmoidoscopy as a screening procedure for neoplasia of the colon. *Surgery Gynec. Obstet.*, **148**, 19–24.

McCallum, R. *et al.* (1977), Flexible fiberoptic proctosigmoidoscopy (f) vs rigid proctosigmoidoscopy (r) as a routine diagnostic procedure (abstract). *Gastrointest. Endosc.*, **23**, 235.

Marks, G. *et al.* (1979), Sigmoidoscopic examinations with rigid and flexible fiberoptic sigmoidoscopes in the surgeon's office: a comparative prospective study of effectiveness in 1012 cases. *Dis. Colon Rect.*, **22**, 162–8.

Overholt, B. F. (1969) Flexible fiberoptic sigmoidoscopy. *Cancer*, **19**, 80–84.

Protell, R. L. (1978), The short colonoscope: computer analysis of a comparison with rigid sigmoidoscopy and hemoccult testing (abstract). *Gastroenterology*.

Rhodes, J. B., Holmes, F. F. and Clark, G. M. (1977) Changing distribution of primary cancers in the large bowel. *J. Amer. Med. Assoc.*, **238**, 1641–3.

Salmon, P. R. *et al.* (1971), Clinical evaluation of fiber-optic sigmoidoscopy employing the Olympus CG-SB colonoscope. *Gut*, **12**, 729–35.

Snyder, D. N., Heston, J. F., Meigs, J. W. and Flannery, J. T. (1977), Changes in site distribution of colorectal carcinoma in Connecticut, 1940–1973. *Am. J. Dig. Dis.*, **22**, 791–7.

Tedesco, F. J. (1979a), Flexible sigmoidoscopy – what is its role? *J. Clin. Gastroent.*, 46.

Tedesco, F. J. (1979b), Twice as many colorectal cancers seen with flexible, 65 cm scope. *Med Trib*, 16.

Winawer, S. J., Leidner, S. D., Boyle, C. and Kurtz, R. C. (1979), Comparison of flexible sigmoidoscopy with other diagnostic techniques in the diagnosis of rectocolon neoplasia. *Dig. Dis. Sci.*, **24**, 277–81.

Winnan, G. *et al.* (1980), Superiority of the flexible to the rigid sigmoidoscope in routine proctosigmoidoscopy. *New Engl J. Med.*, **302**, 1011–12.

CHAPTER ELEVEN

Intraoperative Colonoscopy

KENNETH A. FORDE

'Intraoperative (or peroperative) colonoscopy' refers to the use of a flexible fibreoptic colonoscope introduced per anum during an intra-abdominal surgical procedure without colotomy. Prior to the introduction of colonoscopy, surgeons operated on most lesions of the large bowel without the benefit of preoperative direct visualization and biopsy, except for the rectosigmoid region which has been accessible for inspection since Kelly introduced his rigid sigmoidoscope in 1895. With the introduction of the flexible fibreoptic colonoscope during the past decade, it has been possible for the skilled endoscopist to examine the entire colon preoperatively when it is necessary to do so. Not surprisingly, however, there are limitations to this procedure, and total colonoscopy is occasionally not possible, no matter how experienced the examiner, because of factors such as: excessive colon tortuosity, fixation from postoperative adhesions, pelvic irradiation, or extensive diverticular disease. The luxury of preoperative colonoscopy may not be possible under emergency circumstances. Furthermore, there are unexpected situations that arise in the operating room which make it desirable or necessary to inspect the lumen of the bowel during the conduct of an operative procedure. The concept and practice of inspecting the colonic lumen during an abdominal operation are not new. The first reference to the use of the rigid sigmoidoscope in the operative field at celiotomy was by Klein in 1952 (Klein and Scarborough, 1952). Historically, the technique has been termed 'coloscopy', causing confusion, since some endoscopists have adopted the same term for the use of flexible instruments as well.

11.1 Coloscopy with the rigid sigmoidoscope

While intraoperative rigid sigmoidoscopy (or coloscopy) has been helpful in some situations, it has several disadvantages and hazards. It is awkward for the examiner to maintain sterility, since the unsterile face mask comes near surgical gloves when the short rigid

189

instrument is introduced to its full length. It is necessary to make an opening in the colon, which immediately contaminates the operative field despite the many safeguards employed, such as: good preoperative bowel preparation, isolation of the area of colotomy from the remaining area of the operative field with sterile towels and the use of a purse-string suture to close the bowel around the sigmoidoscope at the colotomy site. Despite attempts to pleat the bowel over the sigmoidscope, its short length permits inspection of only a small segment, and multiple colotomies are necessary for examination of the entire colon. The required manipulation and resultant contamination have been associated with complications, such as local or systemic sepsis, as well as fistula formation (Kleinfeld and Gump, 1960).

11.2 Colonoscopy with the flexible endoscope

The development of flexible fibreoptic colonoscopy has reduced the necessity for multiple colotomies and coloscopy. The technique of intraoperative colonoscopy was described by Marcozzi and Montori (1972) in Europe almost a decade ago and in the United States a year later (Richter, Littman and Levowitz, 1973). Various endoscopists have added modifications to the original techniques (Silverstein, 1974: Eisenberg, 1976; Martin and Forde, 1979; Forde, 1979).

11.2.1 *Preparation*

Whenever possible, plans for intraoperative colonoscopy should be made in advance. Both members of the team, the surgeon as well as the endoscopist, should know the aims of the procedure and their respective roles in achieving the desired results. It must be stated that planning ahead may obviate the need for intraoperative colonoscopy, since many patients could easily undergo routine preoperative colonoscopy the day before an abdominal operation without altering the routine bowel preparation. Unfortunately, there is a misconception among both endoscopists and surgeons of limited experience with these techniques, that examination of the patient under general anaesthesia, and with the abdomen open, is an easier and less risky procedure than routine colonoscopy. This is not at all true, and the examiner and the surgeon must adhere to certain strict principles if the procedure is to be performed efficiently and safely.

Adequate bowel preparation is important for successful intraoperative colonoscopy: additional enemas or colon washouts should be administered a few hours before the procedure. Surgical patients often have their cleansing enemas the evening prior to operation, but this is inadequate for colonoscopy.

Bacteraemia is periodically present with endoscopic instrumentation (Dickman *et al.*, 1976; Norfleet *et al.*, 1976), and perioperative antibiotics should be used under the following circumstances: if the patient has an artificial cardiac valve, pacemaker or vascular prosthesis; if the patient is on steroid therapy or is otherwise immunosuppressed or susceptible to diseases such as endocarditis.

There has been no documentation that carbon dioxide is safer as regards colonic explosions than room air provided the colon is well prepared.

11.2.2 *Equipment*

The endoscopist should be in the operating room prior to the induction of anaesthesia, setting up equipment and making certain that everything is in working order, especially suction apparatus which may also be required by the anaesthetist and the surgical team. Instruments used in the operating room are the same as for colonoscopy performed in the colonoscopy suite. If polypectomy is anticipated, snares (always more than one in case of breakage or mechanical failure) should be available and pretested. The patient should be electrically grounded before the procedure starts. The instruments do not require special cleaning, since the operative field remains isolated by the colonic wall from contamination by the colonoscope.

11.2.3 *Position*

The only *absolute requirements* for positioning are that the endoscopist does not contaminate the operative field, and that there be room to manipulate the shaft of the instrument. The arrangement we have found most convenient is illustrated in Figs. 11.1 and 11.2. After induction of anaesthesia, both thighs are elevated on pillows. The endoscope is introduced 10–12 cm in the rectum and secured on a low table or stool next to or under the operating table and connected to the light source and suction apparatus. The electrocautery grounding plate should be placed in an optimal position at this time. An alternative position is a modified dorsal lithotomy position, with thighs in low stirrups (Fig. 11.3). This is more suitable for a two-person approach when the assistant advances, withdraws or holds the shaft of the instrument while the endoscopist uses both hands for the controls. The lithotomy position may be a disadvantage for the endoscopist who does all the controls and manipulation, since there is no fixed flat surface upon which to rest the bulk of the instrument during insertion.

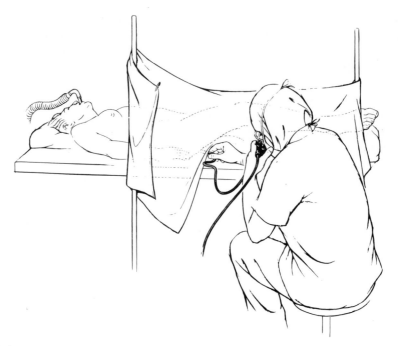

Fig. 11.1 Artist's representation of positioning of the patient for intra-operative colonoscopy.

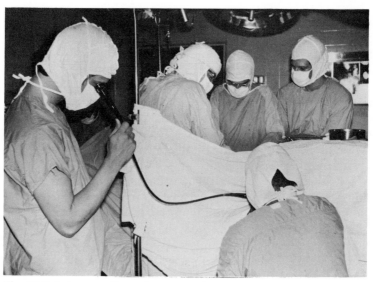

Fig. 11.2 Intraoperative colonoscopy in progress.

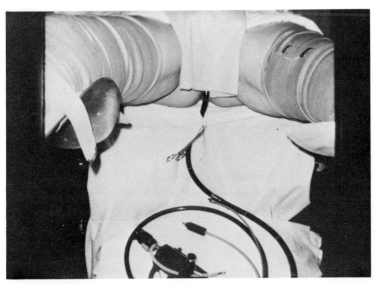

Fig. 11.3 Alternative positioning (low stirrups as for Miles abdomino-perineal resection). Colonoscope inserted in anus and secured although patient draped and abdomen opened.

11.2.4 *Technique*

For the orderly, efficient and safe conduct of peroperative colonoscopy, the endoscopist must be skilled and experienced (Marks, 1974). It is also important for the surgeon to have some concept of endoscopic instrumentation, manipulation and especially the potential hazards. The surgeon should await direction from the endoscopist rather than initiate independent manoeuvres without close co-ordination and communication. We have found that the placement of a non-crushing clamp across the bowel just above the proximal point to be examined is useful in preventing the proximal small intestine from becoming over distended with air, although Sjogren and his colleagues (1978) have felt this undesirable. During intraoperative colonoscopy, as in routine procedures, the chief aim, on introduction of the instrument, is to achieve maximal insertion. In our experience, the usual anatomic landmarks are recognized provided that the colon is not overdistended or over manipulated 'externally' by the surgical team. The surgeon may assist by manually depressing the sigmoid colon to keep it from bowing up once it has lost the tamponade effect of the closed abdominal wall. The surgeon may also redirect the tip so that it is in mid-position in the lumen of the bowel, point out when there is too much air, and pleat the bowel over the endoscope where it is not firmly attached to the parietes. It is easiest to telescope the transverse, and often the ascending colon. The surgeon must be extremely gentle during telescoping manoeuvres lest damage be done to the bowel wall. The endoscopist is more limited than usual in his ability to concertina (pleat) the bowel over the instrument, because the open abdomen permits the air-filled colon to rise out of the confines of the abdominal cavity. Intubation of the ileocaecal valve is usually more difficult when the surgeon attempts to assist the endoscopist. After maximal insertion has been achieved, inspection is performed on withdrawal, insufflating as necessary for visualization, but it is important to aspirate during withdrawal from each segment. If the diagnosis is chronic recurrent bleeding and arteriovenous malformations are being sought, dimming the overhead operating room lights will aid in their detection (see 'Bleeding' below). When a lesion is detected, the surgeon should mark the serosal surface with a suture or haemostatic silver clip. The surgical team must pay careful attention to details such as this and avoid being distracted by watching the path of light as the instrument is being advanced. The average length of a procedure in our hands is currently 15 min for introduction and complete inspection.

Bleeding

When the examination is performed for active massive bleeding, additional aspects of technique should be considered. Clots in the rectum are best removed prior to endoscopy with irrigation through a large rectal tube or a sigmoidoscope. The colonoscope is then advanced by passing it over the meniscus of blood or 'dissecting' between blood clot and colon wall. Blood clots should be fragmented and dispersed, rather than suctioned, to avoid plugging the aspiration channel, rendering the examination impossible. Double-channel instruments may be more efficient in the actively bleeding patient, as well as for the use of additional irrigation aids. We prefer a modification of the dental Water Pik, which delivers rapid periodic pulses of water and can be easily attached to the accessory irrigating channel.

During the examination for acute or chronic bleeding, it is necessary to extend the examination of intraoperative colonoscopy through the ileocaecal valve and into the terminal ileum or above, since arteriovenous malformations may be found in the small bowel. The small bowel is best examined for bleeding sites by having the surgeon hold a 10–12-cm length of intestine so that it can be visualized by the endoscopist and trans-illumination observed from the serosal aspect by the surgeon, who subsequently pleats that segment over the instrument. This procedure is progressively performed until the entire length of the small bowel has been examined.

11.2.5 *Complications*

The hazards of intraoperative colonoscopy can all be avoided by careful technique on the part of both endoscopist and surgeon. Among those described are serosal and mesentric tears with resultant haematoma formation (Sjogren *et al.*, 1978); perforation (both instrumental and secondary to cauterization), and prolonged ileus from over-distension of the small intestine by air. The risk of complication is increased when examining an obviously inflamed bowel.

11.2.6 *Limitations*

Major limitations are the availability of trained personnel, adequate bowel cleansing, and satisfactory equipment. Limitations inherent in the procedure include extensive adhesions and massive bleeding (Bowden, Hooks and Mansberger, 1980; Martin and Forde, 1979). Adhesions may defy surgical attempts at division of scarred tissue, causing the intestine to be so matted that uncoiling of loops of bowel is impossible. This is especially true in the pelvis.

Bleeding may be so rapid as to obscure the endoscopist's view of the lumen, thwarting all attempts at examination of the colon. Usually, however, if specific pathology cannot be seen, it is possible to define the general segment of colon from which the bleeding is arising.

11.2.7 *Indications*

Intraoperative colonoscopy is useful in several situations:

Localization
Lesions noted on previous barium studies or on preoperative endoscopy but not palpable through the bowel wall may be directly visualized (Figs. 11.4 and 11.5).

Previous polyp site
When a polyp that has been excised endoscopically is unexpectedly shown to contain incompletely excised invasive carcinoma, the site must be localized before subsequent colon resection. If the barium enema reveals its location in an area of conventional resection (e.g. a caecal lesion for which right hemicolectomy would ordinarily be per-

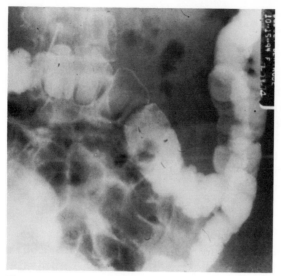

Fig. 11.4 Transverse colon lesion, seen on barium enema but not palpable at operation.

formed), the surgical decision is not difficult. If the polyp was not previously localized by X-ray, it becomes important for the surgeon to remove the appropriate segment of colon. While the practice of marking the polypectomy site endoscopically by submucosal injection of a dye or India ink is a possibility for the future, it is not yet com-

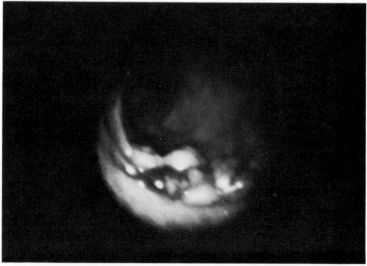

Fig. 11.5 Intraoperative endoscopic appearance of villous adenoma.

monplace practice. In such a situation, intraoperative colonoscopy is a valuable procedure.

Identification of the area of recurrent bleeding
This has been commented on by several authors in the recent literature (Eisenberg, 1976; Martin and Forde, 1979; Hooks, Bowden and Mansberger, 1979; Bowden, Hooks and Mansberger, 1980).

Evaluation of the small intestine
Intraoperative colonoscopy for this indication is most often performed for recurrent bleeding of unknown cause, as above (Bowden, Hooks and Mansberger, 1980).

The difficult polypectomy
For technical or other considerations, a polyp may occasionally prove too difficult to remove by routine colonoscopy, and it may be necessary to resort to intraoperative polypectomy and avoid the potential complications of colotomy (Wilson *et al.*, 1976).

11.3 Conclusions

Intraoperative colonoscopy has been reported to be of value in almost every situation in which it has been employed (Martin and Forde, 1979; Bowden, Hooks and Mansberger, 1980). In our experience, the major clinical advantages have included the avoiding of colotomy or resection, extending or limiting a planned resection, and suggesting unplanned but necessary surgical resection. All endoscopists find a decrease in the necessity for intraoperative procedures as they gain in personal experience and expertise, benefit from improved instrumentation, and an acceptance of the value of colonoscopy by medical and surgical colleagues. However, there remain selected situations in which this technique is both necessary and useful. For these few circumstances, it is important to be acquainted with this variation of colonoscopy technique and to consider its application when confronted with the indications which have been discussed.

References

Bowden, T. A., Hooks, V. H. and Mansberger, A. R. (1980), Intra-operative endoscopy. Gastrointestinal endoscopy. *Ann. Surg.*, **191**, 680.

Dickman, M. D., Farrell, R., Higgs, R. H., Wright, L. E., Humphries, P. J., Wojcik, J. D. and Chappelka, R. (1976), Colonoscopy associated bacteremia. *Surgery Gynec. Obstet.*, **142**, 173–176.

Eisenberg, H. W. (1976), Fiberoptic colonoscopy: intraoperative colonoscopy. *Dis. Colon Rect.*, **19**, 405–406.

Forde, K. A. (1979), Intraoperative colonoscopy. The author replies. *Dis. Colon Rect.*, **22**, 508.

Hooks, V. H., Bowden, T. A. and Mansberger, A. R. (1979), Focal vascular dysplasia in the cecum demonstrated by intra-operative endoscopic transillumination. *Gastrointest. Endosc.*, **25**, 69–71.

Klein, R. R. and Scarborough, R. A. (1952), Diagnosis and treatment of adenomatous polyps of the colon. *Archs Surg.*, **65**, 65.

Kleinfeld, G. and Gump, F. E. (1960), Complications of colotomy and polypectomy. *Surgery Gynec. Obstet.*, **111**, 726.

Marcozzi, G. and Montori, A. (1972), Endoscopy during operation: new diagnostic possibilities. *Chir. Gastroenterol.*, **6**, 23–25.

Marks, G. (1974), Operative coloscopy: a current status appraisal. *Dis. Colon and Rect.*, **17**, 754–758.

Martin, P. G. and Forde, K. A. (1979), Intra-operative colonoscopy: preliminary report. *Dis. Colon Rect.*, **22**, 234–237.

Norfleet, R. G., Mitchell, P. D., Mulholland, D. D. and Philo, J. (1976), Does bacteremia follow colonoscopy? *Gastrointest. Endosc.*, **23**, 31–32.

Richter, R. M., Littman, L. and Levowitz, B. S. (1973), Intra-operative fiber-optic colonoscopy: localization of nonpalpable colonic lesions. *Archs. Surg.*, **106**, 224–228.

Silverstein, F. E. (1974), Tip on avoiding undue bowel distension at intra-operative endoscopy. *Gastrointest. Endosc.*, **21**, 81.

Sjogren, R. W., Johnson, L. F., Butler, M. L., Heit, H. A., Gremillion, D. E. and Cammerer, R. C. (1978), Serosal laceration: a complication of intra-operative colonoscopy explained by transmural pressure gradients. *Gastrointest. Endosc.*, **24**, 239–242.

Wilson, S. M., Poisson, J., Gamache, A., Henderson, M. J. and ReMine, W. H. (1976), Intra-operative fiberoptic colonoscopy – 'The difficult polypectomy'. *Dis. Colon Rect.*, **19**, 136–138.

CHAPTER TWELVE

Therapeutic Colonoscopy

P. FRÜHMORGEN

12.1 Requirements for therapeutic colonoscopy

The endoscopic techniques with which this chapter is concerned are of a therapeutic nature and are frequently referred to as 'operative endoscopy'.

The discussion will include only those therapeutic procedures that have passed from the experimental stage and are now part of the clinical routine.

12.1.1 Technical requirements

Since the establishment of routine diagnostic colonoscopy, the last decade has witnessed the increasing use of therapeutic endoscopy, especially colonoscopic polypectomy and occasionally foreign body removal, both of which had already been performed with the rigid proctosigmoidoscope.

Other techniques used in the broader field of therapeutic endoscopy include the application of drugs (sclerotherapy, injection of vaso-constrictors, acrylic polymers, local pharmacotherapy), mechanical procedures (forceps, baskets, hooks, bougie, clips) as well as the application of thermal snares or probes (polypectomy, electroresection, electrocoagulation, photocoagulation) (Frühmorgen *et al.*, 1980).

In contrast to their widespread application in the upper gastrointestinal tract, the use of sclerotherapy, dilators, baskets, etc., play a much lesser role in the colon or rectum. In order to familiarize the endoscopist with the technical aspects of the diathermy procedures most frequently employed in the colon they will now be described with emphasis on the forms of energy employed.

The physical principle of the thermal techniques is based on the production of heat energy concentrated at a specific site over a defined time interval. In principle, heat may be derived from many sources such as conduction, radiation or convection. Other energy forms, for example electric current or electromagnetic radiation, can be converted into heat energy and the latter method has been so far employed exclusively in therapeutic endoscopy.

(a) *The production of heat using electric current*

When the two poles (electrodes) of a power source are brought into contact with an electrically conductive material to form a circuit, an electric current will flow. If this circuit contains a region of high electrical resistance, heat will be produced at that point. In practice, a high frequency power source (electrosurgical unit) is used in combination with a large-area neutral (indifferent, inactive) patient plate applied to part of the patient's body, and a second, small-area active electrode (therapy electrode). When the active electrode is applied to a part of the body, the intervening tissue completes the circuit, allowing current to flow through the body to the patient plate (Fig. 12.1).

Since the area of contact of the active electrode (snare, coagulation, electrode, hot-biopsy forceps, etc.) is considerably smaller than that of the inactive patient plate, a high current density results which, in turn, generates sufficient heat to vaporize the water in the tissues and destroy the cells, thus achieving a cutting effect with separation of tissue. If the generation of heat is reduced by the application of less current or by allowing it to disperse over larger areas of tissue, this effect can be diminished to produce coagulation.

There are two main reasons for using high-frequency currents: they do not produce any injurious or life-threatening neurophysiological reactions such as cardiac dysrhythmia, and they permit circuits to be made not merely by conductive material (tissue), but also by capacitive coupling (the capacitor effects of neighbouring areas of tissue). This can prevent the production of undesirable thermal effects in other parts of the body due to additional zones of high resistance.

During endoscopic application of a 'blended' current, an undamped oscillating high-frequency current (1.75 MHz tube (valve) current) is used with a superimposed spark gap current. While the pure tube current has a cutting effect, the spark gap current produces

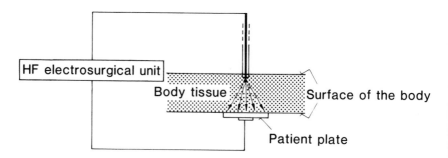

Fig. 12.1 Principle of endoscopic coagulation using a high-frequency (HF) power source.

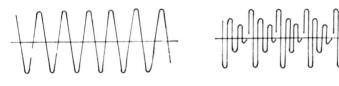

Tube current   Spark-gap current

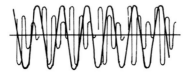

Blended current

Fig. 12.2 Blended current, comprising high-frequency undamped current (tube current) with superimposed high current peaks (spark gap current).

a superficial coagulation effect (Fig. 12.2). Most commercially available high-frequency surgical units permit the selection of either tube or spark gap current or a blend of the two waveforms (blended current).

For endoscopic use, the familiar techniques of electrosurgery are modified to permit the use of flexible active electrodes passed down the instrument channel of the endoscope. Active electrodes are available in the form of flexible snares, probes and hooks. Polypectomy, coagulation and haemostasis can be carried out through the accessory channel of any colonoscope.

In contrast to this high-frequency electrothermal procedure, coagulation and the cutting of tissue can also be achieved with the aid of electromagnetically regulated d.c. current applied in the bipolar mode with current flow only through the tissue to be coagulated (Semm, 1974; 1975). Although theoretically practical for gastrointestinal endoscopic procedures, no clinically relevant application has yet been found for this method.

In addition to these physical methods of heat conduction, further possibilities lie in the principle of heat convection using hot-gas probes, or heat radiation. An endoscopic hot-gas probe has been developed but has not yet been shown to have any clinical value (Bodem *et al.*, 1980).

Heat generated by using infra-red radiation has a haemostatic effect. Devices are already being used intra-operatively and in the treatment of haemorrhoids (Neiger *et al.*, 1977). Guides that transmit this type of radiation through the biopsy channel of an endoscope are available, but an analysis of the problems involved shows that available power sources are unable to produce enough radiation for the fibreendoscopic management of bleeding.

(b) *Production of heat by electromagnetic radiation*
Tissue can also be heated by the influence of electromagnetic wave fields. The heating effect is strongly dependent upon the frequency of the electromagnetic radiation. The spectrum of electromagnetic waves employed extends from relatively low-frequency radio waves to the highest-frequency gamma rays and includes visible light and X-rays. The energy produced in such wave fields is absorbed by the tissue and converted into heat energy. Electromagnetic wave fields in the megahertz and gigahertz ranges have been used in both microwave cookers and short-wave and microwave diathermy units.

Studies of microwave (2.45 GHz) endoscopic coagulation have shown that although local heating can be produced, without tissue contact, its coagulation effect is not adequate for therapeutic purposes (Bodem *et al.*, 1975).

It is possible to use intense light radiation to produce marked coagulation effects in body tissues, but the power has to be conducted to the treatment site through a flexible optical fibre passed through the instrument channel of the endoscope. The demands made on the light source are such that they can be met only by a laser.

Systems employing either a neodymium-YAG laser or an argon ion laser are available for clinical use. The difference in the photocoagulative effect of these two laser systems is due largely to their differing optical wavelengths. The argon laser uses blue-green light of about 0.5μm wavelengths; and the neodymium-YAG laser, invisible infrared light of about 1μm wavelength. Due to differences in radiation absorption within the tissue, the two lasers have different depths of penetration. The depth of penetration of the neodymium-YAG laser is about 4 times greater (approximately 0.8 mm) than the argon laser (approximately 0.2 mm). This means that to achieve identical coagulation effects in the bowel wall with identical exposure time and area exposed, the power density delivered by the neodymium-YAG laser needs to be four times less than that of the argon laser.

The advantages of the laser include no contact with tissue, controlled thermal reaction under direct vision, no current flowing through the patient, a greater therapeutic range compared with electrocoagulation, the selective absorption peculiar to the argon laser, and the self-limiting depth of penetration of the coagulating tissue. These properties all make laser photocoagulation a promising new therapy for endoscopic application, the value of which has already been proved in animal experiments and, at some centres, in clinical application (Brunetaud *et al.*, 1979; Frühmorgen *et al.*, 1975a and b and 1976a and b; Kiefhaber *et al.*, 1977).

The CO_2 laser does not have any endoscopic application at this time.

(c) *Inert gas insufflation*
Many gases are swallowed or produced in the gastrointestinal tract including nitrogen, oxygen, carbon dioxide, hydrogen, methane and hydrogen sulphide. Hydrogen and methane may form an explosive mixture with oxygen when exceeding a critical concentration. These two gases are produced by bacterial fermentation and decomposition within the colon and represent a potential danger during electrosurgery (Engel *et al.*, 1970; Levitt *et al.*, 1968; Newman, 1974). Hydrogen itself is also produced in small quantities during electrosurgical procedures (Galley, 1954).

A number of reports have been published describing the explosion of gases in the bowel during electrosurgical procedures but these incidents can be avoided by insufflating an inert gas such as carbon dioxide during the procedure (Carter, 1952; Levy, 1954; Moutier, 1946). With one exception they have all occurred during rigid proctosigmoidoscopy, where incomplete cleansing of the proximal bowel was an important factor. In only one case has a fatal gas explosion been reported during a colonoscopic polypectomy. This accident may be attributed to the use of mannitol to cleanse the bowel (Bigard *et al.*, 1979; Bond and Levitt, 1979; Williams *et al.*, 1979). This form of bowel preparation (see Chapters 3 and 13) should be avoided or carbon dioxide insufflated when diathermy procedures are to be employed.

The need for the simultaneous insufflation of an inert gas has been assessed (Bond and Levitt, 1979; Frühmorgen and Demling, 1979) to investigate the potential danger of explosion after routine bowel preparation. Gas chromatographic measurements of the luminal hydrogen and methane concentrations have been made (Frühmorgen and Joachim, 1976), and the explosion threshold for hydrogen and methane was found at a concentration of about 4% by volume. The findings demonstrated that after careful cleansing of the bowel by diet, magnesium sulphate and enemas the gas concentrations were less than 0.001%, and no risk of explosion need be feared when electrosurgery is then carried out. If the bowel is not cleansed or if the production of gas is increased there is a distinct danger of an explosive gas mixture forming. Using standard methods of bowel preparation we have experienced no gas explosions in the bowel in a total of 2713 colonoscopic polypectomies. The results of a question-naire distributed (1978) in the Federal Republic of Germany revealed no cases of gas explosion in a total of 7365 polypectomies. At the time of this enquiry only four of 23 centres in Germany routinely insufflated inert gas during endoscopic polypectomy (Frühmorgen and Demling, 1979).

It is our opinion that insufflation of inert gas is only necessary if electrocautery is used when the intestine is inadequately cleansed beforehand, or if mannitol is used. Because mannitol represents a cer-tain risk it is not used in our department at Erlangen.

12.1.2 *Instruments for therapeutic colonoscopy*

(a) *Colonoscopes*

Both single-channel and twin-channel endoscopes of various lengths are available for therapeutic colonoscopy. Clinical experience of twin-channel operating colonoscopes has not shown any particular advantage for use in the colon for polypectomy. Indeed, the greater diameter of this instrument in comparison with the single-channel colonoscopes (a difference of approximately 3 mm) results in a decreased flexibility which makes it more difficult for the examiner to manoeuvre the instrument past 'tight' loops of the colon and renders the examination more painful for the patient. A possible advantage of the twin-channel instrument, however, is that both suction and irrigation are still possible when one channel is blocked by an accessory instrument (forceps, snare, coagulation probe, laser light waveguide). Despite this possible advantage, twin-channel endo-scopes have not found widespread acceptance for routine clinical use. We carry out all our therapeutic colonoscopies using the single-channel instruments that are also used for diagnostic work. In our unit we find that a uniform working length of approximately 130 cm is adequate for all therapeutic examinations and we have found an optical system of between 80° and 90° to be the most satisfactory. Provided that there is no stenosis to obstruct the passage of the instrument, complete inspection of the entire colon and terminal ileum is possible with medium-length instruments. Passage of the colonoscope is facilitated after straightening the sigmoid by providing 'external stiffening' to keep the sigmoid colon straightened by pres-sure from the edge of the hand applied to the abdomen.

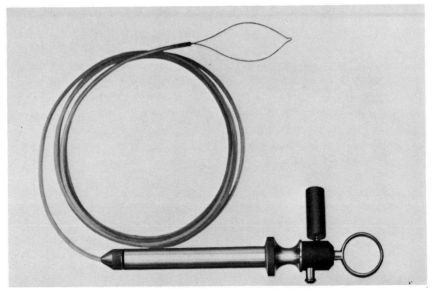

Fig. 12.3 High-frequency diathermy snare (Storz, West Germany).

(b) *Accessories and auxiliary instruments*

Polypectomy. A variety of accessory instruments are available for endoscopic polypectomy, including high-frequency diathermy snares, polyp retrievers, grasping forceps and high-frequency electrosurgical equipment. In our unit we make exclusive use of the various sizes of symmetrical snare developed in our department (Fig. 12.3). A variety of other snares are also available and suitable for polypectomy. The 'home-made' snare may also be used but requires a trained assistant who has experience in the formation of a properly sized snare loop. There are a variety of electrosurgical units available with widely differing power outputs. This makes it impossible to indicate any power setting which is applicable to all units. The optimal settings should be carefully evaluated with any new equipment before endoscopy by testing the effects on a piece of meat or in animal experiments (see Section 12.2.1).

Forceps polypectomy. A wide range of different polypectomy forceps are available for 'hot-biopsy'. They are similar to the biopsy forceps employed in diagnostic endoscopy but are sheathed to provide electrical insulation. Small polypoid lesions can be removed while the base of the polyp is coagulated simultaneously (Williams, 1973; Cotton and Williams, 1980) (see Section 12.2.2).

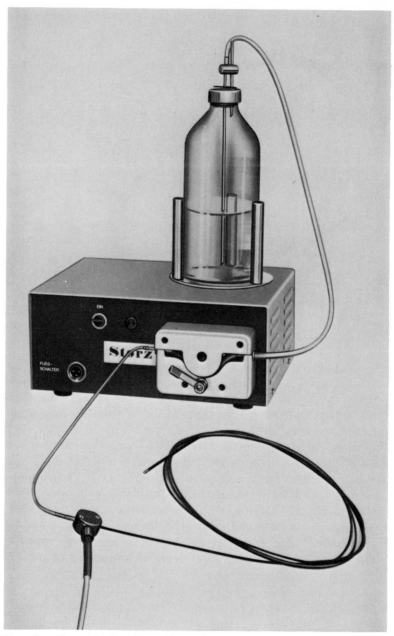

Fig. 12.4 Electro-hydro-thermal probe after Frühmorgen (Storz, West Germany).

Foreign body removal. This therapeutic procedure is rarely required in the colorectal region, but a variety of grasping forceps, snares and hooks are available and can be passed into the colon through the instrument channel of the endoscope (see Section 12.2.4).

Electrocoagulation. For endoscopic haemostasis using high-frequency diathermy current, the same electrosurgical units are used as for polypectomy. Thin flexible button electrodes, some perforated with a flushing or suction facility, are available. An alternative and preferable form of electrocoagulation is that which uses the electro-hydrothermal probe developed by our group (Fig. 12.4) (see Section 12.2.5(a)).

Laser photocoagulation. Two laser systems are available as the sources of energy: the argon ion laser and the neodymium-YAG laser, both of which can be used with a fibreoptic endoscope and a flexible lightguide. While the argon laser can be used with any commercially available endoscope, the neodymium-YAG laser requires a specially modified two-channel endoscope. A recent development is the flexible quartz light guide for use with a single-channel endoscope and which can be used for the neodymium-YAG laser (see Section 12.2.5(b)).

12.2 Techniques of therapeutic colonoscopy

Polypectomy is by far the most important procedure and accounts for about 98% of all the endoscopic therapeutic procedures carried out in the colon. Other techniques such as snare loop biopsy, foreign body removal and endoscopic haemostasis in the colon are all relatively rare indications.

12.2.1 *Snare polypectomy*

Polypoid lesions in the colon can be biopsied using forceps, destroyed using a coagulation electrode or excised using the diathermy snare. The serious disadvantage of bleeding during any mechanical removal and inability to obtain tissue for histological examination after fulguration makes diathermy snare polypectomy the method of choice. Whenever technically possible, this method should always be employed, since a partial forceps biopsy does not always provide a representative histological sample.

(a) *Instrumentation*

The instrumentation for polypectomy comprises a diathermy snare either asymmetrical, or better, symmetrical (Fig. 12.3) and a high-frequency electrosurgical unit. The polyp may be retrieved by aspiration onto the tip of the endoscope, within the polypectomy snare, or by using a polyp retriever (Section 12.1.2(b)).

(b) *Technique*

The polyp to be removed is located using the usual techniques of diagnostic colonoscopy (Cotton and Williams, 1980; Frühmorgen and Classen, 1980) after appropriate bowel cleansing.

Before the procedure, proper functioning of the snare loop and high-frequency electrosurgical unit should be tested. Two snares should always be available for each polypectomy procedure. The back-up snare may be used if the primary snare should break and in the event of complications, such as bleeding, an extra snare may be passed rapidly through the channel if the original snare is difficult to open; this can occur because of coagulated tissue being withdrawn into the snare sheath during the polypectomy procedure.

The assistant must ensure that there is good contact between the patient plate and the skin of the thigh. A polyp may be removed during either intubation or on withdrawal depending upon whether it is in an ideal position for polypectomy when first seen. The polyp head should be snared only when the colonoscope has been optimally positioned in relation to the polyp, and with the instrument shaft free of tension. It may prove helpful to move the patient if the best position of the endoscope to the polyp has not been obtained. To ensnare the head of the polyp, the tip of the endoscope is usually located 2 cm to 3 cm distal to the lesion and the snare is advanced through the instrument channel. The snare loop is then opened in the lumen of the colon, placed over the polyp and manoeuvred to the base of the head (Plates 37–40). During this manoeuvre, it is useful both to manipulate the tip of the colonoscope and partially open and close the snare since repeated movements of the snare may cause flexion of the wire loop enabling it to encircle the polyp head. Some examiners use their right hand to control the colonoscope shaft by torque to right or left, inserting and withdrawing while the assistant opens and closes the snare loop (Waye, 1980). The snare is pulled tight only when it can be seen to be properly positioned at the base of the polyp head. Before closing the loop, the sheath of the snare must always be pushed up against the stalk or base of the polyp. Since the tip of the snare sheath is the fixed point in the system into which the snare loop retracts, if the end of the sheath is positioned several centimetres away from the polyp, closure causes the loop which is already over the polyp to bend the polyp towards the snare sheath, slipping the head out of the wire loop. This is avoided if the tip of

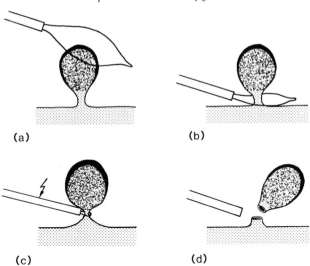

(a)

(b)

(c)

(d)

Fig. 12.5 Schematic representation of the removal of pedunculated polyps.

the sheath is placed against the polyp stalk or base before the snare is closed. If possible, the snare should be tightened by the endoscopist, or by an assistant using the teaching attachment to avoid possible 'guillotining' of the polyp stalk. Once the snare is snugly around the base or stalk of the polyp, and the head becomes 'livid', the snare should not be closed further. Before the application of current the polyp should be drawn into the lumen and towards the tip of the endoscope to avoid thermal damage to the bowel wall. Current is then applied and the snare slowly closed severing the polyp (Fig. 12.5). When placing a snare over a pedunculated polyp which has a stalk of sufficient length it is wise to leave a remnant of the stalk so that this can be re-snared should post polypectomy bleeding occur. In the case of a sessile polyp, the lesion is always snared at the base to include some 2 mm to 3 mm of normal mucosa. After closing the snare, a 'pseudo-stalk' of normal mucosa should be formed by pulling the polyp into the lumen (Fig. 12.6).

Manipulation of the endoscope in the vicinity of the polypectomy site carries the risk of inducing haemorrhage or perforation. When a number of polyps are to be removed, those in the proximal colon should be approached first. Large polyps (greater than 3 cm diameter) may be removed endoscopically in carefully selected cases, since the risk of perforation, haemorrhage, incomplete removal or the presence of malignancy increases with polyps larger than 3 cm to 4 cm (Table 12.1). It is possible to remove such lesions by piecemeal resection,

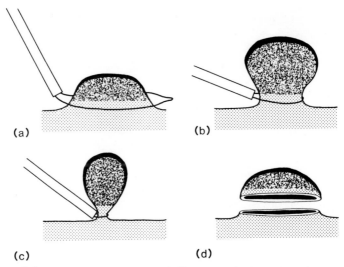

(a)   (b)

(c)   (d)

Fig. 12.6 Schematic representation of the removal of sessile polyps.

and especially important to retrieve all the resected material for histological examination. The piecemeal resection technique is performed by placing the snare loop around a portion of the head of the polyp without attempting to encircle the base completely (Plates 42 and 43). Electrocautery current is applied as the snare is being closed, with removal of a portion of the polyp. The resected portion may be large or small depending upon the position of the snare wire. Piecemeal resection may also be necessary when the snare becomes embedded in the head of a villous polyp and cannot easily be removed. Blood vessels in the head of the polyp are usually rather small, and profuse bleeding is rare during piecemeal polypectomy. Either at the primary

Table 12.1 Size of adenoma and malignancy (n = 1708)
(Erlangen polyp register)

Size	Adenoma with severe cell atypia	Adenoma with adenocarcinoma	n
0–10 mm	13 (1.2%)	7 (0.6%)	1088
11–20 mm	30 (9.4%)	22 (6.9%)	319
21–40 mm	21 (13.0%)	58 (37.0%)	158
41–60 mm	3 (5.0%)	42 (64.0%)	66
>61 mm	2 (6.0%)	24 (69.0%)	35
not measured	1	4	41

or subsequent examinations further portions of the polyp may be removed and large polyps can be reduced to the surface of the colonic wall. Once reduced to about 1 cm diameter the base can be easily snared and the remaining portion removed. The selection of the optimal power setting is adjusted to each situation and requires considerable experience. The settings chosen depend upon the diathermy unit and snare which are used. It is normal to start with a lower power setting and to give short bursts of current under constant observation, increasing the power slowly and stepwise until removal of the polyp is complete. It must again be emphasized that the power steps shown on the electrosurgical unit reveal little about the actual power applied at the snare, since this represents a non-linear function and depends both on the make of the unit and on the changing resistance in the snare at the site of polypectomy. In the case of broad-based polyps, the passage of current through the dried out residuum following partial resection is greatly reduced and this situation invariably requires a high power setting. In the initial years of polypectomy we used the so-called 'blended' current (see Section 12.1.1(a)) but lately we have employed coagulation current almost exclusively. Since changing to coagulation current, we have seen no more cases of bleeding after polypectomy. However, we do not always use coagulation current alone for the removal of broad-based polyps, because dessication of the tissue during removal may cause a change in resistance. In these circumstances 'blended' or pure cutting current may be helpful, especially if the snare wire appears to have stopped cutting through the tissue.

Occasionally despite successful section of the polyp stalk, the head appears to remain *in situ*. Retrieving the polyp directly by aspirating it on to the tip of the colonoscope may conceal bleeding and the polyp should be removed either by pushing with the snare sheath or the polyp grasper. The site of polypectomy should always be inspected immediately after resection so that any bleeding may be detected.

Once severed, polyps can be retrieved with the snare (Plate 41) grasping forceps, retrieval baskets or, most rapidly and reliably, by aspirating the polyp on to the tip of the endoscope. The three or four pronged grasper frequently damages the head of the polyp. Following polypectomy, the patient should be kept under observation overnight at the hospital monitoring both blood pressure and pulse for a 24-hour period.

(c) *Techniques for large sigmoid polyps*
The risk of bleeding or perforation increases with the size of polyps especially if the pedicle is thick. For such polyps, which are less

common above the sigmoid colon, deliberate sigmoid-rectal intussusception has been suggested by some authors as an alternative to piecemeal polypectomy (Gillespie *et al.*, 1978; Strauss, Gordon and Wise, 1978), although we have not practised this in Erlangen.

The polyp is snared using a handleless home-made wire snare which is tightened around the base of the lesion and the colonoscope withdrawn, leaving the snare in place. Later under general anaesthesia the polyp may be intussuscepted to the anal verge by traction, and then be excised and the wound sutured.

This technique provides a safe alternative to piecemeal polypectomy for large broad-based lesions in the sigmoid colon, and may avoid the need for abdominal surgery.

A further technique for medium-sized polyps with a particularly thick stalk has been described using the 'bi-polar' technique (Cotton and Williams, 1980). This approach has not been widely applied and requires a two-channel colonoscope. The polyp is snared in the usual way and then a V-shaped return electrode is passed through the second channel onto the lower part of the stalk; current flows from the snare through the stalk to the return electrode and a lower power setting used, since there is no leakage of current from the polyp head to the contralateral bowel wall. This technique, which is not practised in our department, may occasionally have its place but involves skilled manipulation and the twin-channel colonoscope which is less easy to use.

(d) *Indications*
Because of the well-recognized neoplastic potential of the colonic adenoma and the difficulties of obtaining a representative sample of tissue with the biopsy forceps, all polypoid lesions in the colon and rectum must be totally removed for full histological assessment. This applies both to solitary and multiple polyps, the removal of which involves a certain, but a justifiable, risk. If multiple polyps are too numerous, at least five should be removed in order to establish a correct diagnosis.

The limiting factors of colonoscopic polypectomy using high-frequency current are the experience of the endoscopist on the one hand, and the size of the polyp on the other. Using the snare loop, very tiny polyps having a diameter of 1 mm to 3 mm are either impossible to snare, or are completely destroyed during coagulation, leaving no tissue for histology. In contrast the risk of bleeding perforation or incomplete removal increases considerably in polyps having a base diameter in excess of 3 cm.

There is no indication for proctosigmoidoscopic polypectomy using the rigid instrument since, if a polyp is known to be present in the rectosigmoid, total colonoscopy must be carried out to exclude more proximal pathology. The rectal polyp is then removed during colonoscopy at the conclusion of the examination. Polypectomy with high frequency diathermy current should only be carried out with great care in patients with an implanted cardiac pacemaker, because of the risk of interference with pacemaker function (Mauser, 1971).

(e) *Contraindications*

Informed consent of the patient must first be obtained before endoscopic polypectomy and the complications of the polypectomy procedure should be explained to the patient before any attempt to remove a polyp. If a polyp is discovered fortuitously during a diagnostic colonoscopic examination, in the absence of an 'extended' declaration of consent covering polypectomy, the procedure should be concluded and repeated the following day, after obtaining the patient's informed consent to polypectomy.

Unco-operative patients, those with very active inflammatory large bowel disease, peritonitis, and haemorrhagic conditions are contraindications to polypectomy. In practice, however, in the last 2713 cases, there have been no instances among our patients where polypectomy has not been performed for any of these reasons. Although a polyp base of more than 3 cm in diameter increases the risk associated with endoscopic removal, it does not represent an absolute contraindication.

(f) *Results*

The first colonoscopic polypectomy was carried out in our department in 1970 (Dehyle *et al.*, 1971). In the ten years since then a total of 2713 pedunculated and sessile polyps have been removed from the colon and rectum during colonoscopy. A prospective histological analysis of a subgroup of 2200 polyps removed during 1978 and 1979 in the surgical and medical departments of the University Hospital Erlangen has been undertaken (Hermanek and Frühmorgen, 1980).

Of the 2200 polyps, which were detected in 1042 patients, 52% were pedunculated. The anatomical distribution of the polyps removed is shown in Table 12.2: 70.5% were adenomas, 7.6% carcinomas, with or without adenomatous tissue, and 20.8% were non-neoplastic polyps. Only 0.7% of these polyps were neoplastic polyps other than adenomas and only 0.4% were not retrieved after polypectomy (Table 12.3). Of the 1718 adenomas and carcinomas, 86.2% were adenomas with slight or moderate cell atypia, 4.1% adenomas

Table 12.2 Localization of removed polyps (*n* = 2200)
(Erlangen polyp register)

Rectum	37.5%
Sigmoid	32.3%
Descending colon	9.7%
Left flexure	2.9%
Transverse colon	6.6%
Right flexure	2.7%
Descending colon	5.9%
Caecum	2.2%

with severe cellular atypia and 9.1% adenomas showing adenocarcinoma. An additional 0.6% were polypoid adenocarcinomas without evidence of adenomatous tissue (Table 12.4). Analysis with respect to the size of the adenoma and presence of malignant change shows that, although very rare, adenomas with severe cellular atypia and adenomas with adenocarcinoma are found even in polyps of less than 10 mm in diameter, and confirms that the percentage with malig-

Table 12.3 Histological classification of removed polyps
(*n* = 2200)

Adenomas		1550 (70.5%)
tubular	1262	
tubulo-villous	219	
villous	69	
Carcinomas (with or without		
adenomatous structures)		167 (7.6%)
Other neoplastic polyps		16 (0.7%)
lipoma	8	
leiomyoma	1	
haemangioma	1	
lymphangioma	1	
carcinoid	1	
Non-neoplastic polyps		457 (20.8%)
hyperplastic	382	
juvenile	32	
Peutz-Jeghers	14	
inflammatory	19	
lymphoid	6	
lymphohyperplasia	3	
unclassified	1	
Not retrieved		10 (0.4%)

Table 12.4 Adenoma cancer sequence (*n* = 1718)
(Erlangen polyp register)

Adenomas	1481 (86.2%)
Adenomas with severe cell atypia	70 (4.1%)
Adenomas with adenocarcinoma	157 (9.1%)
Adenocarcinoma, polypoid	10 (0.6%)

nancy (adenoma with adenocarcinoma) increases with increasing size of the polypoid lesion (Table 12.1). Our data also confirms that a variable incidence of malignancy may be observed within adenomas of differing type (Table 12.5). The results of others are essentially similar (Williams *et al.*, 1974; Shinya and Wolff, 1980).

Endoscopic polypectomy may be considered to provide safe removal and cure of an adenoma with adenocarcinoma providing the following criteria are met:

1. The carcinoma is highly differentiated (Grade I or II).
2. The line of endoscopic resection is free of carcinomatous infiltration.
3. The patient will attend for follow-up.

The justification for the endoscopic treatment of an adenoma with adenocarcinoma is that the risk of metastases from such a well-differentiated carcinoma is smaller than the mortality rate of surgery.

(g) *Follow-up after polypectomy*
Follow-up after polypectomy is mandatory. A patient in whom one or more polyps have been found has an increased risk of developing further polyps and those patients in whom adenoma with adenocarcinoma has been removed must clearly be kept under very close surveillance.

Table 12.5 Type of adenoma and malignancy (*n* = 1708)
(Erlangen polyp register)

Histology	Adenoma with severe cell atypia	Adenoma with adenocarcinoma	*n*
Tubular	32 (2%)	63 (5%)	1328
Tubulo-villous	30 (11%)	51 (19%)	268
Villous	8 (7%)	43 (38%)	112
	70	157	1708

Table 12.6 Follow-up schedule after colonoscopic polypectomy (Medical Department of the University, Erlangen, 1st October 1980)

Follow-up (years)	1/4	1/2	1	2	3	5
Adenoma, pedunculated or sessile and removed with margin of healthy tissue					×	
sessile or pedunculated and removed with no margin of healthy tissue	×				×	
Adenoma with severe atypia (focal cancer)						
removed with margin of healthy tissue		×			×	×
removed with no margin of healthy tissue	×				×	×
Adenoma with invasive carcinoma						
removed with margin of healthy tissue, no resection	×	×	×	×	×	×
Non-neoplastic polyps (hyperplastic, lymphoid, juvenile, Peutz-Jeghers)					×	

To date, no confirmed and generally applicable information is available on the optimum intervals between follow-up examination. On the basis of our own experience we have produced a schedule for follow-up after endoscopic polypectomy which is based on the histological assessment of the polyp (Table 12.6). A prospective study will, it is hoped, show whether this schedule is both reasonable and practical with large numbers of patients.

In our own experience of 167 patients followed after polypectomy for a mean period of 1.8 years (1–5 years), it was not possible to identify the actual site of polypectomy in 66%. In 29% a scar or a 'bud' of mucosa was observed and in 3% a remnant of a stalk with normal mucosa was seen. In only three patients (2%) was a local recurrence unequivocally established and each had undergone apparently incomplete removal of a sessile polyp at the initial polypectomy (Frühmorgen *et al.*, 1977).

(h) Complications

Complications are usually the result of improper technique, inadequate skill and training of the endoscopist, or lack of attention to contraindications. The post polypectomy syndrome, bleeding, perforation and gas explosion are possible problems which will be discussed.

Post-polypectomy syndrome. During the course of a careful clinical follow-up after polypectomy, the endoscopist may occasionally observe this rare syndrome which is sometimes also seen after forceps biopsy. It is clinically manifested by abdominal pain, meteorism and a brief period of fever. It is probably caused by local peritoneal irritation resulting from a transmural coagulation. Although these patients require particularly close observation, the symptoms are temporary and usually resolve without the need for further intervention. However, when the clinical course warrants, a 24 to 48-hour period of fasting, and an abdominal X-ray to exclude perforation, is recommended.

Bleeding. Bleeding which requires active treatment can occur, following a polypectomy procedure, due to incomplete coagulation of blood vessels in the polyp stalk or base (Plate 44). Treatments may include endoscopic haemostasis, plasma expanders, blood transfusion or even surgical intervention, and the choice will depend upon the severity of the bleeding, and the endoscopic therapeutic facilities available in the department. The literature (Berci *et al.*, 1974; Frühmorgen and Demling, 1979; Geenan *et al.*, 1974; Rogers *et al.*, 1975; Roseman, 1973; Wolff and Shinya, 1973) reports an incidence of severe bleeding in about 2% of patients following colonoscopic polypectomy (Table 12.7). We have seen no clinically relevant bleeding since instituting the exclusive use of coagulation current for polypectomy.

Treatment of post-polypectomy bleeding. Although a rare occurrence pulsatile massive bleeding may arise from a resected polyp stalk and is not always due to poor electrocoagulation, but may be related to the size of the vessel encountered (Plate 44). A thick stalk supplying a large polyp is more prone to bleed. Bleeding may occur with the very first application of electrocautery current, and this is presumably secondary to blood vessels in the pedicle just under the mucosal surface. If this occurs, the wisest approach is to continue to sever the polyp grasped within the snare in the usual fashion. Following removal of the polyp, the endoscopist should resnare the entire area, including surrounding tissue, and hold it with 'strangulation' pressure for five minutes (Plate 45). After that time, the wire snare may be gently opened, and the stalk observed for further bleeding. If bleeding is seen, the snare should be retightened for an additional

Table 12.7 Complications of polypectomy (collective statistics)

Reference	Polypectomies	Haemorrhage	Perforations	Mortality
Berci et al. (1974)	901	6 (0.67%)	3 (0.22%)	0
Frühmorgen (survey) (1978)	7 365	165 (2.24%)	25 (0.34%)	8 (0.1%)
Geenen et al. (1974)	292	12 (4.10%)	2 (0.68%)	1 (0.34%)
Rogers et al. (survey) (1975)	6 214	115 (1.85%)	18 (0.28%)	0
Roseman (1973)	49	3 (6.12%)	0	0
Wolff and Shinya (1973)	499	1 (0.20%)	1 (0.20%)	0
Total	15 320	302 (1.97%)	49 (0.32%)	9 (0.06%)

five-minute interval. This may require several episodes of 'snare-strangulation'. When normal tissue is bunched up into the snare in this fashion, electrocautery should never be used as an aid to haemostasis, since perforation of the wall may result. Coagulation may be performed when the stalk of a small polyp has been grasped farther towards the wall than the polypectomy site. However, these may also be treated by strangulation for periods of five minutes without further electrocoagulation.

In the case of uncontrolled bleeding it has been suggested that selective arterial catheterization and pitressin infusion can be attempted (Cotton and Williams, 1980). This may achieve sufficient haemostasis to avoid surgical intervention; however, in our opinion it is time consuming and may not be readily available. Alternatively the same authors have suggested the infusion of large volumes of iced water containing epinephrine (5 ml 1:1000 per 50 ml water) through a polyethylene catheter to the bleeding site (Cotton and Williams, 1980).

Our own preference is to use the electro-hydro-thermal probe (Section 12.2.5(a)). The patient should then be kept on bed rest and closely monitored. Repeated tenesmus and the passage of fresh blood clot suggest continued bleeding.

Perforation. Perforation is an extremely serious incident. It may result from forceful passage of the instrument in the absence of a clear view of the lumen especially in a region of diseased bowel wall such as with carcinoma or diverticular disease; or it can be the result of uncontrolled straightening or rotating manoeuvres, prior to polypectomy. Perforation in the region of the polypectomy site may be caused mechanically by the tip of the colonoscope, forceps, snare or grasper or may result from tissue necrosis. Perforation can occur without accompanying acute abdominal pain and is sometimes recognized by the endoscopic appearance (perforated bowel wall, visible fatty tissue, omentum or abdominal organs) and also by the X-ray appearance of free air under the diaphragm. Persistent or subsequent abdominal pain, collapse and peritonitis all suggest a perforation, and a plain abdominal X-ray in the erect or lateral decubitus position should be taken. As a rule, treatment is immediate surgery (Zittel and Boden, 1968). A delay of 12 hours or more in a patient with peritonitis increases the risk of mortality to 75%. In the literature, the risk of perforation associated with polypectomy is about 0.3% (Table 12.7).

Gas explosion. With one exception, the few cases of gas explosion that have been described occurred during electrosurgical procedures carried out through the rigid proctosigmoidoscope. On the basis of experimental studies carried out in our department (Frühmorgen and Joachim, 1976), it seems probable that these were due to inadequate cleansing of the bowel. To date, only one case of a fatal gas explosion occurring during colonoscopic polypectomy has been described (Bigard *et al.*, 1979). This has subsequently been attributed to the use of mannitol for bowel preparation (Chapter 13). The subject of bowel preparation with mannitol is discussed in Chapter 3.

The mortality rate associated with colonoscopic polypectomy is 0.06% (Table 12.7) although the overall complication rate for bleeding and perforation is about 2.3%. These complication rates are well below that of the comparable surgical procedure. Two thirds of our polypectomy patients are aged over 50 and because of the possibility of complications we prefer to keep a patient who has undergone snare polypectomy in hospital and under observation for 24 hours. Ninety-five percent of all complications will become clinically manifest during this time (Frühmorgen and Demling, 1979). Standardized endoscopist training, close observance of recommended contraindications, the avoidance of potent analgesics and general anaesthesia, the use of fluoroscopic control in difficult colonoscopy, and the employment of the best endoscopes and auxiliary instruments available, all serve to keep complications to a minimum. Analysis of 4000 colonoscopies shows that 77% of all complications occur during the first 200 colonoscopies performed by an endoscopist, a further 10% during the next 300 examinations while with still more experience, the complication rate drops to 0.4% (Frühmorgen and Demling, 1979).

12.2.2 *Forceps polypectomy*

Small polyps may be either hyperplastic polyps or small adenomas and it is not possible to differentiate between them visually. Therefore small polyps encountered during colonoscopy should be sampled or removed.

(a) *Cold-biopsy forceps technique*

Now that polypectomy using the high-frequency diathermy snare is possible throughout the entire large bowel, the mechanical removal of polyps using biopsy forceps is seldom used except for very small polyps. Solitary or even multiple biopsy specimens from larger polyps do not provide representative tissue for histological assessment of the polyp as a whole and removal of the entire polypoid lesion is required for diagnosis.

Forceps polypectomy would appear to be justifiable only for the removal of those very small sessile polyps having a diameter of 1 mm to 1.5 mm. One reason for this is that these, often multiple, tiny polyps cannot always be removed, or are destroyed by the high-frequency current, so that no tissue is available for histology. This also applies to the primary coagulation of very small polyps which should, ideally, be removed with large cupped forceps. Several biopsies should be taken to obtain a histological diagnosis of neoplastic or non-neoplastic polyps. The hot-biopsy forceps provide an alternative technique.

(b) *Hot-biopsy forceps*

The hot-biopsy forceps technique (Williams, 1973) has not until now been used in our department but is widely favoured in the UK and USA. The technique involves the use of standard biopsy forceps in an insulated sheath. During biopsy, current is applied, which passes around the cups of the forceps and coagulates the base of the polyp while that part of the polyp grasped by the jaws of the forceps is preserved for histological appraisal. The technique is relatively simple and can be used to biopsy and fulgurate polyps up to 6 mm to 8 mm diameter. In order to prevent coagulation burn of the colonic wall, the polyp is grasped by the forceps and by manipulating the colonoscope or the forceps themselves it is 'tented' away to form a short 'pseudo-pedicle' (Plate 40). Coagulation is applied for two or three seconds, at the same setting as that which is used for routine polypectomy, and the forceps then withdrawn after the coagulation effect is seen. Should any significant portion of polypoid tissue remain, it can be retouched with the forceps still closed and fulgurated. This is usually unnecessary since the coagulation effect will cause any remaining tissue to slough off.

12.2.3 *Snare loop biopsy – tumour resection*

(a) *Snare loop biopsy*

It is possible to remove only superficial tissue with the conventional biopsy forceps and occasionally the use of snare loop biopsy may be useful for lesions in the large bowel. This technique can provide some 200 times more tissue than the biopsy forceps and is similar to polypectomy (Section 12.2.1). The opened snare loop is placed over the area of tissue to be removed and a pseudo-polyp formed by closing the snare. In order to avoid thermal damage to deeper layers of the wall, the base of the pseudo-polyp should be 'tented' into the lumen. Current is then passed and the snare loop closed, thus removing a large biopsy particle. In our own patients we have used this technique for purely diagnostic purposes: to confirm the diagnosis of atypical giant polypoid formations in two cases of Crohn's disease and in 12 patients presenting with partially necrotic tumours where forceps biopsy had already been negative. No complications were observed.

(b) *Tumour resection*

Endoscopic tumour resection using the high-frequency diathermy snare is very similar to snare polypectomy (see Section 12.2.1). Snare loop resection of malignant tumours causing stenosis of the lumen can only be considered as a palliative measure and this procedure would seem to be indicated only in high-risk patients who are unfit for surgery. To date, there has been very little experience of this procedure.

12.2.4 *Foreign body removal*

In contrast to the removal of foreign bodies from the upper gastrointestinal tract, this procedure is only rarely indicated in the colon or rectum, since ingested foreign bodies that have passed the pylorus are usually spontaneously passed through the anus. Foreign bodies that cannot be passed naturally on account of their shape or size, have usually been introduced peranally (Wolff and Geraci, 1977). Such objects include intestinal tubes, vibrators, and in one case, reported by Ottenjann (1978), a hand grenade which had been introduced into the rectum. In a total of 5741 colonoscopies performed in our unit since 1970, only three cases required colonoscopic removal of a foreign body. The objects included a dental prosthesis incarcerated in the sigmoid, an intestinal tube and a transintestinal tube containing mercury which, having been introduced as a guide prior to enteroscopy, had impacted at the splenic flexure. In all three cases it was possible to grasp the foreign body with crocodile forceps or the diathermy snare, and extract them without complication.

12.2.5 *Colonoscopic haemostasis*

Since it first became possible to localize and identify bleeding sites in the gastrointestinal tract, endoscopists have tried to carry out treatment during the emergency endoscopic examination. Since 85% of all acute gastrointestinal bleeding is located in the oesophagus, stomach or duodenum, colonoscopic haemostasis is of only secondary importance. Bleeding in the large bowel is only rarely an indication for

Table 12.8 Results of various working groups with conventional electro-coagulation

Authors	Coagulations (n)	Effective haemostasis	Residual bleeding	Further surgical treatment	
				emergency	elective
Papp (1979)	58	55	6	7	7
Gaisford (1979)	77	71	6	8	?
Sugawa et al. (1975)	6	6	2	2	–
Volpicelli et al. (1978)	12	12	1	–	1
Wara et al. (1980)	50	50	5	5	4

electro- or photocoagulation since bleeding polyps are removed *in toto* with the high-frequency diathermy snare. Haemorrhage from diverticula is rare and usually inaccessible, and diffuse mucosal bleeding, as may be seen in ulcerative colitis, does not constitute an indication for endoscopic haemostasis. The, as yet, small experience with endoscopic haemostasis in the colon involves bleeding after polypectomy, haemorrhage from solitary ulcers, circumscribed bleeding from radiation injury, solitary angioma and acute haemorrhage from angiodysplasia. In this last condition the bleeding lesion may represent merely the 'tip of the iceberg' for the vascular anomalies often extend sub-mucosally. Although local diathermy coagulation for angiodysplasia has been reported (Rogers and Adler, 1976; Hunt, 1980) surgical resection after prior angiography may be necessary for multiple or extensive lesions. In contrast to emergency endoscopy in the upper gastrointestinal tract, massive bleeding from the large bowel causes considerable diagnostic problems, since adequate cleansing of the bowel is difficult and the presence of blood may render vision impossible (see Chapter 15). Despite this, endoscopic haemostasis in the lower GI tract should be discussed since appropriate techniques are available although these have been applied predominantly in upper GI bleeding (Blackwood and Silvis, 1971; Brunetaud *et al.*, 1977 and 1979; Dwyer *et al.*, 1975; Frühmorgen *et al.*, 1976a and 1980; Kiefhaber *et al.*, 1977, 1978 and 1979; Papp, 1979; Sugawa *et al.*, 1975; Volpicelli *et al.*, 1978) (see Table 12.8).

(a) *Electrocoagulation of bleeding*
Flexible button electrodes which can be passed down the instrument channel of any conventional endoscope are available, some with a central hole for use as irrigation or suction electrodes. The high-

frequency diathermy units used for endoscopic polypectomy (see Section 12.2.1(a)) are employed as power sources. For haemostatic procedures the spark gap current is always used for its coagulating properties. There are some disadvantages of conventional electrocoagulation: animal experiments have shown that direct coagulation with a diathermy electrode in the thin-walled sections of the GI tract, in particular the oesophagus and the small and large bowel, carry a considerable risk of perforation (Pesch *et al.*, 1973; Papp *et al.*, 1979). Visualization of the source of bleeding during coagulation is often very difficult. Furthermore, during direct touch coagulation, the electrode adheres to the coagulum which may be 'avulsed' when the electrode is withdrawn causing renewed bleeding. Finally, the electrode itself becomes so contaminated with charred material that it provides an 'unpredictable' depth of coagulation or may even cease to function. In four attempts with this technique to achieve endoscopic haemostasis in the stomach, we were successful in only two cases of polypectomy bleeding and in two further cases we experienced a perforation.

A number of electrodes (Papp *et al.*, 1975) are provided with a central suction channel to improve visualization of the source of bleeding but our own experience suggests that adequate vision is not always achieved. Papp *et al.* (1975) reported more than 58 patients in whom bleeding in the upper gastrointestinal tract has been arrested with this form of electrocoagulation; the only complication reported was re-bleeding in 6 patients. Gaisford (1979) has similarly reported 77 patients with upper gastrointestinal haemorrhage, in 71 of whom (92%) he was able to achieve lasting haemostasis and only six patients suffered re-bleeding. Our own experience highlights the disadvantages of conventional, dry-touch electrocoagulation already described. The ideal technique should combine the advantages of conventional electrocoagulation (low cost, portability) with those of laser coagulation (contact-free coagulation, controlled depth of penetration) while eliminating their respective disadvantages. The most successful technique we have evaluated involves the simultaneous instillation of water through the tip of the electrode prior to and during the coagulation process (Matek *et al.*, 1979). This electro-hydro-thermal probe (EHT) (Fig. 12.4) proved to be both efficient and practical with the following advantages:

1. Water instilled down the electrode before and during coagulation: (a) washes away any blood, permitting optimal visualization of the bleeding site, and (b) prevents the electrode tip from sticking to the coagulum.

Table 12.9 Results of the first EHT coagulations in humans

Coagulations (EHT probe)	Effective haemostasis	Residual bleeding	Further treatment surgical
21	18	3	4 emergencies 1 elective

2. Contamination of the tip of the electrode by charred material is prevented and application of energy to the bleeding site is predictable.
3. Arrest of bleeding is achieved by pure coagulation without charring.
4. The temperature in the region of the electrode is limited to about 100°C.
5. The therapeutic range is wide; within the therapeutic range, neither primary nor secondary perforation is likely.
6. The coagulation system is portable and also economical.

After experimental evidence had demonstrated the efficacy of this method of electrocoagulation, we attempted our first coagulations of bleeding lesions in patients. Twenty coagulations for bleeding lesions were in the upper and a single coagulation in the lower GI tract (Table 12.9). A further case, involved a sigmoid haemangioma which at the time of the examination was not bleeding.

Our experience suggests that it may become a genuine alternative to the costly and non-portable method of laser coagulation. The indications for electrocoagulation in the large bowel using the modified technique described, are identical with those for laser coagulation (see Section 12.2.5(b)). Its use appears justifiable in those cases in which the poor general state of the patient and continued bleeding make surgery impossible, and when no facilities for laser coagulation are available. When employing electrocoagulation in the colon, with which we are specifically concerned here, extreme care must be exercised because of the risk of perforating the relatively thin colonic wall (Papp *et al.*, 1979).

(b) *Photocoagulation of bleeding*
Experience with endoscopic photocoagulation using a laser beam has been restricted to only a few working groups, and has primarily involved its application in the upper gastrointestinal tract. The rare indications for the use of the laser in the colon as with electrocoagulation are due largely to the relative rarity of acute bleeding

in the large bowel, and the technical problems of emergency colonos-copy in the presence of massive haemorrhage. Laser coagulation has, however, been employed in the lower GI tract, and since there are no technical reasons that militate against its use in the colon or rectum, a number of fundamental aspects must be considered. With respect to its clinical applicability, we shall have to consider clinical experience gained in the management of upper gastrointestinal bleeding.

Physical aspects. When biological tissue is irradiated by an intense beam of light, the (light) energy absorbed is converted into heat, which produces an increase in the temperature of the tissue. For endoscopic application of this principle, the following problems need to be taken into account:

1. The intense beam of light must be passed via a flexible light-guide through an instrument channel having a diameter of only a few millimetres.
2. The angle of emergence of the light beam at the distal end of the lightguide must be so small that the spot of light projected onto the gastrointestinal wall at a practical working distance still possesses adequate radiation density to produce a photo-coagulative effect capable of arresting bleeding.

The development of the laser oscillators since 1960 has largely met these criteria (Nath *et al.*, 1973; Reidenbach *et al.*, 1975, 1977, 1978) but only the neodymium (Nd)-YAG and the argon ion laser have been evaluated for gastrointestinal bleeding. The functional difference bet-ween these two types of beam is based on their differing degree of effect on tissue. Blood, or highly vascular tissue absorbs the beam of the argon laser much more strongly than the Nd-YAG laser (Reiden-bach *et al.*, 1975). The resulting different coagulative effect of these two laser beams is shown in the results obtained from animal experiments.

Animal experiments. In animal experiments both lasers can achieve effective haemostasis (Auth *et al.*, 1976; Brunetaud *et al.*, 1977; Frühmorgen *et al.*, 1974, 1975, 1977; Nath *et al.*, 1973; Protell *et al.*, 1978; Silverstein *et al.*, 1976; Waitmann *et al.*, 1975) but acute per-forations were produced by the Nd-YAG (50 W) laser in the therapeutic range. The depth of penetration into blood or highly vas-cular tissue is some four times as great (approximately 0.8 mm) in the case of the Nd-YAG laser, as in the case of the argon ion laser (approximately 0.2 mm). In contrast to the argon laser, it is virtually impossible to limit the photocoagulative effect of the Nd-YAG laser to the submucosa – the most important site of gastrointestinal bleeding – at the power required to achieve haemostasis.

The comparative efficacy of the two laser systems and a greater perforation risk of the Nd-YAG laser have recently been confirmed by Protell and his co-workers (Protell *et al.*, 1978).

We consider that haemostatic effectiveness has been proved for both laser systems; however, it must be emphasized that because of the absorption effect of blood on the argon laser, an absolute pre-requisite is the simultaneous use of a jet of inert gas (e.g. CO_2) to remove blood from the bleeding site, which also helps to improve vision. If the bleeding site remains covered by a pool of blood, this will absorb most of the light energy of either laser system, but particularly that of the argon laser.

Clinical experience and results. The results of investigations in animals indicated that laser coagulation in patients, if carried out by endoscopists with experimental experience, would be justified. We carried out the first successful argon ion laser coagulation in the human gastrointestinal tract in June 1975 (Frühmorgen *et al.*, 1976). This was followed at the end of 1975 by a report from Kiefhaber and his co-workers on the first successful attempts to arrest bleeding in patients using a Nd-YAG laser. Recently, further clinical results have been described (Brunetaud *et al.*, 1977; Ihre and Seligson, 1978; Laurence *et al.*, 1980; Pantsyrev *et al.*, 1978).

Laser coagulation of bleeding lesions may be performed during emergency endoscopy which is, initially, a diagnostic procedure. The contraindications (shock, massive ongoing haemorrhage, non-co-operative patient) are the same as those applicable to emergency endoscopy. A potential source of bleeding such as a haemangioma may be coagulated prior to a first haemorrhage or during the interval between bleeding. Attention has already been drawn to the problems of emergency endoscopy and to the relatively low incidence of acute bleeding in the large bowel. We have coagulated a total of 294 bleeding or potentially bleeding lesions in the gastrointestinal tract, of which 31 were located in the colon or rectum. With the exception of severe arterial bleeding from an inoperable carcinoma of the stomach, a bleeding duodenal ulcer and a gastric ulcer all attempted coagulations were successful. In three patients, recurrent bleeding occurred which proved amenable to repeated coagulation. No perforation or worsening of the haemorrhage was observed.

The results of others have been similar and a review of the literature shows 296 attempted coagulations in 238 patients with the argon ion laser with a success of 84% and that 1776 attempted coagulations have been made in 1533 patients with a neodymium-YAG laser, achieving a success rate of 87% (Table 12.10). Since the majority of cases involve the upper GI tract, no further discussion of the results is given here.

Indications. The indications for laser coagulation in the colon or rectum on the basis of the present limited experience include circumscribed bleeding or potentially bleeding vascular abnormalities (haemangioma, angiodysplasia, Osler–Rendu–Weber disease), bleeding solitary ucler, haemorrhage following therapeutic procedures such as polypectomy and bleeding from inoperable tumour. Diffuse bleeding such as may occasionally be seen in ulcerative colitis is not an indication for photocoagulation.

(c) *Evaluation and limitations*
Any endoscopic technique for arresting bleeding or for the coagulation of potential sources of bleeding in the gastrointestinal tract, must be both effective and free from risk.

   Irrespective of the source of energy employed, deep coagulation in the colon carries the danger of primary or secondary perforation while superficial coagulation can result either in unsuccessful haemostasis, or in re-bleeding. During coagulation, therefore, the endoscopist must judge between, on the one hand, ineffectual coagulation, and on the other, transmural coagulation with subsequent perforation.

   Both laser systems have proved effective in clinical application. In contrast to the Nd-YAG laser, the argon laser is selectively absorbed by blood, and provides self-limitation of the depth of penetration through the tissue to be coagulated – features that make coagulation with the argon laser safer for the patient. Nevertheless, although the efficacy of laser coagulation is now empirically proven, it has not yet been confirmed statistically.

   On the basis of our own comparative investigations of the two laser systems (argon, Nd-YAG) in animal experiments, and the experience of other workers (Protell *et al.*, 1978), and taking into account effectiveness, practicability and risk, we have not been able to decide in favour of the Nd-YAG laser coagulator for clinical application. It remains to be seen whether, through the application of a more powerful laser, coupled with correspondingly shorter exposures, these reservations might be dispelled.

   A comparison of the clinical results obtained at various centres using both laser systems is not really possible, since the patient groups are not comparable. When considering the largely favourable

Table 12.10 Results of laser-coagulation inquiry (Kiefhaber et al., 1979)

Argon laser

Author (country)	Actively bleeding lesions	Patients	Successful %
Brunetaud (F)	87	80	87
Waitmann (USA)	50	20	94
Frühmorgen (D)	43	41	83
Salmon/Bown (GB)	42	42	84
Dwyer (USA)	34	21	70
LeBodic (F)	18	14	82
Laurence (E)	12	10	70
Manegold (D)	10	10	100
	296	238	84

Nd–YAG laser

Author (country)	Actively bleeding lesions	Patients	Successful %
Kiefhaber (D)	587	459	94
Schönekäs (D)	334	298	93
Dwyer (USA)	106	71	87
Pösl/Sander (D)	83	61	97
Rhode (D)	83	61	92
Ramirez (Mex)		80	
Weinzierl (D)	77	70	74
Ghezzi (I)	75	65	87

Nd–YAG laser

Author (country)	Actively bleeding lesions	Patients	Successful %
Vantrappen (B)	53	50	96
Wotzka/Kaes (D)	48	35	81
Ultsch/Bader (D)	37	27	88
Stauber (A)	30	28	80
Fiedler (D)	30	25	80
Kreutzer (A)	29	25	90
Richter (D)	25	20	92
Excourrou (F)	22	20	75
Immig (D)	22	14	82
Knop (D)	22	20	82
Marcon (C)	20	18	75
Ihre (S)	15	15	93
Dixon (USA)	15	12	100
Troidl (D)	12	10	85
Viets (D)	11	11	100
Beckly (GB)	11	9	82
Classen (D)	10	10	100
Zimmermann (D)	5	5	100
Soehendra (D)	3	3	100
Stadelmann (D)	3	3	100
Tytgat (NL)	3	3	75
Deyhle (CH)	3	3	100
Möckel (D)	2	3	100
	1776	1533	87

Organization and Techniques

clinical results so far obtained it must be remembered that they have been gained by groups with considerable technical and experimental experience. Before the widespread use of laser coagulation in the gastrointestinal tract can be advocated, further evaluation of this technique is required.

Laser coagulation, with its acceptable risk of complications, is superior to the alternative, conventional high-frequency coagulation, and to other endoscopic methods involving the use of drugs or mechanical techniques. However, the laser coagulators available at present, are relatively immobile (water connections, three-phase electricity supply, large dimensions, etc.), and cannot be easily transported to the patient in an emergency. The high purchase price, requirement for skilled technical and nursing staff, and need for a large number of patients to justify the cost makes the laser coagulator uneconomical for smaller hospitals with a low incidence of gastrointestinal bleeding.

With the completion of developmental work on the electro-hydrothermal electrode which combines the advantages of the laser (noncontact intermittent coagulation and selectivity) with those of conventional electrocoagulation (low cost, ease of use, mobile, source of energy) but eliminating the disadvantages, we already have an available alternative to photocoagulation with the laser (Reidenbach *et al.*, 1978) (see Section 12.2.5). Since introducing the EHT for clinical application, we now rarely use the laser system.

12.3 Conclusions

Therapeutic colonoscopy has dramatically changed our approach to colonic disease, especially for the diagnosis and treatment of colon polyps where colonoscopic polypectomy has now obviated laparotomy and colotomy. Early experience of haemostasis and the coagulation of vascular lesions has proved promising but the full potential of therapeutic colonoscopy has probably still to be reached. Good training, skillful technique and experience combined with fine clinical judgement will permit the endoscopist to become proficient at these procedures.

References

Auth, D. C., Lam, V. T. Y., Mohr, R. W., Silverstein, F. E. and Rubin, C. E. (1976), A high-power gastric photocoagulator for fiberoptic endoscopy. *IEEE Trans. Biomed. Eng.*, **23**, 129.

Berci, G., Panish, J. F., Schapiro, M. and Corlin, R. (1974), Complications of colonoscopy and polypectomy. *Gastroenterology,* **67**, 584–85.

Bigard, M. A., Gaucher, P. and Lassalle, C. (1979), Fatal colonic explosion during colonoscopic polypectomy. *Gastroenterology,* **77**, 1307–10.

Blackwood, W. D. and Silvis, S. E. (1971), Gastroscopic electrosurgery. *Gastroenterology,* **61**, 305–14.

Bodem, F., Reidenbach, H. D., Nehls, M., Brand, H. and Frühmorgen, P. 1975), Untersuchungen über die Eignung der 2.45 GHz-Mikrowellenerwärmung für eine endoskopische Koagulationstherapie. *Biomed. Technik,* **20**, 238.

Bodem, F., Reidenbach, H. D., Frühmorgen, P. Matek, W. and Kaduk, B. (1980), Investigations on the hemostatic efficacy of the thermocoagulation of gastrointestinal hemorrhages by convective heat transfer via a miniature endoscopic hot gas probe. *Biomed. Technik,* **25**, 179.

Bond, J. F. and Levitt, M. D. (1979), Colonic gas explosion – is a fire extinguisher necessary? *Gastroenterology,* **77**, 1349–50.

Brunetaud, J. M., Roger, J. and Houcke, P. (1979), Laser coagulation: significance for the patient's fate. In: *Operative Endoscopy* (Demling, L. and Rösch, eds), Acron, Berlin.

Brunetaud, J. M., Maffioli, C. and Miro, L. (1977), The laser in digestive endoscopy. *Acta Endoscop. Radiocinemetogr. Tome,* **7**, 69–78.

Carter, H. G. (1952), Explosion in the colon during electrodesication of polyps. *Amer. J. Surg.,* **84**, 514–19.

Cotton, P. B. and Williams, C. B. (1980), *Practical Gastrointestinal Endoscopy,* Blackwell Scientific Publications, Oxford.

Deyhle, P., Seuberth, K., Jenny, S. and Demling, L. (1971), Endoscopic polypectomy in the proximal colon. *Endoscopy,* **2**, 103–05.

Dwyer, R. M., Yellin, A. E., Cherlow, J., Bass, M. and Haverback, B. J. (1975), Laser induced hemostasis in the upper gastrointestinal tract using a flexible fiberoptic. *Gastroenterology,* **68**, 888.

Engel, R. R. and Levitt, M. D. (1970), Intestinal tract gas formation in newborns. *Programs Amer. Ped. Soc. and Soc. for Ped. Res.,* 266.

Frühmorgen, P., Reidenbach, H. D., Bodem, F., Kaduk, B. and Demling, L. (1974), Experimental examinations on laser endoscopy. *Endoscopy,* **6**, 116–22.

Frühmorgen, P., Bodem, F., Reidenbach, H. D., Kaduk, B. and Demling, L. (1975a), The first endoscopic laser coagulation in the human GI-tract. *Endoscopy,* **7**, 156–57.

Frühmorgen, P., Kaduk, B., Reidenbach, H. D., Bodem, F., Demling, L. and Brand, H. (1975b), Long-term observations in endoscopic laser coagulations in the gastrointestinal tract. *Endoscopy,* **7**, 189–96.

Frühmorgen, P., Bodem, F., Reidenbach, H. D., Kaduk, B. and Demling, L. (1976a), Endoscopic laser coagulation of bleeding gastrointestinal lesions. *Gastrointestinal Endoscopy,* **23**, 73–75.

Frühmorgen, P., Bodem, F., Reidenbach, H. D., Kaduk, B. and Demling, L. (1976b), Endoscopic laser coagulation of bleeding gastrointestinal lesions with report of the first therapeutic application in man. *Gastrointest. Endoscopy,* **23**, 73–75.

Frühmorgen, P. and Joachim, G. (1976c), Gas chromatographic analyses of intestinal gas to clarify the question of inert gas insufflation in electrosurgical endoscopy. *Endoscopy,* **8**, 133–36.

Frühmorgen, P., Zeus, J., Phillips, J. and Demling, L. (1977), 5jährige Verlaufsbeobachtungen nach koloskopischer Polypektomie. In: *Fortschritte in der Endoskopie* (Rösch, W. Ed.), Perimed-Verlag, Erlangen, 249.

Frühmorgen, P., Kaduk, B., Reidenbach, H. D., Bodem, F. and Demling, L. (1977), Vergleichende Untersuchungen zur fiberendoskopischen Lichtkoagulation mit einem Argon-Ionen- und einem Neodym-YAG-Laser. In: *Fortschritte der Gastroenterologischen Endoskopoe.* Witzrock-Verlag, Baden-Baden, pp. 219–225 and 233–235.

Frühmorgen, P. and Demling, L. (1979), Complications of Diagnostic and therapeutic colonoscopy in the Federal Republic of Germany (results of an inquiry). *Endoscopy,* **11,** 146–50.

Frühmorgen, P., Bodem, F. and Reidenbach, H. D. (1980), The state of the art of biomedical engineering in the operative-endoscopic treatment of gastrointestinal bleedings. *Hepato-Gastroenterology,* in press.

Frühmorgen, P. and Classen, M. (1980), *Endoscopy and Biopsy in Gastroenterology,* Springer, New York.

Gaisford, W. D. (1979), Endoscopic electrohemostatis of active upper gastrointestinal bleeding. *Amer. J. Surg.,* **137**, 47–53.

Galley, A. H. (1954), Combustible gases generated in alimentary tract and other hollow viscera and their relationship to explosions occurring during anaesthesia. *Brit. J. Anaesth.,* **26**, 189.

Geenen, J. E., Schmitt, M. G. and Hogan, W. J. (1974), Complications of colonoscopy (abstract). *Gastroenterology,* **66**, 812.

Gillespie, P. E., Nicholls, R. J., Thompson, J. P. S. and Williams, C. B. (1978), Snare polypectomy by sigmoid-rectal intussusception. *Brit. Medical J.,* **1**, 1395.

Hermanek, P. and Frühmorgen, P. (1980), *Kolorektale Polypen-Diagnose, Klassifikation, Beziehung zum Karzinom. Zbl. Chir.,* in press.

Hunt, R. H. (1980), Colonoscopy in the diagnosis and management of angiodysplasia. *Abstracts of the IV European Congress of Gastrointestinal Endoscopy,* 97.

Ihre, T. and Seligson, U. (1978), Endoscopic treatment in massive upper gastrointestinal (GI) bleeding. Paper IV. *World Congress of Digestive Endoscopy,* Madrid.

Koch, H., Pesch, H. J., Bauerle, H., Frühmorgen, P., Rösch, W. and Classen, M. (1973), Erste experimentelle Untersuchungen und klinische Erfahrungen zur Elektrokoagulation blutender Läsionen im oberen Gastrointestinaltrakt. In: *Fortschritte der Endoskopie* (Ottenjann, R. ed.), Schattauer-Verlag, Stuttgart, p. 69.

Kiefhaber, P., Nath, G. and Moritz, K. (1977), Endoscopical control of massive gastrointestinal haemorrhage by irradiation with a high power neodymium-YAG laser. *Progress in Surgery,* **15**, 140–55.

Kiefhaber, P., Moritz, K., Schildberg, F. W., Feifel, G. and Herfarth, C. H. (1978), Endosopic Nd-YAG laser irradiation for control of bleeding acute and chronic ulcers. *Langenbecks Arch. Chir.,* **347**, 567–71.

Kiefhaber, P., Moritz, K., Heldwein, W., Lehnert, P. and Weidinger, P. (1979), Endoscopische Blutstillung blutender Ösophagus- und Magenvarizen mit einem Hochleistungs-Neodym-YAG-Laser. In: *Operative Endoskopie* (Demling, L. and Rösch, W. eds), Acron, Berlin.

Kiefhaber, P. (1978), La photocoagulation dans les hémorrhagies digestives. Paper IIc *Symposium International d'Endoscopic Digestive*, Paris.

Laurence, B. H., Vallon, A. G. Cotton, P. B. Armengol Miro, J. R., Salord Oses, J. C., LeBodic, L., Frühmorgen, P. and Bodem, F. (1980), Endoscopic laser photocoagulation for bleeding peptic ulcers. *Lancet*, i, 124–25.

Leheta, F. and Gorsich, W. (1975), Koagulation and Resektion von Blutgefäßen mit dem Argon-Laser. *Fortschr. Med.*, **93**, 653.

Levitt, M. D., French, P. and Donaldson, R. M. (1968), Use of hydrogen and methane excretion in the study of the intestinal flora. *J. Lab. Clin. Med.*, **72**, 988.

Levy, E. I. (1954), Explosions during lower bowel electrosurgery. *Amer. J. Surg.*, **88**, 754–58.

Matek, W., Frühmorgen, P., Kaduk, B., Reidenbach, H. D., Bodem, F. and Demling, L. (1979), Modified electrocoagulation and its possibilities in the control of gastrointestinal bleeding. *Endoscopy*, **11**, 253–58.

Mauser, R. (1971), Störeinflüsse aug Herzschrittmacher durch Elektrochirurgiegeräte. *Elektronik*, **20**, 199.

Moutier, M. F. (1946), Un nouveau cas d'explosion intrarectale au cours d'une electrocoagulation. *Arch. Mal. Appar. dig.*, **35**, 240.

Nath, G., Gorisch, W. and Kiefhaber, P. (1973), First laser endoscopy via a fiberoptic transmission system. *Endoscopy*, **5**, 208–11.

Neiger, A., Moritz, K. and Kiefhaber, P. (1977), Hämorrhoidvenverödungsbehandlung durch Infrarotkoagulation. In: *Fortschritte der Gastroenterologischen Endoskopie* (Henning, H. ed.), Witzstrock, Baden-Baden.

Newman, A. (1974), Breath-analysis tests in gastroenterology. *Gut*, **15**, 308.

Ottenjan, R. (1978), personal communication.

Pantsyrev, Y. and M., Gallinger, Y. and I., Klyaving, Y. and A., Polyvoda, M. D., Krohhin, O. N. Zubarev, I. G., Bocharov, V. V., Mulikov, V. F. and Mikahilov, S. I. (1978), Laser endoscopic coagulation in gastrointestinal hemorrhages. *Laser and Elektro-Optik*, **1**, 32.

Papp, J. P. (1979), State of art. *Amer. J. Gastroenterology*, **71**, 516–21.

Papp, J. P., Fox, J. M. and Wilks, H. S. (1975), Experimental electrocoagulation of dog gastric mucosa. *Gastrointestinal Endoscopy*, **22**, 27.

Papp, J. P., Nalbandian, R. M., Wilcox, R. M. and Ludwig, E. E. (1979), Experimental evaluation of electrocoagulation and fulguration of dog colon mucosa. *Gastrointestinal Endoscopy*, **25**, 140–41.

Pesch, H. J., Koch, H. and Classen, M. (1973), Experimentelle und histologische Untersuchungen zur Elektrokoagulation blutender Läsionen im oberen Gastrointestinaltrakt. *Leber Magen Darm*, **3**, 172–76.

Protell, R. L., Silverstein, F. E., Auth, D. C., Dennis, M. B., Gilbert, D. A. and Rubin, C. E. (1978), The Nd:YAG-Laser is dangerous for photocoagulation of experimental bleeding gastric ulcers when compared with the argon-laser. *Gastroenterology,* **74**, 1080.

Reidenbach, H. D., Bodem, F. Frühmorgen, P., Brand, H. and Demling, L. (1976), The plastic lightguide in endoscopic laser photocoagulation. *Endoscopy*, **8**, 46.

Reidenbach, H. D., Bodem, F. and Frühmorgen, P. (1977), Flexible Lichtleiter für die Laser-Endoskopie- eine vergleichende Zusammenstellung des Standes der Technik. *Laser and Elektro-Optik,* **1**, 11.

Reidenbach, H. D., Bodem, F., Frühmorgen, P., Schroeder, G., Lex, P. and Kaduk, B. (1978), Eine neue Methode zur endoskopischen Hochfrequenzkoagulation von Schleimhautdefekten. *Biomed. Tech. (Berlin),* **4**, 71.

Rogers, B. H. G., Silvis, E., Nebel, O. T., Sugawa, Ch. and Mandelstam, P. (1975), Complications of flexible fiberoptic colonoscopy and polypectomy. *Gastrointestinal Endoscopy,* **23**, 73–75.

Rogers, B. H. G. and Adler, F. (1976), Haemangiomas of the caecum: Colonoscopic diagnosis and therapy. *Gastroenterology,* **71**, 1079–1082.

Roseman, D. M. (1973), Report from San Diego. *Gastrointestinal Endoscopy,* **20**, 36.

Semm, K. (1974), Transabdominale oder transvaginale Eileitersterilisation mit einer neuen Koagulationszange. *Endoscopy,* **6**, 40.

Semm, K. (1975), Elektronisch gesteuerter Schwachstrom als Ersatz des Hochfrequenzstromes in der Endoskopie. In: *Fortschritte der Endoskopie* (Ottenjann, R., ed.), Schattauer, Stuttgart.

Shinya, H. and Wolff, W. I. (1980), Morphology, anatomic distribution and cancer potential of colonic polyps: an analysis of 7000 polyps endoscopically removed. *Amer. J. Surg.,* in press.

Silverstein, F. E., Auth, D. C., Rubin, C. E. and Protell, R. L. (1976), High power argon laser treatment via standard endoscopes. I. A preliminary study of efficacy in control of experimental erosive bleeding. *Gastroenterology,* **71**, 558–61.

Strauss, R. J., Gordon, L. and Wise, L. (1978), Colonoscopic prolapse and sigmoidoscopic removal of pedunculated polyps in the sigmoid colon. *Surgery Gynaecology and Obstetrics,* **48**, 439–440.

Sugawa, Ch., Shier, M., Lucas, C. E. and Walt, A. J. (1975), Electrocoagulation of bleeding in the upper part of the gastrointestinal tract. *Arch. Surg.,* **110**, 975–79.

Volpicelli, N. A., McCarthy, J. D., Barlett, J. D. and Badger, W. F. (1978), Endoscopic electrocoagulation. *Arch. Surg.,* **113**, 483.

Waitman, A. M., Spira, I., Chryssanthou, C. P. and Strenger, R. J. (1975), Fiber-optic-coupled argon laser in the control of experimentally produced gastric bleeding. *Gastrointestinal Endoscopy,* **22**, 78–81.

Wara, P., Højsgaard, A. and Amdrup, E. (1980), Endoscopic electrocoagulation – an alternative to operative haemostasis in active gastroduodenal bleeding? *Endoscopy,* **5**, 237–41.

Waye, J. D. (1980), *Colonoscopy: Techniques, Landmarks and Polypectomy.* MEDC, Inc., Westwood, NJ, USA.

Williams, C. B. (1973), Diathermy-biopsy – a technique for the endoscopic management of small polyps. *Endoscopy,* **5**, 215.

Williams, C. B., Hunt, R. H., Loose, H., Riddell, R. H., Sakai, Y. and Swarbrick, E. T. (1974) Colonoscopy in the management of colon polyps. *Brit. J. Surg.,* 673–82.

Williams, C. B., Bartram, C. I., Bat, L. and Milito, G. (1979), Bowel preparation with mannitol is hazardous. *Gut,* **20**, A933.

Wolf, L. and Geraci, K. (1977), Colonoscopic removal of balloons from the bowel. *Gastrointestinal Endoscopy,* **24**, 41.

Wolff, W. I. and Shinya, H. (1973), A new approach to colonic polyps. *Ann. Surg.,* **178**, 367–78.

Zittel, R. X. and Boden, T. (1968), Jatragene Perforationen von Hohlorganen bei Endoskopie, Sondierung und Bougierung. *Münch med. Wschr.,* **40**, 2265.

CHAPTER THIRTEEN

Complications and Hazards of Colonoscopy

B. H. GERALD ROGERS

The insertion of a 1.8 m colonoscope into a patient followed by its withdrawal together with a colonic polyp is an astounding sight to behold. It looks easy when performed by a skilled colonoscopist in a co-operative patient, but it is probably one of the most difficult and demanding gastrointestinal procedures to perform. Colonoscopy requires a combination of clinical judgement, manipulative skills, anatomical knowledge, patience and sophisticated equipment. Complications are inevitable in this complex situation because the slightest misjudgement, momentary loss of control, malfunction of equipment, anatomical variation or pathological alteration can lead to untoward results. The information and discussions which follow should make the reader aware of potential complications and motivate him to take the necessary precautions to avoid them whenever possible.

13.1 Preparation

The hazards of preparation for colonoscopy include electrolyte imbalance, hypovolemia and dehydration due to catharsis and myocardial infarction during preparation has been reported (Rogers *et al.*, 1975). Good oral hydration should minimize dehydration but electrolyte imbalance should be suspected in those with diarrhoea and corrected prior to colonoscopy. Diuretics should be stopped several days before starting the preparation. It is important to remember that cathartics are contraindicated in those who are suspected of intestinal obstruction and enemas should be used instead.

13.2 Premedication

13.2.1 *Diazepam (Valium)*

Respiratory depression is a common complication of intravenous diazepam which results from giving it too rapidly and can lead to respiratory arrest (Hall and Ovassapian, 1977). Individual sensitivity

237

to intravenous diazepam varies widely and seems to increase with age. Apnea has been reported with as low a dose as 2.5 mg (Del Vecchio, 1978). Rather than giving the drug as a bolus it should be administered slowly while titrating to the desired effect. Equipment for endotracheal intubation and artificial respiration should be available wherever diazepam is being used. One case of diazepam-induced respiratory arrest in an elderly cachetic patient was successfully reversed but later the patient developed severe pneumonia and died (Smith, 1976). Intravenous diazepam should probably be avoided completely in the extremely elderly, cachetic or debilitated patient and in those who already have some degree of central nervous system depression. Thrombophlebitis at the site of injection is a known complication of intravenous diazepam and the reported incidence ranges from 3.5 to 10% (Langdon, 1973; Langdon *et al.*, 1973; Rogers *et al.*, 1975). Usually the phlebitis resolves without further problems but pulmonary embolus after diazepam sedation for endoscopy has been reported (Hoare, 1974). Injecting diazepam into a small vein increases the risk of thrombophlebitis and flushing with 150 ml of saline has been shown to decrease it (Langdon, 1973). It has been possible, in my experience, to avoid diazepam phlebitis completely by injecting the medication slowly in the side arm of a rapidly flowing i.v., thereby delivering a dilute solution. This technique results in visible microprecipitate in the i.v. tubing but does not seem to affect the action of the drug. The injection should be made at the very end of the i.v. tubing where the needle enters the vein because it is known that diazepam is absorbed by plastic tubing (Mac Kichan, Duffner and Cohen, 1979).

13.2.2 *Analgesics*

Adverse reactions to narcotic analgesics such as meperidine/pethidine are not uncommon and include respiratory depression, hypotension, bradycardia, nausea, vomiting and sweating. The nausea, vomiting and sweating will pass without being treated but hypotension and bradycardia are usually treated by placing the patient in the Trendelenberg position and giving i.v. physiological saline. Respiratory depression can be counteracted with naloxone (Narcan). Usually hypotension occurs early in the course of colonoscopy and it is difficult to determine whether it is primarily caused by analgesics, diazepam or the vasovagal reflex. Regardless of the cause, treatment of hypotension is the same and colonoscopy can almost always be completed after a few minutes when blood pressure and pulse have returned to normal.

13.2.3 *Prophylaxis against bacterial endocarditis*

Colonoscopy often results in vigorous and extensive manipulation of the large bowel but the bacteraemia which results is insignificant and most authors who have investigated the problem have not recommended special precautions (Rafoth, Sorenson and Bond, 1975; Norfleet *et al.*, 1976a,b; Dickman *et al.*, 1976; Coughlin, Butler, Alp and Grant, 1977; Hartong, Barnes and Calkins, 1977; Meyer, 1979). These observations may be explained by removal of bacteria by the portal system and no published report of bacterial endocarditis following colonoscopy has appeared. Colonoscopy is not mentioned directly in the publication of the American Heart Association (AHA) concerning prevention of bacterial endocarditis in patients with cardiac disease (Kaplan *et al.*, 1977), but prophylaxis is recommended by the AHA for patients with a prosthetic valve who are undergoing proctosigmoidoscopy and similar recommendations would seem appropriate for colonoscopy. The colonoscopist should bear in mind the risk of bacteraemia and consider the possible need for prophylaxis not only in patients with prosthetic valves but in those who have depressed immune defences and where there is shunting of portal blood as in alcoholic cirrhosis (Dickman *et al.*, 1976).

13.3 Spread of infectious diseases

13.3.1 *Bacterial diseases*

Flexible fibreoptic endoscopic equipment has been implicated in an outbreak of *Salmonella typhimurium* gastroenteritis which occurred in several patients after oesophagogastroduodenoscopy. The organism was subsequently isolated from the cytology brush, the endoscope forceps channel aperture, the lumen of the rubber tubing connecting the suction bottle to the endoscope and the suction collection bottle, which was thought to be the reservoir for the organisms. The instruments had been routinely cleaned with hexachlorophene solution. This outbreak illustrates how bacterial disease can be spread by inadequately cleaned endoscopic equipment (Center for Disease Control, 1977). Gross contamination of instruments was found in all cultures after routine hexachlorophene (pHisoHex) cleansing (Dunkerley, Cromer, Edmiston and Dunn, 1977). Using the same technique with povidone iodine (Betadine) the instruments were found to be sterile. Disinfection of upper gastrointestinal fibreoptic equipment by immersion in gluteraldehyde (Cidex) for two minutes consistently produced sterile cultures (Carr-Locke and Clayton, 1978) and ethylene oxide gas was found to remove bacteria consistently from colonoscopes (Chang, Sakai and Ashizawa, 1973).

Each endoscopy unit must work out its own methods for preventing the spread of disease by bacteria. Numerous effective germicidal solutions are available commercially (Abbott, 1974) but periodic culturing of the endoscope and accessories should be carried out in order to monitor the effectiveness of technique.

13.3.2 *Viral hepatitis*

Viral hepatitis is a constant hazard of colonoscopy since the virus can be found in blood, bile and faeces. Viral hepatitis is a relative contraindication for colonoscopy but occasional cases must be examined and inadvertent examination of a hepatitis patient is not unusual and therefore a method of preventing the transmission of the virus from patient to patient is necessary. Biopsy forceps, snares and other equipment which penetrate tissue should then be steam-sterilized. Flexible fibreoptic endoscopes cannot be autoclaved and therefore must either be cleansed with a germicidal agent or gas-sterilized between patients. Complete removal of hepatitis B surface antigen has been demonstrated by routine cleaning with an iodophor (Betadine) after endoscopic equipment was artificially contaminated by positive blood (Bond and Moncada, 1978). This study agrees with published experience to date which indicates routine cleansing of endoscopic equipment with a germicidal agent is sufficient to prevent the transmission of hepatitis B (McDonald and Silverstein, 1976; Koretz and Camacho, 1979; Hoofnagle, Blake, Buskell-Bales and Seeff, 1980).

Gas sterilization with ethylene oxide is most effective in eradicating all microorganisms, viruses and fungi and is recommended when the entire instrument must be disinfected (Ujeyl, Wurbs, Adam and Classen, 1978) but gas sterilization has its own disadvantages. The process takes about three hours and the sterilized instruments must be exposed to the air for 24 hours before they can be used again. Also, ethylene oxide is mutagenic and has been associated with an increased incidence of leukaemia in workers exposed to the gas (Hogstedt, Malmqvist and Wadman, 1979).

13.4 General anaesthesia

Laceration and perforation of the bowel wall have been reported in patients undergoing colonoscopy with general anaesthesia (Livstone, Cohen, Troncale and Touloukian, 1974; Koyama, 1974; Smith, 1976). Frühmorgen and Demling (1979) advised against it after reviewing colonoscopic complications in West Germany. General anaesthesia eliminates patient discomfort which is an important indicator for safe colonoscopy. General anaesthesia is not indicated unless the patient, e.g. a child or psychotic individual, simply cannot co-operate. It should not be attempted unless the indications are strong and the colonoscopist is experienced.

13.5 Diagnostic colonoscopy

13.5.1 *Mechanical free perforation*

Perforation is the most common major complication of diagnostic colonoscopy occurring in 0.14–0.26% in large surveys (Table 13.1). It frequently requires surgical intervention and can have a fatal outcome. Perforation can be caused by mechanical or pneumatic pressures, or a combination of both. It can be free, as into the peritoneal cavity; closed, as a rupture into the retroperitoneal space; or a subtle leak of gas dissecting its way between the tissues of the bowel wall. The mechanical forces necessary for perforation have been studied in cadaver and surgical specimens by Wu (1978). Mechanical perforation can occur because of lateral bowing of the colonoscope (Smith, 1976), during attempted alpha manoeuvre (Meyers and Ghahremani, 1975), when using the overtube (Roberts, Campbell and Isbister, 1976) or when trying to break up a faecal impaction (Rogers *et al.*, 1975). Several authors mention pain as a limitation to the extent of colonoscopic examination (Sugarbaker and Vineyard, 1973; Dagradi, Alaama and Ruiz, 1975; Britton, Tregoning, Bone and McKelvey, 1977). Even in the patient who has been given moderate doses of analgesics, pain appears to be a reliable warning that pressures being exerted are unsafe. Careful attention to the patient's pain and response patterns should help avoid perforation. When pain occurs, the colonoscope should be withdrawn and a new approach at insertion made. If all attempts at inserting the colonoscope result in significant discomfort, colonoscopy should be stopped or the situation monitored by fluoroscopy, (see Chapter 8), when colonoscopy can usually be completed successfully.

Alternatively the fluoroscope may show a difficult situation imposs-

Table 13.1 Complications of diagnostic colonoscopy in large surveys

Author	Cases	Haemorrhages	Perforations	Mortality
Rogers *et al.*, 1975	25 298	12 (0.05%)	55 (0.22%)	2 (0.008%)
Smith, 1976	12 746	9 (0.07%)	33 (0.26%)	4 (0.03%)
Frühmorgen and Demling, 1979	35 892	3 (0.008%)	51 (0.14%)	7 (0.02%)

ible to overcome thus avoiding needless pain. The importance of fluoroscopic control in avoiding complications has been noted (Graham and Eusebio, 1977; Frühmorgen and Demling, 1979). The diagnosis of overt perforation is usually made immediately by visualization of the peritoneal cavity or by demonstrating intraperitoneal air (Rogers *et al.*, 1975; Roberts, Campbell and Ibister, 1976). Abdominal pain and distention with loss of liver dullness to percussion are usually present and paracentesis should be performed if a tension pneumoperitoneum is present (Jacobsohn and Levy, 1976). Intravenous fluids and antibiotics usually preceed exploratory laparotomy. Aerobic and anaerobic cultures of the peritoneal cavity should be taken. Debridement and primary closure of the perforation with drainage of the peritoneal cavity is indicated if the injured bowel is otherwise healthy. If underlying disease such as diverticular disease or carcinoma is present, then resection may be indicated. Prompt surgical management of colonoscopic perforations can be accomplished with minimal morbidity and mortality (Prorok, Stahler, Hartzell and Sugarman, 1977). Successful non-operative management of colonoscopic perforation has been reported and deserves consideration especially in well-prepared patients with benign colonic disease and medical factors which weigh against surgery (Taylor, Weakley and Sullivan, 1978).

13.5.2 *Pneumatic perforation during diagnostic colonoscopy*

Pneumatic perforation results from over-distension of the bowel wall by insufflated gas. Over-distension is uncommon because excess gas is usually passed per rectum or refluxed into the terminal ileum but when excess pressure cannot be relieved perforation is likely to follow. A review of the original studies of pneumatic rupture of the large bowel is helpful in understanding the mechanism (Burt, 1931). As intraluminal pressure increases the serosa and muscularis rupture first, usually splitting along the tenia of the antimesenteric surface. The mucosa herniates through the opening with increasing pressure and finally bursts with a pop; or the mucosa may gradually thin out into a fine mesh and become permeable so air escapes through it slowly. In a mesenteric perforation air dissects under the serosa for a considerable distance and finally causes rupture at one or more fine points either in the mesentery proper or more commonly along the side of the colon. The rectum was found to be most resistant to rupture, followed by the sigmoid colon, transverse colon and caecum in that order. The caecum is the most likely site for pneumatic rupture because it has both the thinnest wall and the greatest diameter. The tension which is pulling apart the wall of a cylinder is directly related to its radius (La Place's Law) so that even if the pneumatic pressure throughout the large bowel were the same, the greatest strain would be on the caecum.

Early laboratory investigations suggested that pressures ranging up to 570 mm Hg may be produced by colonoscopy equipment (Williams *et al.*, 1973). More recently, however, during routine colonoscopy, intraluminal pressures were found to range only from 9–57 mm Hg when the colonoscope tip was free in the bowel lumen (Kozarek *et al.*, 1980). Maximum pressures occurred when the tip impacted against the bowel wall and rose to 137 mm Hg. Using human cadavers, the cecum was found to rupture at a mean intraluminal pressure of 81 mm Hg, while a pressure of 169 mm Hg was required for disruption of the sigmoid. Therefore enough pressure may occur during colonoscopy to rupture the colon, especially if the wall is already weakened by disease such as a diverticulum, ulceration or carcinoma.

Pneumatic rupture of the colon with blow-out into the peritoneal cavity is diagnosed and treated in the same way as mechanical free perforation. Pneumatic rupture of the large bowel into the retroperitoneal tissues eventually results in subcutaneous emphysema which may distend the scrotum or pass through the mediastinum to the neck (Meyers and Ghahremani, 1975). Plain X-ray films of such patients will help diagnose the site of perforation (Meyers, 1974). Most closed perforations into the extraperitoneal spaces can be managed conservatively with almost always a satisfactory outcome (Lezak and Goldhamer, 1974; Gordon, 1975; Meyers and Ghahremani, 1975).

13.5.3 *Incomplete perforation*

Benign pneumoperitoneum and intramural gas
In a prospective study of 100 patients undergoing colonoscopy only one was found to have intraperitoneal air (Ecker *et al.*, 1977) After colonoscopy, the patient was asymptomatic with stable vital signs and she was successfully treated with complete restriction of oral intake, intravenous fluids and antibiotics. This appears to be correct management because similar patients have been explored and no gross perforation could be identified (Rogers *et al.*, 1975; Kozarek *et al.*, 1980). Leaks which show only intramural gas on X-ray can safely be ignored (Glouberman, Craner, Ogburn and Burdick, 1976).

Serosal laceration

Serosal and seromuscular lacerations can be considered incomplete perforations of the colon and are due to excessive transmural strain caused by mechanical or pneumatic forces. Since the mucosa remains intact the frequency of this complication is not known (Livstone *et al.*, 1974). Most serosal lacerations occur in the sigmoid and are apparently due to mechanical injury (Livstone *et al.*, 1974; Koyama, 1974; Livstone and Kerstein, 1976; Roberts, Campbell and Isbister, 1976; Knoepp, 1977). Those which occur remote from the area of colonoscopy seem to be less frequent and are probably due to distension by air (Wu, 1978). Usually patients with serosal lacerations have discomfort after colonoscopy and distension that may persist for several days whereas others are completely asymptomatic (Graham and Eusebio, 1977). Two cases of serosal lacerations due to over-distension by air during intraoperative colonoscopy have been observed (Sjogren *et al.*, 1978). To determine causative factors, intraluminal and intra-abdominal pressures were measured during routine closed-abdomen colonoscopy. Both pressures were found to be low and to increase with the duration of the procedure. During open-abdomen colonoscopy increases in intraluminal pressure were unopposed by increases in intra-abdominal pressures and probably contributed to the development of serosal lacerations. Cross-clamping the colon to maintain distension was specifically warned against because this seemed to precipitate the tear in one patient. The second patient had a competent ileocaecal valve which may have contributed to the caecal laceration that developed. Extensive adhesion formation has been reported at laparotomy six weeks after documented seromuscular tears and lacerations (Livstone and Kerstein, 1976). However, if serosal laceration is suspected, non-operative conservative management would seem to be indicated.

Serosal and seromuscular lacerations can be prevented by using a gentle technique. The colonoscopist should hold a 6 lb weight in his hand and remind himself that applying pressure greater than this may result in injury even to normal bowel. Any manoeuvre to decrease the strain in passing a redundant loop or flexure is preventive and frequently a simple change in position may facilitate insertion. When passing through the sigmoid colon, changing the patient's position from left lateral decubitus to supine or right lateral decubitus is frequently helpful. Rounding the splenic flexure is often facilitated by having the patient on the right side or even prone. In non-obese patients, manipulation of the colonoscope through the abdominal wall may ease it around the loop of the sigmoid or through a sagging transverse portion. The aim is to convert sharp angulations into gentle curves and the abdomen should be checked frequently to locate the light to assess progress. Spot checks with fluoroscopy are invaluable, especially in obese patients. To avoid damage to the bowel wall colonoscopy should be stopped and the situation evaluated whenever firm resistance is encountered. It is not infrequent for the endoscopist to believe the tip is at the splenic flexure when in fact it is at the descending-sigmoid junction. In such a situation continued insertion may result in a serosal tear or frank perforation.

13.5.4 *Site and underlying conditions related to perforation during colonoscopy*

The sigmoid colon is by far the most common site of perforation during colonoscopy (Rogers *et al.*, 1975; Frühmorgen and Demling, 1979), probably because it is the first challenging segment of colon encountered. Also, it is frequently the site of underlying disease which contributes to perforation, including diverticular disease, carcinoma, radiation colitis, pelvic adhesions or inflammatory bowel disease. Diverticulitis is a perforating condition and should be regarded with caution. Simple filling of the colon during barium examination of patients with acute diverticulitis has resulted in venous intravasation (Nordahl, Silber, Robbins and O'Hara, 1973). Obviously colonoscopy can be hazardous in such patients and should not be performed until abdominal tenderness and systemic symptoms have settled. Two case reports indicate that defunctioned bowel may be more susceptible to perforation (Gordon, 1975; Wu, 1978).

13.5.5 *Haemorrhage*

Most serious haemorrhages which occur during diagnostic colonoscopy are unseen by the endoscopist because they are intra-abdominal (Rogers *et al.*, 1975; Smith, 1976). Such haemorrhage may be completely asymptomatic or manifested by postcolonoscopy abdominal discomfort, hypotension and a falling haematocrit. Without exploratory laparotomy the cause and site of bleeding remain unknown (Wu, 1978). Reported causes of haemorrhages include seromuscular tears (Koyama, 1974), ruptured spleen (Telmos and Mittal, 1977), lacerated mesentery (Smith, 1976), lacerated spleen and lacerated liver (Ellis, Harrison and Williams, 1979). These complications apparently arise from excessive tension on the bowel wall, mesenteric attachments, ligaments and adhesions. Proper management of postcolonoscopy intra-abdominal haemorrhage appears to be careful monitoring of the pulse and blood pressure with transfusions as needed. If bleeding persists, exploratory laparotomy and ligation of bleeding points is indicated. Patients on anticoagulant therapy present a hazard because of the increased risk of intra-abdominal haemorrhage during colonoscopy. It is wise to take patients off anticoagulant therapy and perform coagulation tests which should return to normal before colonoscopy. This is mandatory if biopsy or polypectomy is anticipated.

13.5.6 *Vasovagal reflex*

The vasovagal reflex is characterized by bradycardia, hypotension and a cold, clammy skin. It is caused by stretching the mesentery enough to cause pain and is less likely to occur in those given analgesics as a premedication: a small dose of atropine (0.4 mg) prior to colonoscopy may help prevent it. The symptoms of vasovagal reflex are best treated by putting the patient in the Trendelenberg position, giving i.v. saline and allowing enough time for symptoms to pass when colonoscopy can then be continued.

13.5.7 *Myocardial infarction*

Myocardial infarction has been observed to occur during and shortly after colonoscopy (Rogers *et al.*, 1975). At least one case had a fatal outcome (Smith, 1976). In a series of 23 patients monitored by ECG, one demonstrated ischaemic changes of S-T segment depression, 2 mm below the resting level which persisted during the hour following colonoscopy (Vawter *et al.*, 1975). In a series of 63 patients, 29 developed new or exaggerated ECG abnormalities (Alam, Schuman, Duvernay and Madrazo, 1976). Caution is advised in patients who are known to have heart disease and ECG monitoring should be considered. In addition it may be helpful to administer oxygen by nasal cannula at 4 to 5 l/min. Sublingual nitroglycerine can be used prophylactically and whenever needed for angina.

13.5.8 *Postcolonoscopy distension syndrome*

Several authors have reported the postcolonoscopy distension syndrome which is characterized by an uncomfortably distended abdomen observed towards the end of the procedure (Sugarbaker *et al.*, 1974; Rogers *et al.*, 1975; Smith, 1976). The symptoms can mimic perforation but X-ray will show only distended loops of bowel. Most cases resolve rapidly but at least two have been reported who developed adynamic ileus and required nasogastric suction and intravenous fluids over a period of 48–72 hours (Smith, 1976; Ramakrishnan, 1979). Over-distension of the bowel can be prevented by judicious use of insufflated gas. Particular care should be taken when the colonoscopist is confronted with a stricture or any similar situation where the lumen will not distend. A change in position may be helpful in this situation. Occasional palpitation of the abdomen is useful in judging the amount of insufflated air, and the use of carbon dioxide during colonoscopy will decrease the tendency towards distension because it is absorbed approximately 160 times faster than nitrogen across the mucous membrane (Saltzman and Sieker, 1968).

13.5.9 *Biopsy*

Complications of mucosal biopsy are perforation and haemorrhage, both of which are unusual. The A/S/G/E survey which included 25 298 diagnostic colonoscopies, reported only two perforations and two haemorrhages which were associated with biopsy (Rogers *et al.*, 1975). Both perforations and one of the haemorrhages occurred in patients with inflammatory bowel disease. A perforation was reported following colonoscopic biopsy at the splenic flexure in a patient with Crohn's disease (Abrams, 1977). This apparent increased risk in patients with inflammatory bowel disease is probably related to the inflamed, hyperaemic and ulcerated mucosa. It seems wise to take biopsies from intact mucosa or margins of ulcers rather than from an ulcer base.

13.5.10 *Miscellaneous*

Dissection of an aortic aneurysm in a 50-year-old woman has been reported (Rogers *et al.*, 1975). Partial colonic obstruction has been converted to complete obstruction apparently by insufflating too much air (Rogers *et al.*, 1975). Colonic obstruction developed in the sigmoid in a patient with extensive diverticular disease after colonoscopy. The incipient and partial obstruction was thought to be rendered complete by the trauma of colonoscopic manipulation (Graham and Eusebio, 1977).

There have been reports of colonoscopy inducing volvulus and a sigmoid volvulus was created by an alpha manoeuvre. It was treated by repeating colonoscopy and then reducing the volvulus by clockwise rotation (Smith, 1976). A transverse colon volvulus was reported in a patient who developed large bowel obstruction after colonoscopy. The volvulus apparently occurred when insufflated air was trapped by the acute angles of the hepatic and splenic flexures. Laparotomy, decompression of the bowel and relief of the volvulus produced uneventful recovery (Britton *et al.*, 1977). A caecal volvulus occurred after colonoscopy and at surgery a right hemicolectomy was necessary because the caecum was found to be gangrenous (Smith, 1976).

A delayed perforation occurred in a patient in whom a volvulus was reduced by colonoscopic technique (Wertkin, Wetchler, Waye and Brown, 1976), and a biopsy taken at the point of the volvulus ahead of the colonoscope on insertion may have contributed. Incarceration of a previously freely reducible long-standing incisional hernia after colonoscopy occurred in a 65-year-old man. At operation a knuckle of small bowel was found to be caught in the hernia which was reduced and repaired. The authors blamed the complication on over-insufflation because of a technically difficult colonoscopy and warn others to keep this hazard in mind when patients with hernia are undergoing colonoscopy (Rees and Williams, 1977). Impaction of the colonoscope in the hernia sac has also been reported but fortunately, it was extricated without damage to patient or instrument (Waye, 1975). Pulmonary embolus has been reported to follow colonoscopy (Smith, 1976) and good hydration, early ambulation and avoidance of over-sedation should help prevent this complication.

13.6 Colonoscopic polypectomy

13.6.1 *Perforation*

Perforation associated with colonoscopic polypectomy is one of the major complications with a frequency that ranges from 0.29% to 0.42% in large surveys (Table 13.2). It can be caused by cutting through the bowel wall which has been pulled into the snare loop, application of too much power with eventual necrosis of a transmural burn, and by mechanical or pneumatic pressures acting on the bowel wall already weakened by electrocoagulation.

There is increased risk of perforation during removal of sessile polyps (Smith, 1976). This is probably related to the close proximity of the polypectomy site to the bowel wall which makes transmural coagulation more likely. When a pseudopedicle is made to remove a sessile polyp, it is important not to place too much traction on it because doing so will thin it out and cause the electrosurgical effect to be close to the bowel wall and not at the intended site of transection.

Table 13.2 Complications of colonoscopic polypectomy in large surveys

Author	Cases	Haemorrhages	Perforations	Mortality
Rogers *et al.*, 1975	6214	115 (1.85%)	18 (0.29%)	0
Smith, 1976	9238	71 (0.77%)	39 (0.42%)	1 (0.01%)
Frühmorgen and Demling, 1979	7365	165 (2.24%)	25 (0.34%)	8 (0.1%)

If a polyp is not freely moveable over the underlying submucosa a polypoid carcinoma with infiltration should be suspected and only biopsy is indicated. A piecemeal method of removing large broad-based polyps has been described but it should be used only when the indications are strong and certainly not by a novice (Shinya and Wolff, 1975). One-step electrosurgical removal of a sessile polyp with a diameter between 1 and 1.5 cm is possible, but the larger the polyp the more likely there will be a perforation. A sessile polyp with a diameter greater than 1.5 cm is beyond the capabilities of the electrosurgical snare and one-step removal should not be attempted.

Perforation after colonoscopic polypectomy may be immediate, delayed for days or weeks and may never become clinically evident. The signs and symptoms of immediate perforation are similar to those of mechanical perforation which has already been described. There are some unique features of delayed perforation which deserve mention. Pain at the time of polypectomy is an ominous sign and suggests a transmural burn (Sugarbarker *et al.*, 1974) which can be followed by a delayed perforation (Meyers and Ghahremani, 1975). Abdominal pain which is slow in onset (Graham and Eusebio, 1977) or fever and leukocytosis on the day following polypectomy may mean perforation (Meyers and Ghahremani, 1975). Symptoms of perforation may be minimal or absent so that only if the patient is explored for other reasons will a silent perforation be discovered (Overholt, Hargrove, Farris and Wilson, 1976). A postpolypectomy perforation usually occurs at the site of the polypectomy and if more than one polyp is removed, it is most likely to be found at the site of the largest (Meyers and Ghahremani, 1975). An unusual exception is a remote electrical perforation of the ileum during polypectomy from the left colon (Erdman, Boggs and Slagle, 1979). This disturbing complication is probably due to concentration of the field of electrical current because of inhomogeneity of the patient's tissue. Fortunately this unpredictable and unpreventable complication is very rare.

Exploratory laparotomy and closure is the preferred method of therapy for free perforation and should be performed as soon as the diagnosis is established (Prorok, Stahler, Hartzell and Sugarman, 1977). However, each case must be evaluated individually since at least one postpolypectomy perforation has been managed successfully without exploration (Taylor, Weakley and Sullivan, 1978). Retroperitoneal perforations which are manifested by extraperitoneal gas only respond well to conservative therapy (Meyers and Ghahremani, 1975; Yassinger *et al.*, 1978). When extraluminal gas is found at the end of colonoscopy and polypectomy, it is usually impossible to know whether it is due to mechanical damage, pneumatic pressure or the effects of electrocoagulation. In order to avoid unnecessary exploration, conservative management could be continued as long as the patient remains asymptomatic, the inflammation appears to remain localized and extraluminal gas is gradually resolving.

13.6.2 *Transmural burn*

When a patient who has undergone polypectomy develops abdominal pain, leukocytosis and fever without evidence for perforation, a diagnosis of transmural burn is presumed (Rogers *et al.*, 1975). The presumptive diagnosis is strengthened if the patient experienced pain at the time of polypectomy or electrocoagulation (Sugarbaker *et al.*, 1974). Conservative therapy is indicated.

13.6.3 *Haemorrhage*

The most common major complication of colonoscopic electrosurgical snare polypectomy is haemorrhage with a frequency that ranges from 0.77% to 2.24% in the large surveys (Table 13.2). Postpolypectomy haemorrhage is caused by inadequate coagulation of the blood vessels within the pedicle. Inadequate coagulation can be caused by mechanically cutting the pedicle while applying too little power and conversely by applying too much power which results in electrocutting without electrocoagulation. Ideally polypectomy is performed with just the right blend of cutting and coagulating power which will transect the pedicle completely while simultaneously coagulating the blood vessels within it. Most postpolypectomy haemorrhages occur immediately after transection of the pedicle (Rogers *et al.*, 1975; Frühmorgen and Demling, 1979) and most delayed haemorrhages manifest themselves within the first 24 hours although some occur as much as 21 days later (Norfleet, 1974).

Analysis of the data collected during the 1974 A/S/G/E complication survey showed that there was an increased incidence of postpolypectomy haemorrhage reported by inexperienced colonoscopists who had performed less than 25 polypectomies (Rogers *et al.*, 1975). The same survey showed an increased incidence of postpolypectomy haemorrhage reported by those using the Cameron–Miller electrosurgical unit and snare. This increased bleeding was probably related to the very thin wire of the Cameron–Miller snare loop which has a tendency to cut before coagulation is complete. If the operator is aware of this tendency and uses the equipment according to the manufacturer's instructions postpolypectomy haemorrhage should be rare.

Treatment of postpolypectomy haemorrhage is primarily expectant. Most bleeding will cease spontaneously as the severed blood vessels go into spasm and contract. Tissue thromboplastin and oedema produced in the stump by the electrosurgical burn also contribute to haemostasis. If postpolypectomy bleeding persists, the patient should be kept on absolute bed rest and intravenous saline administered. The haemoglobin, haematocrit, pulse and blood pressure must be monitored and transfusions given if needed and surgery considered if four or more units of blood are required.

The colonoscopic management of postpolypectomy haemorrhage requires a cool head and calm nerves. Brisk bleeding will obscure the field of view and swamp the polypectomy site with blood within minutes of transection of the pedicle. The endoscopist should be prepared for a postpolypectomy haemorrhage whenever removing a polyp with a thick pedicle (8–15 mm), since it is the larger pedicle which is most likely to bleed. Leave at least 1 cm of pedicle behind and more if possible. As soon as the polyp has been severed, reopen the snare and pass the loop over the stump of the pedicle. Close the snare loop around the stump only if an arterial pumper is seen and apply enough pressure to stop the bleeding. The snare should then be left and current is not applied unless bleeding continues after ten minutes hold. If current is applied the snare wire is likely to become embedded in the stump and if not easily removed, it should then be left in place. This can be accomplished by disassembly of the snare handle from the tubing and then withdrawing the colonoscope over it leaving the snare in place. The snare will then pass spontaneously after a few days. If resnaring is impossible and bleeding continues, try to change the position of the patient in such a way that blood drains away from the polypectomy site so that a further attempt at resnaring the pedicle can be made. Attempts to aspirate the blood usually fail because clots occlude the suction channel and render it useless. Electrocoagulation of a bleeding polypectomy site has been reported to be successful (Spencer, Coates and Anderson, 1974) but it should be applied judiciously since overcoagulation could result in perforation (Geenen, Schmitt, Wu and Hogan, 1975). One of the problems of electrocoagulating a bleeding point is the presence of blood itself which interferes with coagulation of the vessel wall. The blood vessel will be easier to electrocoagulate if the bleeding can be stopped or slowed by the injection of a vasoconstrictor solution such as epinephrine 1:10 000, through an endoscopic catheter. If it becomes clear that the bleeding cannot be controlled at colonoscopy, a serious attempt should still be made to locate and retrieve the head of the polyp before withdrawing the scope.

There are several other methods available for managing persistent postpolypectomy haemorrhage. Successful angiographic management of severe postpolypectomy haemorrhage with selective intra-arterial vasoconstrictor infusion has been reported and seems ideally suited to this complication (Carlyle and Goldstein, 1975). In one of this author's patients, postpolypectomy haemorrhage occurred when a large sessile polyp was removed from the sigmoid colon at 18 cm insertion. Because of persistent bleeding, the patient was given general anaesthesia and the anus was dilated so the bowel could be pulled down until the polypectomy site came into view. It was oversewn even though it had stopped bleeding by that time. Transabdominal surgical therapy will be necessary if bleeding continues and angiography is not available or unsuccessful and if the polypectomy site cannot be oversewn transanally.

The experience of postpolypectomy haemorrhage which can be gleaned from the literature will be helpful to those who must deal with this complication. In the 1974 A/S/G/E survey (Rogers et al., 1975), there were 115 haemorrhages associated with 6214 polypectomies (1.9%). Immediate haemorrhage out-numbered delayed haemorrhage by a ratio of 3:1. Delayed bleeding occurred from as little as twenty minutes after polypectomy to as long as nine days. Most delayed haemorrhages occurred in the first 24 hours and stopped spontaneously. About half required blood transfusions. Only one case was reported in which the pedicle was still bleeding at repeat colonoscopy and it was stopped by repeat coagulation of the bleeding stalk. Most postpolypectomy haemorrhages did not require surgical intervention and there were no deaths.

In the Wisconsin survey (Geenen et al., 1975), five haemorrhages occurred after 292 polypectomies (1.7%). Four occurred in the first 24 hours and one after eight days. Three patients required blood transfusions. One patient with immediate bleeding and another with bleeding after eight days required operative intervention and all patients with postpolypectomy haemorrhage recovered.

The German survey (Frühmorgen and Demling, 1979), included 7365 polypectomies and 165 associated haemorrhages (2.24%): 91

required no therapy, 50 were treated conservatively and 24 required surgery. Among the 165 haemorrhages, there were three deaths. In a series of 53 polypectomies in 43 patients, one fatality was reported (Moldow and McGregor, 1974). It occurred in a 78-year old insulin dependent diabetic woman who had mild postpolypectomy bleeding over a six-hour period. Her haemoglobin never fell below 10% but she developed severe metabolic acidosis with a pH of 6.9. She died within hours following surgery to stop her colonic bleeding.

13.6.4 *Incomplete polypectomy*

Incomplete polypectomy is a distressing and time-consuming complication as the following example will show. An attempt was made to remove a large polyp on a short pedicle which had a diameter of 2 cm (Dagradi, Riff, Norum and Juler, 1976). The snare became fused to the pedicle and could not be removed. Consequently the polypectomy could not be completed in spite of the application of maximum power and firm traction on the snare wire. An attempt at resnaring the polyp was unsuccessful because of the inability to extrude the snare after the colonoscope had been passed to the caecum. Eventually the patient went to surgery where the polyp was removed through a caecotomy. As a result of their experience, the authors recommended piecemeal polypectomy for such large lesions.

Another case of incomplete polypectomy was solved by pulling out the snare tube and handle leaving the wire in place (Stearns *et al.*, 1975). Another snare was inserted and the polyp was removed piecemeal fashion down to the first snare. I had one experience of an incomplete polypectomy with a large sigmoid polyp which had a short thick pedicle. At maximum power no tissue effect could be observed. Firm traction on the snare wire was avoided because under these circumstances in the past, too rapid transection of the pedicle resulted in postpolypectomy haemorrhage. The polyp in my patient was located just around the bend in the sigmoid and piecemeal polypectomy would have been hazardous. I elected to send the patient directly to surgery after withdrawing the tube and the snare handle leaving the bare wire in place. A few hours later, the polyp was out and the patient made an uneventful recovery. Even if the snare can be removed after an incomplete polypectomy, promptness in sending such patients to surgery is necessary in order to preserve the polyp for histological examination. I have two cases in which large colonic polyps disappeared after attempts at snare removal were unsuccessful. Evidently, enough current was applied to cause necrosis of the pedicle and eventual sloughing of the polyp.

A more common occurrence which is not discussed in the literature is an incomplete transection of the pedicle. In this situation the snare wire cuts through part of the coagulated pedicle but stops short of complete transection. The colonoscopist finds that the polyp is still firmly attached to the bowel wall and the snare handle has been closed completely. Under these circumstances unless the current density is increased significantly at the pedicle, further application of power will simply desiccate tissue rather than cut it. The current density can be increased by either turning up the power or putting more tension on the snare wire. In order to increase tension on the snare wire it should be adjusted by shortening the point of attachment in the handle. (This is easy to do with the Cameron–Miller handle but in order to accomplish this with the ACMI handle, a relief hole must be drilled.) Sometimes a gentle pull is all that is necessary to complete a polypectomy but forceful pulling should be avoided because it may result in perforation due to traction on the bowel wall. If a gentle pull, increasing power or increasing tension on the snare does not complete the polypectomy it is best to leave it in place and start again with a new snare.

13.6.5 *Pacemaker patients*

The patient with a demand cardiac pacemaker presents a hazard because the high frequency current from the electrosurgical equipment may suppress the pacemaker and cause asystole (O'Donoghue, 1973). Some pacemakers have been shielded to prevent interference by electrosurgical currents (Fein, 1967). Even so, it appears wise to take special precautions in patients with pacemakers. The patient return plate should be positioned under the buttocks or thigh so that the distance of the electrical field is as far as possible from the pacemaker. The patient should be monitored and substitute pacing equipment available. Interference on the cardiac monitor during the application of current indicates that the pacemaker is not properly shielded. Electrosurgery should be limited to not more than two or three seconds if any pacemaker suppression is produced, or the pacemaker should be converted to a fixed-rate modality using the magnet provided.

13.6.6 *Explosion of flammable gases*

All who perform colonoscopic electrosurgery must be aware of the hazard of combustible gases (hydrogen and methane), which are produced by bacterial fermentation under anaerobic conditions and found in the colon in varying concentrations. The production of methane and hydrogen appears to be completely unrelated. Hydrogen can be detected in almost all colons under normal non-fasting conditions whereas only about one third of the population are methane producers (Levitt, 1971).

In the past, explosions during electrosurgery with the rigid proctosigmoidoscope led to the recommendation for the use of CO_2 under positive pressure in order to prevent such disasters (Becker, 1953). These recommendations appealed to me and during my first colonoscopic polypectomy in 1971, CO_2 was insufflated throughout the procedure to prevent any possible explosion simply by excluding the oxygen from room air. This technique did not result in significant alterations of the pCO_2, HCO_3^- or pH (Rogers, 1974). Since that time I have used this technique in thousands of patients without untoward effect and the only contraindication to its use is CO_2 retention in patients with severe pulmonary disease.

It has been shown that standard preparation for total colonoscopy reduces colonic hydrogen to undetectable levels (Ragins, Shinya and Wolff, 1974). Fasting or the ingestion of an elemental diet lowers hydrogen formation to negligible levels by 12 to 16 hours (Bond and Levitt, 1975). Methane production is less affected by fasting and even persists after thorough bowel cleansing. In order to reduce residual methane to well below its explosive range it must be diluted by repeatedly insufflating and aspirating air (Ragins, Shinya and Wolff, 1974). The only explosion during colonoscopic polypectomy was reported from France (Bigard, Gaucher and LaSalle, 1979). The patient had a polyp in the caecum. The preparation comprised two days of non-residue diet and isotonic 4% mannitol lavage on the evening before the examination. At colonoscopy, the large bowel was found to be very clean with no faecal matter. No inert gas was insufflated. After application of 8–10 s of coagulating current, there was an explosion which was audible in the endoscopy room. The patient jerked upwards off the endoscopy table and the colonoscope was completely ejected. The patient immediately showed clinical signs of shock and complained of generalized abdominal pain. He was quickly transferred to the operating theatre and laparotomy was carried out 15 min after the explosion. There were numerous full-thickness lacerations in the right colon and the transverse colon as far as the splenic flexure and multiple bleeding points were visible around these perforations. In addition the spleen was found to have numerous capsular lacerations. An extended right hemicolectomy was performed. The patient received 45 U of blood during the procedure but it proved impossible to achieve haemostasis and he died. The authors blamed the use of mannitol for the explosion and advised against using it since metabolism of unabsorbed mannitol by colonic bacteria probably resulted in the production of hydrogen. On the basis of this disastrous explosion, routine insufflation of CO_2 for polypectomy was recommended and this is now the official policy of the French Endoscopic Society. Obviously great care is required with all non-absorbed carbohydrates like mannitol which should probably be avoided when preparing a patient for colonoscopic electrosurgery.

Ideally, total colonoscopy should be performed to confirm a well prepared colon and three or four gas exchanges with room air at the polypectomy site should reduce combustible gases to below their explosive range. For added safety, CO_2 can be insufflated at the site prior to electrosurgery.

Insufflation of an inert gas such as CO_2 throughout colonoscopy remains the only sure method of avoiding explosion and is easily done with most modern instruments.

13.6.7 *Miscellaneous complications*

Accidental removal of the stoma of a ureterosigmoidostomy (Plate 184) has been reported (Williams and Gillespie, 1979). The stoma presented as a polypoid mass that appeared at endoscopy to be a malignant polyp. Removal resulted in renal sepsis and unilateral nephrectomy.

A recurrence of diverticulitis after polypectomy had been reported (Sugarbaker *et al.*, 1974). However, the diagnosis of recurrent diverticulitis is presumptive since it would seem difficult to differentiate it from a transmural burn.

13.6.8 *Prevention of complications*

Only a qualified endoscopist should undertake electrosurgery during colonoscopy and skill in diagnostic colonoscopy is acknowledged as a prerequisite in undertaking colonoscopic surgery (Shinya and Wolff, 1975). This is necessary for locating the lesion, obtaining the best view and then being able to respond appropriately to any untoward circumstances. The colonoscopist must be thoroughly conversant with the principles of electrosurgery (Curtiss, 1973). It is extremely important for the physician to be familiar with the electrosurgical equipment used and accessories and the equipment should be maintained in good condition.

It is wise to check the patient's coagulation profile beforehand. A postpolypectomy haemorrhage has been reported in one patient who had a factor VII deficiency (Smith, 1976). The endoscopist should remember that a patient who is a poor surgical risk will probably not do well after a complication which requires exploratory laparotomy (Moldow and McGregor, 1974).

The snare should work freely enough so the operator can sense the pressure being applied in order to avoid premature transection of the pedicle. The snare loop must be closed snugly around the pedicle so the protruding wire will not burn the adjacent mucosa. A grazing or contralateral burn can be avoided by making sure that the head of the polyp is either free in the lumen or in contact with the mucosa over a large area. Application of low power for long periods can result in widespread electrical burns not appreciated endoscopically. Application of power for two seconds is usually adequate to determine whether or not local tissue effect is being obtained. If no effect is seen then the power setting is increased and current applied for two more seconds. It is not safe to transect the pedicle until tissue effect has been seen, which includes swelling, bubbling and changing of tissue colour from pink to white. The patient return plate should be positioned so that there is broad surface contact to a smooth soft area of skin in order to avoid a burn.

At the end of any electrosurgical procedure in the colon, the patient should be warned about the possibility of delayed perforation or haemorrhage. It takes approximately three weeks for the mucosa to heal and a low roughage diet, the avoidance of vigorous exercise and the use of a softening agent like Metamucil may be helpful in avoiding postpolypectomy complications. Certainly, the patient should be instructed to seek medical help if rectal bleeding or abdominal pain develops.

13.6.9 *Colonoscopic versus transabdominal polypectomy*

In spite of all the above mentioned complications, removal of colonic polyps at colonoscopy is clearly the method of choice when compared to transabdominal colotomy and polypectomy. The published complication rates for the transabdominal approach show a morbidity of 20% and a mortality of 1.3% (Kleinfield and Gump, 1960). The published complication rates for the colonoscopic approach show a morbidity of 2.3% and a mortality of 0.06% when results from several large series are combined (Frühmorgen and Demling, 1979). So the introduction of colonoscopic polypectomy has reduced the associated morbidity by a factor of 10 and the associated mortality by a factor of 20.

13.7 Electrocoagulation

13.7.1 *Perforation*

In the A/S/G/E series there were two perforations which followed electrocoagulation of small polyps (Rogers *et al.*, 1975). In the Wisconsin series a perforation resulted from excessively high current used during ball-tip coagulation of a bleeding biopsy site (Geenen *et al.*, 1975). Fulguration of a 2-mm polyp in the sigmoid resulted in a perforation that required surgery (Nivatvongs and Goldberg, 1979). Transmural electrocoagulation is a hazard of the ball-tip coagulator because during use it is pressed against the bowel wall thereby thinning it out and making injury more likely. Transmural electrocoagulation is less likely with the Williams' forceps because the lesion is pulled away from the underlying muscularis propria (Williams, 1973).

13.7.2 *Haemorrhage*

Two cases of haemorrhage following biopsy and electrocoagulation of 7-mm polyps with the Williams' forceps have been reported (Rand, 1977). Surgery was required in both cases to control bleeding. In both cases the polyps were located behind a fold in the caecum and therefore poorly accessible to snare removal. The bleeding sites were pinpointed by superior mesenteric angiograms. No complications were encountered by Rand in removing polyps up to 6 mm in size using the same technique. Eight hundred 'hot biopsies' for destruction of small polyps or telangiectases without subsequent haemorrhage have been reported by Williams and Tan (1979) and this technique has been associated with few reported complications.

13.8 Mechanical equipment failure

Mechanical equipment failure is common but rarely results in patient injury and therefore is reported infrequently in the literature. Colonoscope failure and fracture of snare wires during polypectomy have been reported (Smith, 1976). In one case where the snare loop became disengaged from the pull wire, it was eventually retrieved by using the biopsy forceps (Corlin, 1972). Good maintenance of endoscopic equipment should minimize equipment failure but it cannot be eliminated completely. Therefore, in order to avoid inconvenience, back-up equipment should always be available.

13.9 Flexible fibreoptic sigmoidoscopy

The resurgence of interest in flexible fibreoptic sigmoidoscopy introduces the possibility of increased complications because of its more widespread use by the occasional examiner. In the original series of over 500 cases only one complication was reported and that was toxic megacolon which developed 48 hours after endoscopy (Overholt,

1971). In the German survey 77.7% of the complications reported occurred in the sigmoid (Frühmorgen and Demling, 1979) and thus, the hazards of flexible fibreoptic sigmoidoscopy would appear to be very similar to those of colonoscopy. There are two notable exceptions which relate to position and preparation. There may be an increased risk of injury to the sigmoid colon when passing the flexible instrument with the patient in the knee–elbow position because there is less latitude for making a gentle curve as the tip is advanced. If flexible sigmoidoscopy is started with the patient on the left side then changes in position and external compression can be used to facilitate passage. There may be an increased risk of explosion since present advocates of flexible sigmoidoscopy emphasize the minimal preparation required (Manier, 1978; Winawer, Leidner, Boyle and Kurtz, 1979; Marks *et al.*, 1979). Under these circumstances preparation of the large bowel is incomplete. The chances for residual explosive gases to be present are similar to those undergoing open-tube rigid sigmoidoscopy (Becker, 1953; Levy and Levitt, 1976). During electrosurgery in the incompletely prepared patient electrosurgery should be avoided altogether unless a protective gas is used (Rogers, 1974).

13.10 Conclusions

Diagnostic colonoscopy is a relatively safe procedure with a very low morbidity and insignificant mortality. However, complications can occur, the most serious of which is usually perforation.

Colonoscopic polypectomy is the method of choice when compared with transabdominal colotomy and polypectomy, although haemorrhage may be expected in about 2% of such cases.

Used with thought and care the colonoscope can dramatically alter the approach to diagnosis and management of colonic disease.

References

Abbott, J. P. (1974), Are there methods of sterilization to destroy hepatitis B virus? *J. Am. Med. Ass.*, **229**, 579.

Abrams, J. S. (1977), A hard look at colonoscopy. *Am. J. Surg.*, **133**, 111–15.

Alam, M., Schuman, B. M., Duvernoy, W. F. C. and Madrazo, A. C. (1976), Continuous electrocardiographic monitoring during colonoscopy. *Gastrointest. Endosc.*, **22**, 203–5.

Becker, G. L. (1953), The prevention of gas explosions in the large bowel during electrosurgery. *Surgery Gynec. Obstet.*, **97**, 463–7.

Bigard, M. A., Gaucher, P. and LaSalle, C. (1979), Fatal colonic explosion during colonoscopic polypectomy. *Gastroenterology*, **77**, 1307–10.

260 *Organization and Techniques*

Bond, J. H. and Levitt, M. D. (1975), Factors affecting the concentration of combustible gases in the colon during colonoscopy. *Gastroenterology,* **68,** 1445–8.

Bond, J. H., Levy, M. and Levitt, M. D. (1976), Explosion of hydrogen gas in the colon during proctosigmoidoscopy. *Gastrointest. Endosc.,* **23,** 41–42.

Bond, W. W. and Moncada, R. E. (1978), Viral hepatitis B infection risk in flexible fibreoptic endoscopy. *Gastrointest. Endosc.,* **24,** 225–30.

Britton, D. C., Tregoning, D., Bone, G. and McKelvey, S. T. D. (1977), Colonoscopy in surgical practice. *Br. Med. J.,* **1,** 149–51.

Burt, C. A. (1931), Pneumatic rupture of the intestinal canal with experimental data showing the mechanism of perforation and the pressure required. *Archs. Surg.,* **22,** 875–902.

Carlyle, D R. and Goldstein, H. M. (1975), Angiographic management of bleeding following transcolonoscopic polypectomy. *Dig. Dis.,* **20,** 1196–201.

Carr-Locke, D. L. and Clayton, P. (1978), Disinfection of upper gastrointestinal fibreoptic endoscopy equipment: an evaluation of a cetrimide chlorhexidine solution and glutaraldehyde. *Gut,* **19,** 916–22.

Center for Disease Control (1977), *Morbid. Mortal. Wkly Rep.,* **26,** 266.

Chang, F. M., Sakai, Y. and Ashizawa, S. (1973). Bacterial pollution and disinfection of the colonofiberscope. II: Ethylene oxide gas sterilization. *Dig. Dis.,* **18,** 951–8.

Corlin, R. F. (1972), Snare wire fracture during colonic polypectomy. *Gastrointest. Endosc.,* **19,** 90.

Coughlin, G. P., Butler, R. N., Alp, M. H. and Grant, A. K. (1977), Colonoscopy and bacteremia. *Gut,* **18,** 678–9.

Curtiss, L. E. (1973), High frequency currents in endoscopy: a review of principles and precautions. *Gastrointest. Endosc.,* **20,** 9–12.

Dagradi, A. E., Alaama, A. and Ruiz, R. (1975), Clinical experiences with colonoscopy: a review of 100 cases. *Am. J. Gastroent.,* **63,** 408–13.

Dagradi, A. E., Riff, D. S., Norum, T. M. and Juler, G. (1976), A complication of colonoscopic (caecal) polypectomy. *Am. J. Gastroent.,* **65,** 449–53.

Del Vecchio, P. J. (1978), Apnea after intravenous diazepam administration (Letter to the editor), *J. Am. Med. Ass.,* **239,** 614.

Dickman, M. D., Farrell, R., Higgs, R. H., Wright, L. E., Humphries, T. J., Wojcik, J. D. and Chappelka, R. (1976), Colonoscopy associated bacteremia. *Surgery Gynec. Obstet.,* **142,** 173–6.

Dunkerley, R. C., Cromer, M. D. Edmiston, C. E. Jr. and Dunn, G. D. (1977), Practical technique for adequate cleansing of endoscopes: a bacteriological study of pHisoHex and Betadine. *Gastrointest. Endosc.,* **23,** 148–9.

Ecker, M. D., Goldstein, M., Hoexter, B., Hyman, R. A., Naidich, J. B. and Stein, H. L. (1977), Benign pneumoperitoneum after fiberoptic colonoscopy: a prospective study of 100 patients. *Gastroenterology,* **73,** 226–30.

Ellis, W. R., Harrison, J. M. and Williams, R. S. (1979), Rupture of spleen at colonoscopy. *Br. Med. J.,* **1,** 307–8.

Erdman, L H., Boggs, H. W. Jr. and Slagle, G. W. (1979), Electrical ileal perforation: an unusual complication of colonoscopy. *Dis. Colon Rec.,* **22,** 501–2.

Fein, R. L. (1967), Transurethal electrocautery procedures in patients with cardiac pacemakers. *J. Am. Med. Ass.,* **202,** 101–3.

Frühmorgen, P. and Demling, L. (1979), Complications of diagnostic and therapeutic colonoscopy in the Federal Republic of Germany. Results of an inquiry. *Endoscopy,* **2,** 146–50.

Geenen, J. E., Schmitt, Jr. M. G., Wu, W. C. and Hogan, W. J. (1975), Major complications of colonoscopy: bleeding and perforation. *Am. J. Dig. Dis.,* **20,** 231–5.

Glouberman, S., Craner, G. E., Ogburn, R. M. and Burdick, G. E. (1976), Radiologic survey for extraluminal air following gastrointestinal tract fiberendoscopy. *Gastrointest. Endosc.,* **22,** 165–7.

Gordon, M. J. (1975), Retroperitoneal emphysema from colonoscopy of the distal limb of a Hartmann colostomy. *Gastrointest. Endosc.,* **22,** 101–2.

Graham, J. and Eusebio, E. B. (1977), Complications of colonoscopy. *Illinois Med. J.,* **152,** 39–42.

Hall, S. C. and Ovassapian, A. (1977), Apnea after intravenous diazepam therapy. *J. Am. Med. Ass.,* **238,** 1052.

Hartong, W. A., Barnes, W. G. and Calkins, W. G. (1977), The absence of bacteremia during colonoscopy. *Am. J. Gastroent.,* **67,** 240–4.

Hoare, A. M. (1974), Pulmonary embolus after diazepam sedation. (Letter to editor.) *J. Am. Med. Ass.,* **230,** 210.

Hogstedt, C., Malmqvist, N. and Wadman, B. (1979), Leukemia in workers exposed to ethylene oxide. *J. Am. Med. Ass.,* **241,** 1132–3.

Hoofnagle, J. H., Blake, J., Buskell-Bales, Z. and Seeff, L. B. (1980), Lack of transmission of type B hepatitis by fiberoptic upper endoscopy. *J. Clin. Gastroent.,* **2,** 65–69.

Jacobsohn, W. Z. and Levy, A. (1976), Colonoscopic perforation: its emergency treatment. *Endoscopy,* **8,** 15–17.

Kaplan, E. L. *et al.* (1977), Prevention of bacterial endocarditis. *Circulation,* **56,** 139A.

Kleinfield, G. and Gump, F. E. (1960), Complications of colotomy and polypectomy. *Surgery Gynec. Obstet.* **111,** 726–8.

Knoepp, L. F. (1977), Colonoscopy in clinical practice. *South. Med. J.,* **70,** 526–30.

Koretz, R. L. and Camacho, R. (1979), Failure of endoscopic transmission of hepatitis B. *Dig. Dis. Sci.,* **24,** 21–24.

Koyama, Y. (1974), Fiberscopic examination of colo-rectal diseases. *Am. J. Proctol.,* **25,** 51–58.

Kozarek, R. A., Earnest, D. L., Silverstein, M. E. and Smith, R. G. (1980), Air-pressure-induced colon injury during diagnostic colonoscopy. *Gastroenterology,* **78,** 7–14.

Langdon, D. E. (1973), Thrombophlebitis following diazepam. *J. Am. Med. Ass.,* **225,** 1389.

Langdon, D. E., Harlan, J. R. and Bailey, R. L. (1973), Thrombophlebitis with diazepam used intravenously. *J. Am. Med. Ass.,* **223,** 184–5.

Levitt, M. D. (1971), Volume and composition of human intestinal gas determined by means of an intestinal washout technic. *New Engl. J. Med.,* **284**, 1394–8.

Lezak, M. G. and Goldhamer, M. (1974), Retroperitoneal emphysema after colonoscopy. *Gastroenterology,* **66**, 118–20.

Livstone, E. M., Cohen, G. M., Troncale, F. J. and Touloukian, R. J. (1974), Diastatic serosal lacerations: an unrecognized complication of colonoscopy. *Gastroenterology,* **67**, 1245–7.

Livstone, E. M. and Kerstein, M. D. (1976), Serosal tears following colonoscopy. *Arch. Surg.,* **111**, 88.

Mac Kichan, J., Duffner, P. K. and Cohen, M. E. (1979), Adsorption of diazepam to plastic tubing. (Letter to the editor.) *New Engl. J. Med.,* **301**, 332–4.

McDonald, G. B. and Silverstein, F. E. (1976), Can gastrointestinal endoscopy transmit hepatitis B to patients? *Gastrointest. Endosc.,* **22**, 168–70.

Manier, J. W. (1978), Fiberoptic pansigmoidoscopy: an evaluation of its use in an office practice. *Gastrointest. Endosc.,* **24**, 119–20.

Marks, G., Boggs, W., Castro, A. F., Gathwright, J. B., Ray, J. and Salvati, E. (1979), Sigmoidoscopic examinations with rigid and flexible fiberoptic sigmoidoscopes in the surgeon's office: a comparative prospective study of effectiveness in 1012 cases. *Dis. Colon Rect.,* **22**, 162–8.

Meyer, G. W. (1979), Prophylaxis of infective endocarditis during gastrointestinal procedures: report of a survey. *Gastrointest. Endosc.,* **25**, 1–2.

Meyers, M. A. (1974), Radiological features of the spread and localization of extraperitoneal gas and their relationship to its source. An anatomical approach. *Radiology,* **111**, 17–26.

Meyers, M. A. and Ghahremani, G. G. (1975), Complications of fiberoptic endoscopy. II. Colonoscopy. *Radiology,* **155**, 301–8.

Moldow, R. E. and McGregor, J. J. (1974), Transcolonic polypectomy. *Arizona Med.,* **31**, 267–9.

Nivatvongs, S. and Goldberg, S. M. (1979), Experience with colonoscopic polypectomy; review of 700 polyps. *Minnesota Med.,* **62**, 197–9.

Nordahl, D. L., Silber, F. J., Robbins, A. H. and O'Hara, E. T. (1973), Nonfatal venous intravasation from the site of diverticulitis during barium enema examination. *Dig. Dis.,* **18**, 253–6.

Norfleet, R. G. (1974), Colonoscopy experience in 100 examinations. *Wisconsin Medical Journal,* **73**, 66–68.

Norfleet, R. G., Mitchell, P. D., Mulholland, D. D. and Philo, J. (1976a), Does bacteremia follow colonoscopy? *Gastrointest. Endosc.,* **23**, 31–32.

Norfleet, R. G., Mulholland, D. D., Mitchell, P. D., Philo, J. and Walters, E. W. (1976b), Does bacteremia follow colonoscopy? *Gastroenterology,* **70**, 20–21.

O'Donoghue, J. K. (1973), Inhibition of a demand pacemaker by electrosurgery. *Chest,* **64**, 664–6.

Overholt, B. F. (1971), Flexible fiberoptic sigmoidoscopy: technique and preliminary results. *Cancer,* **28**, 123–6.

Overholt, B. F., Hargrove, R. L., Farris, R. K. and Wilson, B. (1976), Colonoscopic polypectomy: silent perforation. *Gastroenterology,* **70**, 112–13.

Prorok, J. J., Stahler, E. J., Hartzell, G. W. Jr. and Sugarman, H. J. (1977), Surgical management of colonoscopic perforation (abstract). *Gastrointest. Endosc.,* **23**, 238.

Rafoth, R. J., Sorenson, R. M. and Bond, J. H. Jr. (1975), Bacteremia following colonoscopy. *Gastrointest. Endosc.,* **22**, 32–33.

Ragins, H., Shinya, H. and Wolff, W. I. (1974), The explosive potential of colonic gas during colonoscopic electrosurgical polypectomy. *Surgery Gynec. Obstet.,* **138**, 554–6.

Ramakrishnan, T. (1979), Adynamic ileus complicating colonoscopy. *South. Med. J.,* **72**, 92–93.

Rand, A. A. (1977), Hemorrhage following coagulation biopsy of larger than diminutive polyps of the cecum: report of 2 cases (abstract). *Gastrointest. Endosc.,* **23**, 239.

Rees, B. I. and Williams, L. A. (1977), Incarceration of hernia after colonoscopy. *Lancet,* **1**, 371.

Roberts, R., Campbell, C. B. and Isbister, W. H. (1976), Two complications of diagnostic colonoscopy. *Med. J. Aust.,* **2**, 793–4.

Rogers, B. H. G. (1974), The safety of carbon dioxide insufflation during colonoscopic electrosurgical polypectomy. *Gastrointest. Endosc.,* **20**, 115–17.

Rogers, B. H. G., Silvis, S. E., Nebel, O. T., Sugawa, C. and Mandelstam, P. (1975), Complications of flexible fiberoptic colonoscopy and polypectomy. *Gastrointest. Endosc.,* **22**, 73–77.

Saltzman, H. A. and Sieker, H. O. (1968), Intestinal response to changing gaseous environments: normobaric and hyperbaric observations. *Ann. N.Y. Acad. Sci.,* **150**, 31–39.

Shinya, H. and Wolff, W. I. (1975), Colonoscopic polypectomy: technique and safety. *Hosp. Pract.,* **10**, 71–78.

Sjogren, T. W. Jr., Johnson, L. F., Butler, M. L., Heit, H. A., Gremillion, D. E. and Cammerer, R. C. (1978), Serosal laceration: a complication of intraoperative colonoscopy explained by transmural pressure gradients. *Gastrointest. Endosc.,* **24**, 239–42.

Smith, L. E. (1976), Fiberoptic colonoscopy: complications of colonoscopy and polypectomy. *Dis. Colon Rect.,* **19**, 407–12.

Spencer, R. J., Coates, H. L. and Anderson, M. J. (1974), Colonoscopic polypectomies. *Mayo Clinic Proc.,* **49**, 40–43.

Stearns, M., Williams, C., Hoexter, B., Anderson, M. and Gathright, B. (1975), Symposium: Evaluation of colonoscopic examination. *Dis. Colon Rect.,* **18**, 365–85.

Sugarbaker, P. H. and Vineyard, G. C. (1973), Fiberoptic colonoscopy. A new look at old problems. *Am. J. Surg.,* **125**, 429–31.

Sugarbaker, P. H. Vineyard, G. C., Lewicki, A. M., Pinkus, G. S., Warhol, M. J. and Moore, F. D. (1974), Colonoscopy in the management of diseases of the colon and rectum. *Surgery Gynec. Obstet.,* **139**, 341–9.

Taylor, R., Weakley, F. L. and Sullivan, B. H. Jr. (1978), Non-operative management of colonoscopic perforation with pneumoperitoneum. *Gastrointest. Endosc.,* **24**, 124–5.

Telmos, A. J. and Mittal, V. K. (1977), Splenic rupture following colonoscopy. (Letter to editor.) *J. Am. Med. Ass.,* **237**, 2718.

Ujeyl, A. K., Wurbs, D., Adam, W. and Classen, M. (1978), Gas sterilization of fiber endoscopes. *Endoscopy,* **10**, 71–74.

Vawter, M., Ruiz, R., Alaama, A., Aronow, W. S. and Dagradi, A. E. (1975), Electrocardiographic monitoring during colonoscopy. *Am. J. Gastroent.,* **63**, 155–7.

Waye, J. D. (1975), Colonoscopy: a clinical view. *Mt Sinai J. Med.,* **41**, 1–34.

Wertkin, M. G., Wetchler, B. B., Waye, J. D. and Brown, L. K. (1976), Pneumotosis coli associated with volvulus and colonoscopy. *Am. J. Gastroent.,* **65**, 209–14.

Williams, C. B. (1973), Diathermy-biopsy: a technique for endoscopic management of small polyps. *Endoscopy,* **5**, 215–18.

Williams, C. B. and Gillespie, P. E. (1979), Accidental removal of ureteral stoma at colonoscopy. *Gastrointest. Endosc.,* **25**, 109–10.

Williams, C. B. *et al.* (1973), Colonoscopy: an air pressure hazard. *Lancet,* **2**, 729.

Williams, C. B. and Tan, G. (1979), Complications of colonoscopy and polypectomy (abstract). *Gut,* **20**, A903.

Winawer, S. J., Leidner, S. D., Boyle, C. and Kurtz, R. C. (1979), Comparison of flexible sigmoidoscopy with other diagnostic techniques in the diagnosis of rectocolon neoplasia. *Dig. Dis.,* **24**, 277–81.

Wu, T. K. (1978), Occult injuries during colonoscopy: measurement of forces required to injure the colon and report of cases. *Gastrointest. Endosc.,* **24**, 236–8.

Yassinger, S., Midgley, R. C., Cantor, D. S., Poirier, T. and Imperato, T. J. (1978), Retroperitoneal emphysema after colonoscopic polypectomy. *West. J. Med.,* **128**, 347–50.

PART TWO

Clinical Practice

CHAPTER FOURTEEN

Rectal Bleeding

EDWIN T. SWARBRICK and RICHARD H. HUNT

14.1 The problem

14.1.1 *The size and nature of the problem*

Intestinal bleeding is a common clinical problem whether it presents as anaemia with occult blood loss, minor rectal bleeding or more acutely as haematemesis, melaena or massive rectal bleeding. The problems of management in these cases are well known and the mortality from massive bleeding is high. This chapter concerns the place of colonoscopy in the diagnosis and treatment of lower gastrointestinal bleeding. Because rectal bleeding frequently reflects the presence of treatable organic disease, it should always be investigated promptly and thoroughly.

The exact prevalence of minor rectal bleeding or occult blood loss in the general population is unknown but it is a common presenting feature in gastrointestinal clinics. In 440 consecutive cases referred to St. Mark's Hospital by family practitioners for the investigation of probable colorectal disease, 311 (71%) complained of rectal bleeding (Williams and Thompson, 1977). In a further series of 183 similar patients referred to a general hospital, 66 (36%) complained of frank rectal bleeding and 27 (15%) had occult blood in the stool as determined by Haemoccult testing (Hunt *et al.*, 1980).

14.1.2 *The causes of rectal bleeding*

The persistence of rectal bleeding in the absence of any other symptoms may not immediately be recognized as a sign of serious disease and the diagnosis of haemorrhoids or anal fissure may be made too readily; other important causes are listed in Table 14.1.

Colorectal cancer commonly presents with rectal bleeding which can occur in up to 80% of patients with a carcinoma of the rectum, gradually decreasing with more proximal tumours to 30% in patients with caecal or ascending colon lesions (Staniland, Ditchburn and

267

Table 14.1 Causes of rectal bleeding

Haemorrhoids	Diverticular disease
Anal fissure	Vascular abnormality
Polyps	Angiodysplasia
	Angioma
Carcinomas	Varices
Inflammatory bowel disease	Causes above the ileocaecal value
Ulcerative colitis	Meckels diverticulum, etc.
Crohn's disease	
Ischaemic colitis	Causes of upper gastrointestinal
Infective	bleeding
Solitary ulcer syndrome	
Radiation colitis	

de Dombal, 1976). Right-sided lesions, however, commonly present with anaemia due to occult bleeding (Plate 108).

The diagnosis of a carcinoma leading to elective surgery is preferable to emergency surgery for obstruction or perforation which carries a high morbidity and mortality (Holliday and Hardcastle, 1979). Whether colonoscopy or indeed any other technique will lead to the diagnosis of 'early' carcinoma and a reduced mortality remains to be seen; if so, it will be in conjunction with an increased clinical suspicion or in the screening of asymptomatic subjects. It is not yet clear if colorectal cancer is ever 'early' in terms of patient survival. Current evidence suggests that the prognosis of a tumour depends upon its biology while its differentiation and staging at diagnosis, based on its spread, are only a reflection of this.

Rectal bleeding commonly occurs in up to 50% of patients with colorectal polyps and colonoscopic polypectomy is both diagnostic and curative (Williams *et al.*, 1974). Most carcinomas of the rectum and colon arise from a benign adenoma and the removal of a benign polyp from the rectum will decrease the risk of rectal cancer (Gilbertsen, 1974). Whether removal of polyps will contribute to a reduction in the incidence of colonic as well as rectal carcinoma is not yet known (see Chapter 10) but early evidence suggests that this will be so (Gilbertsen *et al.*, 1979). Rectal bleeding is also a prominent presenting symptom of inflammatory bowel disease and may be present in up to 90% of patients with ulcerative colitis and more than 60% of patients with Crohn's disease of the colon (Staniland, Ditchburn and de Dombal, 1976).

Although rectal bleeding is most often chronic, it may also be acute, massive and dangerous. Colonoscopy has been considered by some authors to be an unsuitable investigation in these patients (Hedberg, 1974; Sivak, Sullivan and Rankin, 1974), but we and others (Rossini and Ferrari, 1976; Hunt and Buchanan, 1979; Forde, 1980) have found it useful and the subject is discussed in more detail in this book (Chapter 15).

Slow occult blood loss often contributes to anaemia and may be the only sign of carcinoma or vascular abnormality of the right side of the colon. The causes of upper gastrointestinal blood loss should be excluded first by barium meal, oesophagogastroduodenoscopy and if this does not reveal the cause, by barium follow-through examination or small bowel enema.

14.2 The approach to the problem

14.2.1 *Approach by the primary care physician*

Rectal bleeding must be taken seriously by the family practitioner and promptly investigated if patients are to be treated properly. A history should be taken with particular attention being paid to the patient's age, sex and past medical history. There is an increased incidence of colorectal cancer in people over the age of 40, in women who have also had carcinoma of the breast or genitalia, and in those patients who have a family history of colorectal cancer, familial polyposis or previous colorectal neoplasm (Winawer *et al.*, 1976). Particular attention must be paid to the colour of blood being passed, whether it is mixed in with the stools or merely on the lavatory paper and whether it is associated with an alteration in bowel habit, appetite or weight. Abdominal pain, particularly if this is a new symptom, may be highly significant and attention should be paid to the site of pain, its radiation and relationship to eating, defaecation and passage of flatus. General symptoms such as lethargy, fatigue and weight loss may be important pointers to significant disease.

A full physical examination must be carried out with particular attention being paid to the external examination of the anal canal; the examination glove should be inspected for the presence of blood.

Proctoscopic examination of the anal canal can be performed with ease by any doctor and is the only way to diagnose haemorrhoids which are not prolapsed. Haemorrhoids, even if present, may not be the cause of bleeding and the decision to investigate further demands clinical judgement. Sigmoidoscopy is the next investigation of choice and should be performed before the barium enema to exclude the presence of rectal disease and it is at this stage that the decision to seek specialist advice must be taken.

14.2.2 *Approach by the hospital specialist*

In addition to taking a careful history and performing a full general examination, the specialist must perform a proctosigmoidoscopy on all patients with rectal bleeding, however firmly the clinical evidence points to the diagnosis of haemorrhoids or anal fissure. It is most important that patients should first be sigmoidoscoped without any form of preparation or wash-out. Such preparation may wash away luminal contents including stool, blood or pus and may change the appearances of the rectal mucosa preventing the clinician from observing early changes of inflammatory bowel disease. Furthermore, some bowel preparations produce a non-specific increase in inflammatory cells in the mucosa which may mislead both the histologist and the clinician. The examination may be repeated after a wash-out to enable the sigmoidoscope to be passed to its fullest extent when the lumen of the bowel above the rectosigmoid junction may be seen and biopsy readily performed when necessary. Although many colorectal cancers are within the reach of the rigid sigmoidoscope, adenomatous polyps are a more common finding than carcinoma and are seen in between 4.7% and 9.7% of asymptomatic patients undergoing routine sigmoidoscopy (Wilson, Dale and Brines, 1955; Hertz, Deddish and Day, 1960; Moertel, Hill and Dockerty, 1966). Expertise in the technique of sigmoidoscopy is readily learned but Madigan and Halls (1968) have stressed the importance of experience. They showed that in 58% of their patients the sigmoidoscope did not reach more than the last few centimetres of the distal sigmoid colon, when the position of the sigmoidoscope was checked by radiology. Stretching of the rectum often accounted for an apparently greater insertion of the instrument.

Flexible fibreoptic sigmoidoscopes with a working length of 55–65 cm are increasingly widely available, relatively easy to use and give an excellent view of the left side of the colon. They may be passed as far as the splenic flexure (Bohlman *et al.*, 1977; Winnan *et al.*, 1980) (see also Chapter 10).

If there is a history of diarrhoea or a suggestion of inflammatory bowel disease, rectal biopsies should be taken as there is often macroscopic sparing of the rectum which may nevertheless show histological abnormalities.

14.2.3 *The relationship of barium enema to colonoscopy*

The standard barium enema was described by Haenisch in 1911 and air contrast studies remain the principal investigation in the diagnosis of colonic disease despite the advent of colonoscopy (Chapter 7). These can provide an accurate picture of the whole colon, especially demonstrating mass lesions and strictures and the newer techniques are sensitive enough to show minor mucosal abnormalities. Although there is little difference between colonoscopy and barium enema from the point of view of patient preference, time spent and the bowel preparation required, colonoscopy is usually performed with some sedation and a period of recovery is necessary. There is also a definite risk of complications such as perforation or even death (Rogers *et al.*, 1975; Smith and Nivatvongs, 1975; Colin-Jones, Cockel and Schiller, 1978), as a result of colonoscopy; in contrast the risks of barium enema are negligible.

Barium enema may fail unavoidably to demonstrate some lesions such as those which are sessile and flat and even the best double contrast studies can fail to detect mild but often extensive inflammatory bowel disease (Williams, C. B., personal communication) or mucosal vascular abnormalities. The results are also difficult to interpret in diverticular disease or after colonic surgery where lesions may be missed whether at the region of the anastamosis or in those patients who have a colostomy.

While colonoscopy can detect mucosal lesions which are not seen by the best radiological techniques, the avoidable failures of the barium enema are usually due to the errors of technique and interpretation. This occurs either because the correct films have not been taken or have not been scrutinized carefully, because of poor bowel preparation or because of a tortuous sigmoid colon. Failures may also occur with overfilling of the terminal ileum, where there is a particularly long colon with overlapping flexures or in patients where there is spasm or residue in the caecum. In a small group of patients where a carcinoma was detected by colonoscopy following a normal barium enema, it was found that almost all the patients had presented with rectal bleeding or anaemia and none with unexplained mucous discharge or a change in bowel habits (Williams, Swarbrick and Hunt, 1975). Commonly these lesions were undiagnosed because of poor reading of the barium enema films, most of which had been performed at the referring hospitals. Nevertheless, the missed lesions were frequently detectable on review of the barium enema.

The lesion demonstrated in the single contrast barium enema in (Fig. 14.1) was present on all views of the sigmoid colon but was not reported by the radiologist or the clinician who referred the patient for colonoscopy. A large pedunculated polyp (Fig. 14.2) was found at colonoscopy and removed. In the double contrast study (Fig. 14.3) an overlying loop of bowel obscures the annular carcinoma in the sigmoid colon which was missed prior to colonoscopy. Whereas colonoscopy

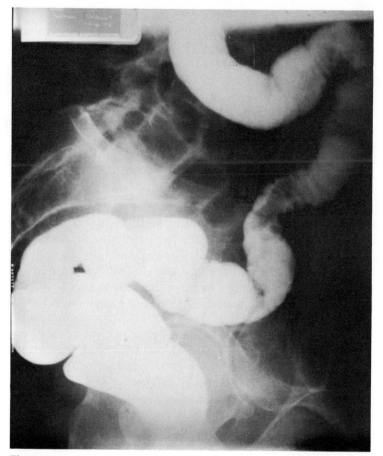

Fig.14.1 A single-contrast barium enema. The lesion (arrowed) was present in three views but not reported by the radiologist or the referring clinician.

would have been indicated in the first case even if the lesion had been seen, it might have been avoided in the second, if the films available had been carefully scrutinized or the correct film, i.e. the opposite oblique view, taken.

A decision that is sometimes difficult to make is whether to repeat an unsatisfactory barium enema during the investigation of intestinal bleeding. It is often more expedient to proceed straight to colonoscopy since a polyp found on X-ray will require removal, a suspicious area may require biospsy and a further unsatisfactory enema will, in any case, be an indication for colonoscopy. Furthermore, colonoscopy can detect those mucosal lesions which are undetectable by the best double contrast barium enemas.

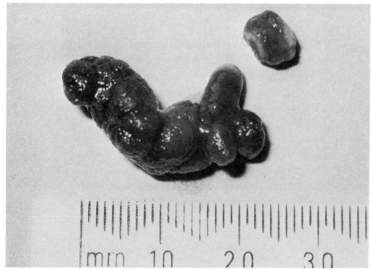

Fig. 14.2 An irregular pedunculated polyp and stalk removed at colonoscopy from the patient whose barium enema is shown in Fig. 14.1.

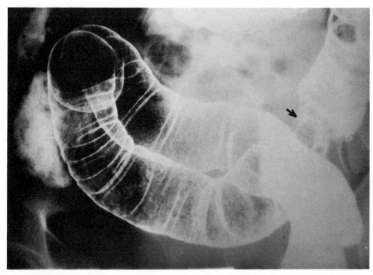

Fig. 14.3 The oblique pelvic view of a double-contrast barium enema. The radiologist did not take the opposite oblique film and missed the annular carcinoma (arrowed).

14.3 The findings on colonoscopy

It is in the investigation of unexplained rectal bleeding that colonoscopy has proved to be a most accurate and valuable investigative technique. In an early study reported from St. Mark's Hospital (Swarbrick *et al.*, 1976), 239 patients with persistent unexplained rectal bleeding were examined by colonoscopy. Local anorectal conditions had been excluded by digital rectal and proctosigmoidoscopic examination and the patients had all had a barium enema, many of which had used double contrast techniques. In all patients the barium enema had been reported as being normal. The whole colon was examined in 95% of patients and a causative lesion was found in 95 patients (40%). Of these 95 patients, 39 had polyps which were removed by diathermy snare. Twenty-four patients had inflammatory bowel disease and nine had miscellaneous conditions such as diverticular disease or vascular abnormalities etc. Most important however were the 23 patients (10%) who had carcinoma which had been missed at the original barium examination. The results of the study were in close agreement with those of others (Table 14.2) and in these reported series a probable cause of bleeding was found in 582 of 1456 (40%) patients; carcinomas were found in 153 (10.5%). These results do not suggest that colonoscopy is better than barium enema at diagnosing such lesions since the clinical suspicion in all these series was high and the investigations were performed by enthusiastic colonoscopists. Indeed in one series (Hunt, 1980) almost 50% of 'missed' carcinomas were identifiable on subsequent careful review of the X-ray films: furthermore, many of the films were of poor quality and in some, single contrast only. However, for reasons of expediency and those discussed previously, colonoscopy was performed rather than a further barium enema.

14.3.1 *Colorectal cancer*

Colorectal cancer is the most important cause of rectal bleeding and is responsible for over 16 000 deaths per annum in England and Wales (OPCS Mortality Statistics, 1976) and second only to carcinoma of the lung and bronchus as a cause of death from malignant neoplasms. In the United States it is the commonest malignant disease responsible for 100 000 deaths per annum (Winawer, Melamed and Sherlock, 1976). If half to two thirds of colorectal cancers present with rectal bleeding (Staniland, Ditchburn and de Dombal, 1976) up to 11 000 patients per year in England and Wales who suffer from this condition will report rectal bleeding to their doctor.

Fifty per cent of all colonic carcinomas have been said to occur in the

Table 14.2 Colonoscopy in barium enema-negative rectal bleeding

Author	Number of patients	Carcinoma	Polyp	Inflammatory bowel disease	Other	Total
Hunt et al. (1980)	698	67 (10%)	110	60	55	292 (42%)
Penfold (1975)	71	12 (17%)	11	1	2	26 (36%)
Waye (1976)	93	15 (16%)	14	10	17	56 (60%)
Britton et al. (1977)	30	5 (16%)	8	1	0	14 (47%)
Tedesco et al. (1978)	258	29 (11%)	39	19	15	102 (39.5%)
Brand et al. (1980)	306	25 (8.2%)	43	11	13	92 (30%)
Total	1456	153 (10.5%)	225	102	102	582 (40%)

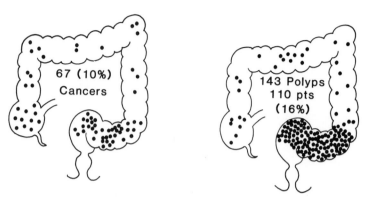

Fig. 14.4 The sites of 67 cancers and 143 polyps in 110 patients detected at colonoscopy from a group of 698 patients who had persistent rectal bleeding and otherwise normal investigation (Hunt *et al.*, 1980).

descending or sigmoid colon (Aylett, 1968) and 55% of colorectal cancers to be within reach of the conventional 30 cm rigid sigmoidoscope (Winawer, Melamed and Sherlock, 1976). Recent reports however suggest that more cases are occurring above the rectosigmoid junction and these are less easily detected at sigmoidoscopy (Cady *et al.*, 1974; Wolff *et al.*, 1975; Snyder, Heston and Meigs, 1977; Rhodes *et al.*, 1977). As might be expected those carcinomas found at colonoscopy are above the rectosigmoid junction and furthermore are distributed throughout the colon (Fig. 14.4) which underlines the importance of a total colonoscopic examination for patients presenting with rectal bleeding.

It is not yet known if the diagnosis of colon cancer by colonoscopy can improve the prognosis of an individual patient but it is of interest that of 51 such patients in whom accurate staging was possible (Buchanan *et al.*, 1980) 15 (29%) were classified as being Dukes' A, 25 (50%) Dukes' B, 9 (18%) Dukes' C and 2 (4%) Dukes' D. Thus 79% of patients had between 70% and 100% chance of a complete cure compared with 50% of patients in previously reported operative series (Morson and Dawson, 1979).

14.3.2 *Polyps*

Adenomatous polyps have been found in approximately 16% of patients who present with rectal bleeding and who undergo colonoscopy (Table 14.2). It is not known why a polyp should bleed but it probably does so due to infarction and resulting necrosis. The tendency for a polyp to bleed does not appear to be related to its size and even small adenomas may be responsible for considerable blood loss (Plate 61).

The real importance of colonic polyps, however, lies in their potential for malignant change (see Chapter 16). A significant number of polyps greater than 1 cm are malignant, with up to a 40% risk of malignancy if the polyp exceeds 2 cm and there is a widely held belief that most, if not all, carcinomas develop in adenomatous tissue (Morson, 1974; 1976). The appearance of a polyp either on barium enema or on direct vision at endoscopy gives no information about its nature and histological examination is essential. Since simple forceps biopsy of such lesions provides an inadequate specimen for histological appraisal (Hellwig and Barbosa, 1952), they should be removed by diathermy snare. Diagnosis and treatment are therefore effected simultaneously, quickly and safely and there is a significant reduction in the cost, period of hospitalization and the patient's absence from work.

It must always be remembered that the patient who has one adenomatous polyp or carcinoma has an increased risk of having a second simultaneous lesion (Morson, 1974), either further polyps or a second cancer and this possibility must always be excluded. Similarly, metachronous lesions may develop in patients who already have a history of one or more colonic neoplasms (Morson, 1976) and colonoscopy may play an important part in the long-term follow-up of such patients as will be discussed in Chapter 17.

14.3.3 *Diverticular disease*

Diverticular disease is a common condition probably occurring in 10% of patients over the age of 40 and 35% of patients over the age of 60 (Morson and Dawson, 1979). Severe distortion of the sigmoid colon with local contraction of circular muscle prevents even high quality barium studies from adequately displaying the diseased segment of colon. Localized strictures are common and present considerable diagnostic difficulties for both the clinician and radiologist; in the past, the cause of such strictures was often found only at laparotomy. Similarly, it is often difficult to demonstrate the presence of a carcinoma, polyp or inflammatory bowel disease in the diverticular segment.

Bleeding may occur from diverticula themselves and lead to mild, moderate or massive blood loss. Rigg and Ewing (1966) reviewed more than 5000 patients with diverticular disease and only 15% showed evidence of haemorrhage. In their extensive review of the literature they found that bleeding was reported in 5% to 41% of all such patients.

In five reported studies where colonoscopy has been used to evaluate complicated diverticular disease (Dean and Newell, 1973; Greene, Livstone and Troncale, 1974; Sugarbaker *et al.*, 1979; Hunt *et al.*, 1975; Hunt, 1979), the results show that 26 carcinomas (15%) were found in 169 patients with severe diverticular disease.

At colonoscopy, the site of bleeding may be localized to a particular diverticulum although the bleeding point itself is rarely seen (Plate 59). In some patients with diverticular disease there may be areas where the vascular pattern of the mucosa has disappeared and the mucosa itself is hyperaemic and friable. These areas tend to occur on the prominent mucosal fold within the diverticular segment (Plate 34). The histological appearances are those of non-specific inflammation, with some dilated veins and increased amounts of stainable iron in the lamina propria and submucosa. These histological appearances suggest local congestive ischaemia possibly resulting from compression of the folds within the lumen (Morson, personal communication, 1980).

Massive rectal bleeding which may occur more frequently from the right side of the colon (Casarella, Kanter and Seaman, 1972) may be caused by recurrent diverticula damage leading to the sudden asymmetric rupture of a submucosal artery towards the lumen of the diverticulum at the antemesenteric margin (Meyers, Alonso and Gray *et al.*, 1976). However, angiodysplasia is being found more frequently and diverticular disease less frequently in patients with massive rectal bleeding.

14.3.4 *Inflammatory bowel disease*

Ten per cent of patients undergoing colonoscopy for barium enema negative rectal bleeding may be found to have unsuspected inflammatory bowel disease at colonoscopy (Table 14.2). In patients with histologically proven ulcerative colitis, bleeding may be seen from wide areas of the colonic mucosa which is friable but in Crohn's disease friability is less common and bleeding may be seen coming from individual ulcers. Postinflammatory or pseudopolyps are an unusual site of bleeding but adenomatous polyps, although uncommon, occur more frequently than in the general population (Teague and Read, 1975). Since it is impossible to distinguish either on X-ray or by visual appearances between a large pseudopolyp and an adenomatous polyp it is probably wise to biopsy all large polyps in patients with inflammatory bowel disease. Whether an adenomatous polyp in a patient with ulcerative colitis represents premalignant change in an unstable mucosa is unknown but it would seem prudent to follow such patients carefully with frequent rectal biopsies.

The clinician should ensure that patients are not suffering from severe attacks of colitis when considering colonoscopy because this is a contraindication to the procedure (see Chapter 2). This is unlikely to be so in patients being investigated for colonic bleeding only.

A number of other inflammatory conditions of the large bowel which may present with rectal bleeding, pose difficulties in differential diagnosis and may be missed on the barium enema examination.

Amoebic and schistosomal colitis
Infective conditions are generally a contraindication to colonoscopy but amoebic colitis may be diagnosed in the absence of barium enema changes when the characteristic ulceration may be seen in those areas difficult for the radiologist to display clearly such as the caecum and sigmoid colon. In acute disease, the mucosa is inflamed and friable and resembles that seen in acute radiation colitis (Plate 171). In chronic disease, however, the ulceration may be localized but usually consists of discrete small punched out ulcers with a rolled oedematous margin (Plate 172).

The colon may be very abnormal after a long history of infection with *Schistosoma mansoni*. The changes may be those of a stricture or colonic polyposis and although patients may have a normal sigmoidoscopy the polyps may be seen at colonoscopy (Plate 176) (Wright, Renton and Swarbrick, 1976). The diagnosis can be confirmed by the presence of viable schistosome ova in the stools of a patient who gives a history of possible exposure (Nebel *et al.*, 1974).

Antibiotic (pseudomembranous) colitis
Colitis is a well-recognized complication of antibiotic therapy (Scott, Nicholson and Kerr, 1973; Beavis, Parsons and Salfield, 1976). Rectal bleeding alone is unusual in this condition and the patients usually present with diarrhoea. The diagnosis is most frequently made at sigmoidoscopy but the rectum may be spared and the barium enema normal. The mucosa is hyperaemic and friable and often studded with the characteristic creamy plaques of pseudomembrane (Plate 168). Biopsies will usually show acute non-specific inflammation without goblet cell depletion but the 'explosive' plaque-like lesions show typical appearances (Plate 169) (De Ford, Molinaro and Daly, 1974).

Ischaemic colitis
An episode of ischaemic colitis may occur without abdominal pain and patients may present with fresh bleeding. Endoscopy within hours of such an event may show fresh blood in the lumen and superficial serpiginous ulceration in a hyperaemic friable mucosa. There is often a sharp demarcation between normal and abnormal mucosa at each end of the

ischaemic segment (Plates 157, 159, 160, 162 and 165). Biopsies at this stage will show clearly demarcated ulceration of the mucosa with oedema and dilated capillaries packed with blood (Plate 161) (Hunt and Buchanan, 1979). Healed ischaemic strictures may be diagnosed at colonoscopy, when the histology shows haemosiderin deposition within macrophages; these findings carry considerable diagnostic weight (Morson and Dawson, 1979).

Solitary ulcer

Solitary ulcer of the rectum is well recognized (Plate 183) and the histology diagnostic (Madigan and Morson, 1969; Rutter and Riddell, 1975). Solitary non-specific ulcers have also been reported in the colon and may present with rectal bleeding. In one such patient who had a normal barium enema and otherwise normal mucosa two isolated ulcers were observed at the splenic flexure (Kurtz, 1976). Solitary ulcers elsewhere than in the rectum are probably ischaemic in origin.

Radiation colitis

Radiation damage may occur to either large or small intestine and may present with rectal bleeding. A history of radiation therapy usually points to the diagnosis but it must be remembered that such damage may occur 20–30 years after therapy (Morson and Dawson, 1979). Typically, in acute stages, the mucosa is friable but in the healing stage there are usually multiple telangiectasia (Plates 166 and 167); the fusiform stricturing is usually late. Making the correct diagnosis in a female patient who has had irradiation for a pelvic carcinoma excludes the possibility of a recurrence or a second primary tumour.

14.3.5 *Vascular abnormalities*

Angiodysplasia and haemangiomas

Vascular abnormalities of the colon, first described by Phillips in 1839, are an uncommon but increasingly well-recognized cause of colonic bleeding. They are important to recognize, as a cure may be readily effected. Vascular abnormalities, particularly angiodysplasia have been diagnosed more frequently since the development of colonoscopy and the nature of these lesions has been clarified recently (Boley *et al.*, 1979). Angiodysplasia may take several forms (see Plates 48, 49, 52 and 54), the typical lesion being a small mesh of mucosal vessels, sometimes very like the spider naevus seen in the skin of patients with chronic liver disease. These vascular ectasias are now considered to be degenerative in nature and quite separate from constitutional or neoplastic angiomatous malformations; in the past this distinction has not been clear (Bartelheimer, Remele and Ottenjann 1972; Richardson, McInnis and Ramos *et al.*, 1975; Rogers and Adler, 1976; Skibba *et al.*, 1976; Wolff, Grossman and Shinya, 1977).

Angiodysplasia is more common in the elderly and may be a significant cause of blood loss and anaemia (Hunt, 1980). The lesions occur most frequently in the caecum and the ascending colon but may be found elsewhere. They have been reported in association with aortic valvular stenosis and sclerosis (Williams, 1961; Boss and Rosenbaum, 1971; Rogers and Adler, 1976).

In the investigation of rectal bleeding from a suspected vascular abnormality, a plain abdominal X-ray may show calcification of a large haemangioma but this is rare. A barium enema is seldom helpful as the lesions are flat and mucosal or submucosal.

Angiodysplasia may be demonstrated by angiography but smaller lesions may require subtraction or magnification techniques (Galloway, Casarella and Shimkin 1974; Tarin *et al.*, 1978). They may also be demonstrated at colonoscopy; this technique offers therapeutic benefits as the small lesions can be fulgurated by diathermy using insulated biopsy forceps (Williams, 1973; Rogers and Adler, 1976; Hunt, 1980; Rogers, 1980). The mucosa is pulled away from the underlying muscularized mucosa before coagulation is attempted (see Fig. 14.5).

Argon ion laser photocoagulation has been used successfully in the treatment of nine vascular malformations of the colon (Frühmorgen

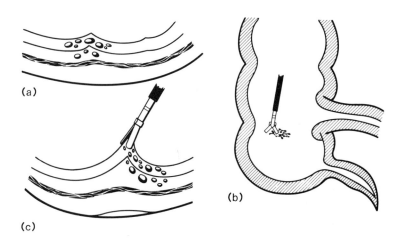

Fig. 14.5 The technique of diathermy biopsy for small angiodysplasia lesions which lie in the mucosa and submucosa (a). The edge of the lesion is picked up in the diathermy forceps (b), and tented away from the thin walled caecum as diathermy is applied (c).

et al., 1976). Electrosurgical and laser techniques are likely to come into more prominence during the next decade for the treatment of these vascular abnormalities (see Chapter 12).

Varices
Varices of the colon (Plate 58) are a rare cause of rectal bleeding but one case has been diagnosed at colonoscopy following a normal barium enema (Geboes, Broeckaert and Vantrappen, 1975).

14.4 The problem in special circumstances

14.4.1 *Acute massive bleeding*

Rectal bleeding may sometimes present as an acute emergency and once the patient has been resuscitated, it is important to identify the site of bleeding. Colonoscopy has been considered an unsuitable investigation in patients with massive colonic haemorrhage (Hedberg, 1974; Sivak, Sullivan and Rankin, 1974) and selective angiography has been recommended as an appropriate first investigation (Reuter and Bookstein, 1968; Nusbaum, Baum and Blakemore, 1969; Giacchino *et al.*, 1979). However, others have found colonoscopy very useful and the subject is reviewed more fully in Chapter 15 of this book. The development of therapeutic procedures for such lesions as angiodysplasia means that colonoscopy must be considered early in the patient's management. It is always important to exclude causes of upper gastrointestinal haemorrhage by endoscopy in these circumstances before proceeding to colonoscopy or angiography.

14.4.2 *Intraoperative colonoscopy*

In some patients a source of gastrointestinal bleeding cannot be found in spite of all investigative measures. Laparotomy may be considered in these circumstances and peroperative endoscopy may be useful (Espiner, Salmon and Teague, 1973; Greenberg *et al.*, 1976; Forde, 1980). For full discussion of this subject, see Chapter 11.

The endoscope may be passed either anally or orally and the whole of the intestine is effectively examined. In this way it is possible to avoid performing enterostomies which carry a high morbidity. Not only can the lumen be effectively examined during this procedure but the intestinal wall is transilluminated and can be examined by the surgeon.

14.4.3 *Colonoscopy in children*

This subject is discussed in detail elsewhere in this book (Chapter 20), but many paediatricians now consider that colonoscopy is a primary investigation for suspected colonic disease in children (Habr-Gama *et al.*, 1979). The commonest indication will probably be rectal bleeding and even large polyps (3–4 cm) can be successfully removed from the small colon without the need for general anaesthetic (Laage *et al.*, 1980).

14.4.4 *Flexible sigmoidoscopy*

This technique is increasingly available and most gastroenterologists will soon be using it as an office or out-patient clinic procedure. This may significantly reduce the number of barium enemas or total colonoscopic examinations required and many of the conditions responsible for bleeding, or indeed other symptoms which would be beyond the reach of the rigid sigmoidoscope will be diagnosed at fibre sigmoidoscopy (Winnan *et al.*, 1980). The subject is discussed fully in Chapter 10.

14.4.5 *Colonoscopy in the investigation of anaemia and occult faecal blood loss*

Colonoscopy is proving to be very useful in the investigation of anaemia and should be considered in those anaemic patients in whom upper intestinal barium studies and endoscopy as well as barium enema and proctosigmoidoscopy have failed to demonstrate a cause. In 59 such patients we have found undiagnosed cancer in 8 (14%) and a definitive diagnosis in a further 20 (34%) (Hunt *et al.*, 1979).

14.4.6 *The limitations of colonoscopy*

Effective colonoscopy depends upon adequate preparation and even the slightest faecal soiling may obscure vascular lesions and small polyps. Significant amounts of fresh or altered blood may also present a problem. Certain areas such as the acute flexures or the proximal surface of a mucosal fold are frequently 'blind spots' and great care and attention should be paid to them. The newer colonoscopes will permit full flexion of the tip and should reduce the incidence of missed lesions at these sites.

Colonoscopy may be impossible in certain patients, notably those who have had previous abdominal or pelvic surgery, irradiation therapy and those with strictures or severe diverticular disease, but in most situations, persistent and careful technique will reduce the number of failures to a minimum.

14.5 Conclusions

Patients who present with persistent rectal bleeding may be suffering from serious treatable disease. While double-contrast barium enema studies remain the investigation of choice in such patients, the results of these investigations may be uncertain or unhelpful. Colonoscopy has revolutionized the investigation and treatment of such patients. Colonic polyps and some vascular abnormalities may be diagnosed and treated simultaneously using this technique, inflammatory bowel disease may be diagnosed and treated appropriately at a time when it is not recognizable by even the best of barium studies and the presence of suspected malignancy may be confirmed or refuted. A negative endoscopy is often a positive contribution to a patient's management. Colonoscopy must be considered in all patients who have rectal bleeding with a normal barium enema and protosigmoidoscopy.

References

Aylett, S. O. (1978), Rectal bleeding with special reference to cancer of the large intestine. *Brit. Med. J.*, **3**, 103–106.
Bartelheimer, W., Remmele, W. and Ottenjann, R. (1972), Coloscopic recognition of hemangiomas in the colon ascendens. *Endoscopy*, **4**, 109–114.
Beavis, J. P., Parsons, R. L. and Salfield, J. (1976), Colitis and diarrhoea, a problem with antibiotic therapy, *Brit. J. Surgery*, **63**, 299–304.
Bohlman, T. W., Katon, R. M., Lipshutz, G. R., McCool, M. F., Smith, F. W. and Melnyk, C. S. (1977), Fiberoptic pansigmoidoscopy. An evaluation and comparison with rigid sigmoidoscopy. *Gastroenterology*, **72**, 644–649.
Boley, S. J., Sammartano, R., Brandt, L. J. and Sprayregen, S. (1979), Vascular ectasias of the colon. *Surg. Gyn. & Obs.*, **149**, 353–359.
Boss, E. G. and Rosenbaum, J. M. (1971), Bleeding from the right colon associated with aortic stenosis. *Am. J. Dig. Dis.*, **16**, 269–275.
Brand, E. J., Sullivan, B. H., Sivak, M. V. and Rankin, G. B. (1980), Colonoscopy in the diagnosis of unexplained rectal bleeding. *Annals of Surgery*, in press.
Britton, D. C., Tregoning, D., Bone, G. and McKelvey, S. T. D. (1977), Colonoscopy in surgical practice. *Brit. Med. J.*, **1**, 149–151.
Buchanan, J. D., Lightfoot, N. L., Thurston, J. R., Teague, R. H., Williams, C. B., Milton-Thompson, G. J. and Hunt, R. H. (1980), Prognosis of colonic carcinomas diagnosed by colonoscopy. *Gut* A454.
Cady, B., Persson, A. V., Morson, D. L. and Maunz, D. C. (1974), Changing patterns of colorectal carcinoma. *Cancer*, **33**, 422–426.
Casarella, W. J., Kanter, I. E. and Seaman, W. B. (1972), Right sided colonic

diverticula as a cause of acute rectal haemorrhage. *N. Engl. J. Med.,* **286**, 450–453.

Colin-Jones, D. G., Cockel, R. and Schiller, K. F. R. (1978), Current endoscopic practice in the United Kindom. *Clin. Gastroentol.* **7**, 775–786.

Dean, A. L. and Newell, J. P. (1973), Colonoscopy in the differential diagnosis of carcinoma from diverticulitis of the sigmoid colon. *Brit. J. Surg.,* **60**, 633–635.

De Ford, J. W., Molinaro, J. R. and Daly, J. J. (1974), Lincomycin- and clindamycin-associated colitis. *Gastrointest. Endosc.,* **21**, 19–21.

Espiner, H. J., Salmon, P. R., Teague, R. H. and Read, A. E. (1973), Operative colonoscopy. *Brit. Med. J.,* **1**, 453–454.

Forde, K. A. (1980), Colonoscopy in acute rectal bleeding. *Congress Forum III 2nd Int. Congression: Colonoscopy and disease of the large bowel.*

Frühmorgen, P., Bodem, F., Reidenbach, H. D., Kaduk, B. and Demling, L. (1976), Endoscopic laser coagulation of bleeding gastrointestinal lesions with report of the first therapeutic application in man. *Gastrointest. Endosco.,* **23**, 73–75.

Galloway, S. J., Casarella, W. J. and Shimkin, P. M. (1974), Vascular malformations of the right colon as a cause of bleeding in patients with aortic stenosis. *Radiology,* **113**, 11–15.

Geboes, K., Broeckaert, L. and Vantrappen, G. (1975), Varices of the colon: Diagnosis by colonoscopy. *Gastrointest. Endosc.,* **22**, 43–45.

Giacchino, J. L., Geis, W. P., Pickleman, J. R., Dado, D. V., Hadcock, W. E. and Freeark, R. (1979), Changing perspectives in massive lower intestinal haemorrhage. *Surgery,* **86**, 368–76.

Gilbertsen, V. A. (1974), Proctosigmoidoscopy and polypectomy in reducing the incidence of rectal cancer. *Cancer,* **34**, 936–939.

Gilbertsen, V. A., Williams, S. E., Schuman, L. and McHugh, R. (1979), Colonoscopy in the detection of carcinoma of the intestine. *Surg. Gynaec. Obs.,* **149**, 877–878.

Greene, F. L., Livstone, E. M. and Troncale, F. J. (1974), Fiberoptic colonoscopy in the managment of colonic disease. *South. Med. J.,* **67**, 105–110.

Greenberg, G. R., Phillips, M. J., Tovee, E. B. and Jeejeebhay, K. N. (1976), Fiberoptic endoscopy during laparotomy in the diagnosis of small intestinal bleeding. *Gastroenterology,* **71**, 133–135.

Habr-Gama, A., Alves, P. R. A., Gama Rodriguez, J. J., Teixeira, M. G. and Barbieri, D. (1979), Paediatric Colonoscopy. *Dis. Col. & Rect.,* **22**, 530–535.

Haenisch, F. (1911), The value of the röentgen ray in the early diagnosis of carcinoma of the bowel. *Am. Q. Roentgenol.,* **3**, 175–183.

Hedberg, S. E. (1974), Endoscopy in gastrointestinal bleeding: A systematic approach to diagnosis. *Surg. Clin. North Am.,* **54**, 549–559.

Hellwig, C. A. and Barbosa, E. (1952), How reliable is biopsy of rectal polyps. *Cancer,* **12**, 620–624.

Hertz, R. E., Deddish, M. R. and Day, E. (1960), Value of periodic examination in detecting cancer of the rectum and colon. *Postgrad. Med.,* **27**, 290–294.

Holliday, H. W. and Hardcastle, J. D. (1979), Delay in diagnosis and treatment of symptomatic colorectal cancer. *Lancet,* **i,** 309–311.

Hunt, R. H. (1978), Colonoscopy in clinical practice. Experience of techniques and clinical application. (Thesis for Gilbert Blane Medal) Royal College of Surgeons of London.

Hunt, R. H. (1979), The role of colonoscopy in complicated diverticular disease. *Acta Chirurgica Belgia,* **6,** 349–353.

Hunt, R. H. (1980), Angiodysplasia – an important cause of gastrointestinal bleeding in the elderly. *Gut,* **21** A460.

Hunt, R. H. and Buchanan, J. D. (1979), Transient ischaemic colitis – Colonoscopy and biopsy in diagnosis. *J. R. Nav. Med. Serv.,* **65(1),** 15–19.

Hunt, R. H., Lightfoot, N. L., Miller, J., Colin-Jones, D. G. and Milton-Thompson, G. J. (1980), Evaluation of the haemocult test in the symptomatic patient. *Hepato Gastroenterology,* Suppl. 1., p. 98, E.15.4.

Hunt, R. H., Swarbrick, E. T., Teague, R. H., Thomas, B. M., Thornton, J. R. and Williams, C. B. (1979), Colonoscopy for unexplained rectal bleeding. *Gastroenterology,* **76(5),** part 2, 1158.

Hunt, R. H., Teague, R. H., Swarbrick, E. T. and Williams, C. B. (1975), Colonoscopy in the management of colonic strictures. *Br. Med. J.,* **2,** 360–1.

Kurtz, M. D. (1976), Colonoscopic diagnosis of non-specific ulcer of the colon. *Gastrointest. Endosc.,* **23** 90–91.

Laage, N. J., Campbell, C. A., Douglas, J. R., Walker-Smith, J. A., Boothe, I. W., Harries, J. T. and Williams, C. B. (1980), *Total colonoscopy in children,* in press.

Madigan, M. R. and Halls, J. M. (1968), The extent of sigmoidoscopy shown on radiographs with special reference to the recto-sigmoid junction. *Gut,* **9,** 355–362.

Madigan, M. R. and Morson, B. C. (1969), Solitary ulcer of the rectum. *Gut,* **10,** 871–881.

Meyers, M. A., Alonso, D. R., Gray, G. F. and Baer, J. W. (1976), Pathogenesis of bleeding colonic diverticulosis. *Gastroenterology,* **71(4),** 577–583.

Moertel, C. G., Hill, J. R. and Dockerty, M. B. (1966), The routine proctoscopic examination: a second look. *Mayo Clin. Proc.,* **41,** 368–374.

Morson, B. C. (1974), The polyp cancer sequence in the large bowel. *Proc. R. Soc. Med.,* **67,** 451–457.

Morson, B. C. (1976), Genesis of Colorectal Cancer. *Clin. Gastroenterol.,* **5(3),** 505–525.

Morson, B. C. and Dawson, I. M. P. (1979), *Gastrointestinal pathology.* Blackwell Scientific Publications, Oxford, 2nd edition.

Nebel, O. T., El-Masry, N. A., Castell, D. O., Farid, Z., Fornes, M. F. and Sparks, H. A. (1974), Schistosomal colonic polyposis: Endoscopic and histologic characteristics. *Gastrointest. Endosc.,* **20,** 99–101.

Nusbaum, M., Baum, S. and Blakemore, W. S. (1969), Clinical experience with the diagnosis and management of gastrointestinal haemorrhage by selective mesenteric catheterisation. *Ann. Surg.,* **170,** 506–514.

Office of Population Censuses and Surveys (1977), *Mortality Statistics for England and Wales 1974,* Series DH 2, no. 1, Table 2 p. 12.

Penfold, J. C. (1975), The results of diagnostic colonoscopy in the management of unexplained bleeding from the rectum. *Aust. N.Z. J. Surg.*, **45(4)**, 361–363.

Phillips, B. (1839), Surgical cases. *London Med. Gas.*, **23**, 514–517.

Reuter, S. R. and Bookstein, J. J. (1968), Angiographic localization of gastro-intestinal bleeding. *Gastroenterology*, **54**, 876–883.

Rhodes, J. B., Holmes, F. F. and Clark, G. M. (1977), Changing distribution of primary cancers in the large bowel. *J. Amer. Med. Assoc.*, **238**, 1641–3.

Richardson, J. D., McInnis, W. D., Ramos, R. and Aust, J. B. (1975), Occult gastrointestinal bleeding: an evaluation of available diagnostic methods. *Arch. Surg.*, **110(5)**, 661–665.

Rigg, B. M. and Ewing, M. R., Current attitudes on diverticulitis with particular reference to colonic bleeding. *Arch. Surg.*, **92**, 321–332.

Rogers, B. H. G. (1980), Endoscopic diagnosis and therapy of mucosal vascular abnormalities of the gastrointestinal tract occurring in elderly patients and associated with cardiac, vascular and pulmonary disease. *Gastrointest. Endosc.*, **26**, 134–38.

Rogers, H. G. and Adler, F. (1976), Hemangiomas of the cecum. Colonoscopic diagnosis and therapy. *Gastroenterology*, **71**, 1079–1082.

Rossini, F. P. and Ferrari, A. (1976), Emergency colonoscopy. *Acta Endosc. Radiochim.*, **6**, 165–168.

Rutter, K. R. P. and Riddell, R. K. (1975), The solitary ulcer syndrome of the rectum. *Clin. Gastroenterol.*, **4(3)**, 505–530.

Scott, A. J., Nicholson, G. I. and Kerr, A. B. (1973), Lincomycin as a cause of pseudomembranous colitis. *Lancet*, **i**, 1232–34.

Sivak, M. V., Jr., Sullivan, B. H., Jr. and Rankin, G. B. (1974), Colonoscopy: a report of 644 cases and review of the literature. *Am. J. Surg.*, **128(3)**, 351–357.

Skibba, R. M., Hartong, W. A., Mantz, F. A., Hinthorn, D. R. and Rhodes, J. B. (1976), Angiodysplasia of the cecum: colonoscopic diagnosis. *Gastrointest. Endosc.*, **22**, 177–179.

Smith, L. E. and Nivatvongs, S. (1975), Complications in colonoscopy. *Dis. Colon Rectum*, **18(3)**, 214–220.

Snyder, D. N., Heston, J. F., Meigs, J. W. and Flannery, J. T. (1977), Changes in site distribution of colorectal carcinoma in Connecticut 1940–1973. *Am. J. Dig. Dis.*, **22(9)**, 791–797.

Staniland, J. R., Ditchburn, J. and de Dombal, F. T. (1976), Clinical presentation of diseases of the large bowel. (A detailed study of 642 patients) *Gastroenterology*, **70(1)**, 22–28.

Sugarbaker, P. H., Vineyard, G. C., Lewicki, A. M., *et al.* (1974), Colonoscopy in the management of diseases of the colon and rectum. *Surg. Gynaecol. Obstet.*, **139**, 341–349.

Swarbrick, E. T., Hunt, R. H., Fevre, D. I. and Williams, C. B. (1976), Colonoscopy for unexplained rectal bleeding. *Gut*, **17**, 823.

Tarin, D., Allison, D. J., Modlin, I. M. and Neale, G. (1978), Diagnosis and management of obscure gastrointestinal bleeding. *Brit. Med. J.*, **2**, 751–754.

Teague, R. H. and Read, A. E. (1975), Polyposis in ulcerative colitis. *Gut*, **161(10)**, 792–795.

Tedesco, F. J., Waye, J. D., Rasin, J. B., Morris, S. J. and Greenwald, R. A.

(1978), Colonoscopic evaluation of rectal bleeding – a study of 304 patients. *Ann. Intern. Med.,* **89(6)**, 907–909.

Waye, J. D. (1976), Colonoscopy in rectal bleeding. *S. Afr. J. Surg.,* **147(3)**, 143–149.

Williams, C. B. (1973), Diathermy biopsy: a technique for the endoscopic management of small polyps. *Endoscopy,* **5**, 215–18.

Williams, C. B., Hunt, R. H., Loose, H., Riddell, R. H., Sakai, Y. and Swarbrick, E. T. (1974), Colonoscopy in the management of colon polyps. *Br. J. Surg.,* **61(9)**, 673–682.

Williams, C. B., Swarbrick, E. T. and Hunt, R. H. (1975), unpublished data.

Williams, J. T. and Thomson, J. P. S. (1977), Ano-rectal bleeding: a study of causes and investigative yields. *The Practitioner,* **219**, 327–331.

Williams, R. C. (1961), Aortic stenosis and unexplained gastrointestinal bleeding. *Arch. Intern. Med.,* **108**, 859–863.

Wilson, G. S., Dale, E. H. and Brines, O. A. (1955), An evaluation of polyps detected in 20 847 routine sigmoidoscope examinations. *Am. J. Surg.,* **90**, 834–840.

Winawer, S. J., Melamed, M. and Sherlock, P. (1976), Potential of endoscopy, biopsy and cytology in the diagnosis and management of patients with cancer. *Clin. Gastroenterology,* **5(3)**, 575–595.

Winawer, S. J., Sherlock, P., Schottenfeld, D. and Miller, D. G. (1976), Screening for colon cancer. *Gastroenterology,* **70**, 783–789.

Winnan, G., Berci, G., Panish, J. *et al.* (1980), Superiority of the flexible to the rigid sigmoidoscope in routine proctosigmoidoscopy. *New Engl. J. Med.,* **302**, 1011—1012.

Wolff, W. I., Grossman, M. B. and Shinya, H. (1977), Angiodysplasia of the colon: diagnosis and treatment. *Gastroenterology,* **72**, 329–33.

Wright, S. G., Renton, P. and Swarbrick, E. T. (1976), Stricture of the descending colon due to schistosomiasis. *Postgrad. Med. J.,* **52**, 601–604.

CHAPTER FIFTEEN

Emergency Colonoscopy

F. P. ROSSINI and A. FERRARI

The massive loss of blood from the large intestine presents several diagnostic and therapeutic problems involving several specialists: internist, radiologist, angiographer, gastroenterologist/endoscopist, and surgeon. Whenever gastrointestinal bleeding occurs, whether from the upper or lower tract, the problem is always the same: identification of the source of haemorrhage. The physician must decide which diagnostic procedures should be undertaken and their appropriate order to provide the most reliable diagnosis on which to plan effective therapy. The emergency diagnostic procedures which are available for the investigation of haemorrhage from the colon are listed in Table 15.1.

15.1 Upper gastrointestinal haemorrhage

When upper gastrointestinal haemorrhage is massive, causing a rapid transit of fresh blood through the intestinal tract, red bleeding may occur from the anus although its origin is from the upper digestive tract. Whenever gastrointestinal bleeding is considered as a cause of rectal bleeding, an oesophagogastroduodenoscopy should be performed (Retzlaff, Hagedorn and Bartolomew, 1961; Bartelheimer, Remmele and Ottenjahn, 1972; Crespon et al., 1973; Deyhle et al., 1974; Hedberg, 1974; Feiber, Jewel and Boden, 1975; Gaisford, 1975; Skiba et al., 1976; Swarbrick et al., 1976; Waye, 1976; Hunt, 1978). Upper gas-

Table 15.1 Emergency diagnostic procedures for haemorrhage

Proctoscopy
Barium enema
Selective arteriography
Diagnostic endoscopy
Exploratory laparotomy
Intraoperative endoscopy

trointestinal endoscopy has a high diagnostic accuracy and is more useful to exclude a bleeding lesion in the stomach or duodenum than is gastric aspiration with a nasogastric tube.

15.2 Proctoscopy

The traditional rigid proctosigmoidoscope is used to exclude a lesion causing bleeding in the anorectal region. The large proctosigmoidoscope, with an auxillary suction pump, is particularly useful to clear thick clots which often collect in the region of the rectal ampulla.

15.3 Barium enema

The barium enema is no longer considered a useful diagnostic investigation because of the poor results which are usually obtained in acute massive bleeding, and because of the difficulties encountered in performing the procedure in patients who are often in poor physical condition. Although claims have been made for a hypothetical haemostatic effect of barium sulphate (Adams, 1974), there is no evidence that it is of any clinical benefit for stopping acute colonic bleeding.

15.4 Emergency selective arteriography (ESA)

The diagnostic technique of choice in the investigation of massive haemorrhage from the lower intestinal tract is emergency selective angiography (ESA), which can provide the exact location of a bleeding point in about 80% of cases (Reuter and Bookstein, 1968; Nusbaum, Baum and Blakemore, 1969; Frey, Reuter and Bookstein, 1970; Genant and Ranninger, 1972; Baum, Athanasoulis and Waltman, 1974; Casarella, Kanter and Seaman, 1972; Galloway, Casarella and Shimkin, 1974). Although emergency angiography may identify the site of bleeding, it seldom allows the radiologist to determine the nature of the bleeding lesion. A successful diagnostic examination requires the mobilization of an entire angiographic or radiographic team which includes an expert radiologist (Eisenberg, Laufer and Skillman, 1973). The angiographic examination has several drawbacks: there is a high incidence of complications, with a mortality of 0.03%, and a morbidity of 1.41% (Wenz, 1974; Sigstedt and Lunderquist, 1978); the procedure itself induces a degree of discomfort for the patient, many of whom already have a compromised circulation; the radiation exposure is high and the cost of the procedure itself is expensive. Angiography is only of benefit during active bleeding, requiring a blood loss flow of about 0.5–1.0 ml/min. When ESA is unsuccessful, and the source of bleeding remains unidentified, the search for a diagnosis must continue. Before the clinician requests a surgical exploratory laparotomy, it is important to consider the role of emergency colonoscopy.

15.5 Emergency colonoscopy

Colonoscopy may be used to reveal the source of haemorrhage from the colon in the same way as emergency oesophagogastroduodenoscopy is employed to locate the bleeding site in the upper gastrointestinal tract. Emergency colonoscopy is considered a routine investigation for colonic bleeding in several centres and should be performed as soon as possible, either during acute bleeding or as soon as is practical after bleeding has stopped.

Emergency colonoscopy is considerably easier and more diagnostically rewarding than most endoscopists realize. Successful emergency colonoscopy requires more than good instrumentation, for the endoscopist must have patience and determination to persist with the examination in spite of the difficulties encountered. Endoscopic instruments with sophisticated optical systems, a greater degree of tip deflection, larger suction channels, and systems for flushing water onto the colonic walls have all made emergency endoscopy of the large intestine an exciting, as well as feasible, approach to the diagnosis of colonic haemorrhage.

15.5.1 *Intraoperative emergency colonoscopy*

When all diagnostic methods have failed to locate the site of bleeding, it may be necessary to proceed to an emergency exploratory laparotomy. Even during surgery, however, endoscopy may be of considerable benefit. At laparotomy, the colonoscope may be inserted into the anus after the abdomen has been opened. Close co-operation between the surgeon and the endoscopist is necessary for this technique. Using the diagnostic procedure described in Chapter 11, it is possible to demonstrate small lesions which may be responsible for bleeding. Transillumination of the bowel wall with the brilliant cold light from the endosocope tip permits close study of the vascular network, an observation which may be of extreme importance in the diagnosis of vascular ectasias. Intraoperative emergency colonoscopy can, therefore, be of great help to the surgeon in providing information on the site of a haemorrhage, thereby avoiding a useless colotomy, or perhaps helping to define the limit of colonic resection if that is indicated (Marcozzi and Montori, 1971; Marcozzi, Montori and Crespi, 1972; Marcozzi and Montori, 1972).

Occasionally, when a previous endoscopic diagnostic procedure has localized the site of pathology, such as an arteriovenous malformation, a bleeding polyp, or a small tumour, the surgeon may have difficulty in identifying that area, even with the abdomen open. In these circumstances, intraoperative colonoscopy will almost always be successful in identifying the site of the original lesion.

In some instances, emergency colonoscopy may be unsuccessful and yet, at subsequent exploratory laparotomy, the surgeon may still fail to delineate the area of bleeding. When this occurs, it is sometimes helpful to re-endoscope the patient during exploratory laparotomy with the endoscopist and surgeon working as a team to attempt together to identify the bleeding site.

15.5.2 *Indications and contraindications to emergency colonoscopy*

Emergency colonoscopy should be performed as soon as possible in all patients with massive loss of blood from the colon (Kirkpatrick, 1969; Rossini, 1973; Rossini, 1975). The definition of massive haemorrhage is a clinical evaluation which includes evidence of an acutely contracted blood volume – pallor, diaphoresis, tachycardia, hypotension and thready pulse in a patient passing copious quantities of bright red blood with a haemoglobin less than 10 g/dl. The procedure should be attempted at the time of rectal bleeding, rather than delay the procedure until bleeding has ceased. The only contraindication is severe haemorrhage with cardiovascular shock. Emergency colonoscopy is not indicated in those patients in whom a diagnosis has already been made, and in whom there is already an explanation for the loss of blood.

15.5.3 *Choice of instruments for emergency colonoscopy*

A single-channel colonoscope is preferred during emergency endoscopy, since these instruments are more flexible and permit easier intubation. Although the twin-channel instruments permit much better suction of residual stool and blood clot from the lumen, they have a larger diameter and are stiffer, hence more difficult to pass into the colon. The best results have been obtained with a single-channel medium-length fibrescope, which allows a comfortable and rapid examination of the large bowel at least as far as the splenic flexure, and often beyond.

15.5.4 *Technique of emergency colonoscopy*

Before beginning emergency colonoscopy, the patient's cardiovascular and respiratory status must be stabilized. The rigid proctosigmoido-scope is used initially to survey the rectum to exclude lesions that may be bleeding at the anorectal level and is frequently helpful for evacuating large clots from the rectal ampulla. The fibrescope, how-ever, has many advantages over the traditional rigid proctosigmoido-scope, even for the evaluation of lesions in the rectum. These advan-tages include ease of handling, which makes for a rapid and accurate exploration; the elimination of blind spots due to the polydirectional flexibility of the endoscope tip; and the capability of air insufflation to tense the walls of the rectum during biopsy, cytology or polypectomy. The flexible endoscope provides magnification of small lesions and permits the endoscopist to localize lesions at various levels of the colon (Rossini *et al.*, 1979). Awkward patient positions may be avoided during colonoscopy, since the entire examination is performed with the patient either supine or in the left lateral position.

The technique employed for emergency colonoscopy is the same as that for routine endoscopy but with some precautions. As always, the endoscopist must visualize the colonic lumen, and over-insufflation must be avoided because distension of the colon can worsen the haemorrhage. The endoscopist should avoid coarse manoeuvres which may cause pain and during intubation the instrument should be kept as straight as possible. The use of fluoroscopy can be most helpful (Rossini and Ferrari, 1976).

In patients with torrential bleeding, no preparation is required, since the bleeding itself purges the bowel of faeces (Rossini and Ferrari, 1980), but tap water enemas may occasionally be required to remove blood clots. Premedication is seldom used, since patients usually wil-lingly co-operate with the endoscopist in the belief that the examin-ation will provide the answer to their problem. Sedative medication is also avoided during emergency colonoscopy to avoid respiratory depression in a patient whose cardiovascular system is already com-promised. The restless attitude of patients during emergency colonos-copy may be due to insufficiency of the cerebral circulation rather than to instrument manoeuvring. In order to reduce bowel motility and avoid concentric spasm which may prevent colonic distension (making insertion slower), an antispasmodic such as prifinium bromide (7.5 mg) can be given i.v.

Total colonoscopy is usually not necessary, since most lesions responsible for bleeding are found on the left side of the large bowel. Flushing water on the colonic wall with a forceful injection of water via the biopsy channel will often remove blood and clot to allow the endoscopist to see whether mucosal ulceration is responsible for haemorrhage. Although blood may coat the lens and obscure vision, this problem can usually be solved by using the technique of holding the lens-washing button down while simultaneously depressing the suction button.

Summary
1. Stabilize cardiovascular and respiratory status.
2. Visualize lumen.
3. Avoid over-insufflation.
4. Insert instrument as straight as possible.
5. Stop when lesion is identified.
6. Stop when instrument enters a blood-free area.

15.5.5 *Failure of emergency colonoscopy*

Improvement in instrumentation and in endoscopic techniques has decreased the number of failures during emergency colonoscopy. One cause for its failure may be the long and tortuous loops of the sigmoid which can make insertion into the descending colon impossible. Another cause of failure to make a diagnosis is the presence of thick clots or coarse faecal residues, preventing adequate examination of the bowel lumen. However, when stool is present in the bowel, it usually indicates that the situation is not one of massive haemorrhage, and colonoscopy may actually be a 'delayed' procedure rather than an emergency one. If the lesion which is causing haemorrhage is identified, immediate full investigation of the entire large bowel is not required. If the endoscopist should locate an isolated ulcerated bleeding diverticulum (Plate 60), which may be a cause of severe haemorrhage (Casarella Kanter and Seaman, 1972; Behringer and Albright, 1973; Debray *et al.*, 1974; Hunt, 1979), the examination should be discontinued at that point. Once the colonoscope is advanced to an area where there is no further blood in the colonic lumen, this should be the end-point of intubation at emergency colonoscopy, and withdrawal should then be started, looking carefully for the cause and site of bleeding.

15.5.6 *Results of emergency colonoscopy in 335 cases*

In the past seven years, 335 emergency colonoscopies have been performed at Ospedale Maggiore di S. Giovanni Battista e della Città di Torino, and the diagnoses are listed in Table 15.2. Emergency colonoscopy was the first diagnostic examination in patients presenting to the emergency room with acute massive bleeding. After institution of initial supportive therapy, endoscopy was performed without waiting

Table 15.2 Clinical diagnosis at emergency colonoscopy, 1972–79*

	Number of cases
Diverticular disease	48
Solitary diverticulum of right colon	4
Ulcerative colitis	45
Ulcerative colitis plus carcinoma or polyp	2
Radiation colitis	15
Ischaemic colitis	14
Ulcerated carcinoma	57
Polyp	23
Angioma	2
Solitary ulcer	5
Angiodysplasia of right colon	4
Anastomotic recurrence of carcinoma	22
Recurrence of Crohn's disease (ileotransversostomy)	4
Endometriosis	3
Postpolypectomy haemorrhage (6–8 days after)	9
Lymphoma	1
Ureterosigmoidostomy plus ulcerated carcinoma	1
Total	259

*Only results of emergency colonoscopy performed with fibrescope above the rectosigmoid junction are reported.

for eventual improvement of the clinical status or for cessation of haemorrhage. In most of the patients, the bleeding site was identified in the left colon (Table 15.3), and in 77.3% of all patients examined, a correct diagnosis was made by emergency colonoscopy (Table 15.4). This series contains a high proportion of diagnoses of carcinoma and ulcerative colitis, since patients in our catchment area seek medical attention late in the course of their disease and frequently only when a medical catastrophe occurs. In 55 patients (16%), identification of the bleeding site was not achieved. These procedures are considered to be failures of the emergency technique. Following endoscopic diagnosis,

Table 15.3 The localization of bleeding areas at emergency colonoscopy

Site	*Number of cases*	%
Left portion of large bowel	221	85.3
Transverse colon	11	4.3
Right portion of large bowel	27	10.4

Table 15.4 The results of emergency colonoscopy, 1972–79

	Number of cases	%
Correct diagnosis	259	77.3
Diagnostic failures	55	16.4
No lesions up to the caecum	21	6.3
Total	335	

surgical resection was performed in eight patients (3%) to control massive bleeding, and at laparotomy in these cases the diagnostic accuracy of emergency colonoscopy was confirmed and in this group of patients, preoperative localization of a bleeding lesion was considered important for planning the correct surgical approach. The findings in these eight patients are shown in Table 15.5.

Emergency endoscopic treatment was performed in five patients (1.9%). These included four polypectomies using the wire snare and fulguration of one angioma. The literature cites numerous instances of electrofulguration technique for angiomas, vascular ectasias or hemangiomas, such as those seen in Osler–Rendu–Weber disease (Plate 47), as well as in non-specific ulcers of the colon (Fruhmorgen, Zeus and Demling, 1975; Rogers and Adler, 1976; Montori *et al.*, 1976; Wolff, Grossman and Shinya, 1977). During removal of a bleeding polyp, visualization can be difficult due to continued bleeding, and this can often be overcome by advancing the endoscope beyond the bleeding point and placing the snare under visual control as the instrument is withdrawn. Even when technical difficulties are encountered in such a therapeutic procedure, every effort at success should be made because it offers the possibility of rapidly solving the problem of haemorrhage. During emergency colonoscopy, a worsening of haemorrhage was encountered in only two patients. One patient had inflammatory bowel disease (ulcerative colitis) (Plate 63), and the other patient was elderly, with severe diverticular disease. They were both operated upon as emergency situations.

Table 15.5 Diagnosis at laparotomy in eight cases following emergency colonoscopy

Diverticular disease	2
Ulcerative colitis	2
Carcinoma	1
Polyp	1
Angioma	1
Angiodysplasia	1

15.5.7 *Benefits of emergency colonoscopy*

1. It is possible to identify the source of haemorrhage in over 75% of cases and this result is almost as good as emergency selective angiography.

2. The procedure has little risk for the patient over and above routine colonoscopy. These risks are less than those of emergency selective angiography and of surgical exploratory operations.

3. Snare polypectomy and endoscopic electrocoagulation may control haemorrhage directly.

4. Localization of the bleeding site may avoid exploratory laparotomy. The results of emergency colonoscopy in localizing the bleeding site is superior to that of primary exploratory laparotomy alone.

5. Intraoperative colonoscopy may offer assistance to the surgeon and avoid multiple colotomies during surgical exploration and may help to delineate a line of resection.

6. In the future, the treatment of massive haemorrhage of the large bowel may be helped by the use of laser therapy (Frühmorgen *et al.*, 1975; 1976).

Because of the advantages listed above, and the ability to locate the source of bleeding in a high percentage of cases, emergency colonoscopy may be suggested as the method of choice in the diagnosis of massive haemorrhage in the colon; the procedure meets all the requirements of a diagnostic technique. Both therapeutic and diagnostic emergency colonoscopy have a promising future; and these procedures are often very rewarding to perform.

References

Adams, J. T. (1974), The barium enema as treatment for massive diverticular disease. *Dis. Colon Rect.,* **17**, 439–41.

Bartelheimer, W., Remmele, W. and Ottenjahn, R. (1972), Coloscopic recognition of hemangiomas in the colon ascendent. Case report of so called cryptogenic gastrointestinal bleeding. *Endoscopy,* **4**, 100–14.

Baum, S., Athanasoulis, C. A. and Waltman, A. C. (1974), Angiographic diagnosis and control of large-bowel bleeding. *Dis. Colon Rect.,* **17**, 447–53.

Behringer, G. E. and Albright, N. L. (1973), Diverticular disease of the colon. A frequent cause of massive rectal bleeding. *Am. J. Surg.,* **125**, 419–23.

Casarella, W. J., Kanter, I. E. and Seaman, W. B. (1972), Right-sided colonic diverticula as a cause of acute rectal hemorrhage. *N. Engl. J. Med.,* **286**, 450–3.

Crespon, B., Housset, P., Campora, A., Paolaggi, J. A. and Debray, Ch. (1973), Apport de la coloscopie d'urgence dans les hémorragies digestives basses. *Acta Endosc. Radiocm.,* **11**, 133–4.

Debray, Ch., Leymarios, J., Crespon, B., Nardi, C. and Martin, E. (1974), Hémorragie massive par diverticulose colique (intérêt de l'artériographie – image en anneau – et de la coloscopie). *Nouv. Presse Méd.*, **3**, 715–20.

Deyhle, P., Blum, A. L., Nuesch, H. J. and Jenny, S. (1974), Emergency coloscopy in the management of the acute peranal hemorrage. *Endoscopy*, **6**, 229.

Eisenberg, H., Laufer, I. and Skillman, J. J. (1973), Arteriographic diagnosis and management of suspected colonic diverticular hemorrhage. *Gastroenterology*, **64**, 1091.

Feiber, S. S., Jewel, K. L. and Boden, R. (1975), Arteriovenous malformation of the colon, a source of massive low intestinal hemorrage. *J. Med. Soc. New Jersey*, **72**, 34.

Frey, C. F., Reuter, S. R. and Bookstein, J. J. (1970), Localization of gastrointestinal hemorrage by selective angiography. *Surgery, Gynec. Obstet.*, **67**, 549.

Frühmorgen, P., Bodem, F., Reidenbach, H. D., Kaduk, B., Demling, L. and Brand, H. (1975), The first endoscopic laser coagulation in the human GI tract. *Endoscopy*, **7**, 156–7.

Frühmorgen, P., Bodem, F., Reidenbach, H. D., Kaduk, B. and Demling, L. (1976), Endoscopic laser coagulation of bleeding gastrointestinal lesions with report of the first therapeutic application in man. *Gastrointest. Endosc.*, **23**, 73–75.

Frühmorgen, P., Zeus, J. and Demling, L. (1975), New aspects of therapeutic coloscopy. *Endoscopy*, **7**, 59.

Gaisford, W. D. (1975), Emergency colonoscopy in acute hemorrage per rectum. *Gastrointest. Endosc.*, **21**, 187.

Galloway, S. J., Casarella, W. J. and Shimkin, P. M. (1974), Vascular malformations of the right colon as a cause of bleeding in patients with aortic stenosis. *Radiology*, **113**, 11–15.

Genant, H. K. and Ranninger, K. (1972), Vascular dysplasias of the ascending colon. *Am. J. Roentg.*, **115**, 34–91.

Hedberg, S. E. (1974), Endoscopy in gastrointestinal bleeding: a systematic approach to diagnosis. *Surg. Clinics N. Am.*, **54**, 549–59.

Hunt, R. H. (1978), Rectal bleeding. *Clinics Gastroent.*, **3**, 719–40.

Hunt, R. H. (1979), The role of colonoscopy in complicated diverticular disease. A review. *Acta Chir. Belg.*, **6**, 349–53.

Kirkpatrick, J. P. (1969), Massive rectal bleeding in the adult. *Dis. Colon Rect.*, **12**, 248–52.

Montori, A., Messinetti, S., Viceconte, G., Miscusi, G., Viceconte, G. W. and Pastorino, C. (1976a), Diagnostic and operative colonoscopy in emergency disease of the colon. *Surg. Italy*, **6**, 1.

Marcozzi, G. and Montori, A. (1971), Utilità dell'endoscopia digestiva peroperatoria nelle sindromi di difficile diagnosi. *Min. Gastroent.*, **17**, 139–41.

Marcozzi, G. and Montori, A. (1972), Endoscopy during operation: new diagnostic possibilities. *Chir. Gastroent.*, **6**, 23.

Marcozzi, G., Montori, A. and Crespi, M. (1972), Intra-operative endoscopy:

new diagnostic possibilities. Urgent endoscopy of digestive and abdominal diseases. *Int. Symp. Prague,* Carlsbad, 244–7.

Montori, A., Viceconte, G., Miscusi, G., Viceconte, G. W. and Pastorino, C. (1976b), Therapeutic colonoscopy. *Endoscopy,* **8**, 81–84.

Nusbaum, M., Baum, S. and Blakemore, W. S. (1969), Clinical experience with the diagnosis and management of gastrointestinal haemorrage by selective mesenteric catheterization. *Ann. Surg.,* **170**, 506–14.

Retzlaff, J. A., Hagedorn, A. B. and Bartolomew, L. G. (1961), Abdominal exploration for gastrointestinal bleeding of obscure origin. *J. Am. Med. Ass.,* **177**, 104.

Reuter, S. R. and Bookstein, J. J. (1968), Angiographic localisation of gastrointestinal bleeding. *Gastroenterology,* **54**, 876–83.

Rogers, B. H. G. and Adler, F. (1976), Hemangiomas of cecum: colonoscopic diagnosis and therapy. *Gastroenterology,* **71**, 1079–82.

Rossini, F. P. (1973), La coloscopia d'urgenza nelle enterorragie. *Acta Endosc. Radiochim.,* **3**, 131–3.

Rossini, F. P. (1975), *Atlas of Coloscopy.* Piccin Medical Books, Padova.

Rossini, F. P. and Ferrari, A. (1976), Emergency coloscopy. *Acta Endosc. Radiochim.,* **2**, 165–8.

Rossini, F. P. and Ferrari, A. (1980), *Slide Atlas of Coloscopy.* Piccin Medical Books, Padava.

Rossini, F. P., Ferrari, A., Mezzedimi, R. and Massa, F. (1979), Use and advantages of flexible sigmoidoscopy in the early detection of tumours and high risk lesions. *Acta Endosc. Radiochim.,* **3**, 193–9.

Sigstedt, B. and Lunderquist, A. (1978), Complications of angiographic examinations. *Am. J. Roentg.,* **130**, 455–60.

Skiba, R. M., Hartong, W. A., Mautz, F. A., Hinthorn, D. R. and Rhodes, J. A. (1976), Angiodysplasia of cecum. *Gastrointest. Endosc.,* **22**, 177.

Swarbrick, E. T., Hunt, R. H., Fevre, D. I. and Williams, C. B. (1976), Colonoscopy in unexplained rectal bleeding. *Gut,* **17**, 823.

Waye, J. D. (1976), Colonoscopy in rectal bleeding. *S. Afr. J. Surg.,* **14**, 143–9.

Wenz, W. (1974), *Abdominal Angiography.* Springer Verlag, New York, 1974.

Wolff, W. I., Grossman, M. B. and Shinya, H. (1977), Angiodysplasia of the colon: diagnosis and treatment. *Gastroenterology,* **72**, 329–33.

CHAPTER SIXTEEN

The Polyp Problem

DAVID W. DAY and BASIL C. MORSON

The term polyp is used to describe any circumscribed lesion that projects above the surface of the surrounding mucosa. Polyps vary in their shape, size and surface appearances and may be sessile or pedunculated. Although the macroscopic appearances of some polyps are reasonably characteristic it is only by microscopic examination that the nature of any particular polyp can be determined. The several types of polyp differ in their clinical significance and particularly in their malignant potential so that accurate histological diagnosis is 'of major importance in the management of the individual patient.

From a practical point of view, therefore, it is important that all removed polyps should be submitted to the histopathologist for microscopic examination, together with adequate clinical details including colonoscopic findings. Obviously, whenever possible, polyps should be removed in their entirety. The stalk of a pedunculated polyp should be identified by a thread, and sessile polyps should be placed with their submucosal side downwards on a suitable surface such as a ground-glass slide, to which they will adhere, before being placed in fixative. These procedures facilitate proper orientation of the polyp in the laboratory so that sections can be cut in the right plane. This is necessary not only for diagnosis of the type of polyp but, in the case of neoplastic polyps, assumes crucial importance in the assessment of whether the polyp has been completely removed, whether or not malignant change has occurred, and if it has, where the malignant tissue is in relation to the line of excision.

The vast majority of polyps of the large bowel encountered in clinical practice can be assigned to one of four categories (see Table 16.1): the neoplastic group, comprising adenomas with or without malignant change and polyps composed entirely of malignant tissue; inflammatory polyps; hamartomatous polyps; and metaplastic or hyperplastic polyps. Other less common types of polypoid lesion that can occur will be mentioned after a discussion of these four principal classes.

Table 16.1 Histological classification of the common types of large bowel polyp

---

Neoplastic: adenoma with/without invasive carcinoma
                adenocarcinoma
Inflammatory: e.g. ulcerative colitis or Crohn's disease
                benign lymphoid polyps
Hamartomatous: Peutz-Jeghers'
                juvenile
Unclassified: metaplastic (hyperplastic)

16.1 Hamartomatous polyps

Hamartomas are malformations composed of an abnormal mixture of tissues normally found in the affected part of the body, often with an excess of one particular tissue type. In the large bowel the two types encountered with any frequency are the juvenile polyp and the Peutz-Jeghers' polyp.

Juvenile polyps are usually single or few in number and the majority occur in the rectum in children and adolescents. Rarely, multiple lesions may be present in the large bowel or elsewhere in the gut in the form of a gastrointestinal polyposis. Grossly, the juvenile polyp is characteristically round and smooth with a bright red surface (Plate 88), deep to which are paler areas representing mucin-filled cysts. Histologically, a large proportion of the polyp consists of fine

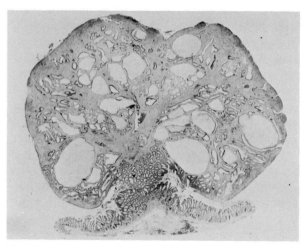

Fig. 16.1 Juvenile polyp. Cystically dilated glands are separated by an excess of lamina propria. H & E × 4.4.

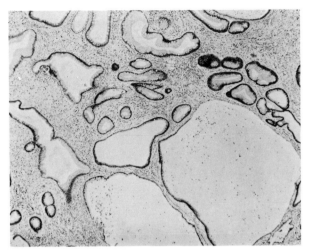

Fig. 16.2 Juvenile polyp. Glands are lined by normal colonic epithelium. H & E × 24.5.

connective tissue in which there are some inflammatory cells and capillaries and which closely resembles the structure of the lamina propria of the normal mucous membrane. Interspersed in the connective tissue are glands which are lined by normal colonic epithelial cells and which not infrequently are cystically dilated (Figs 16.1 and 16.2). The polyps may become infected and ulcerate and if this occurs it may be difficult to differentiate them from inflammatory polyps. Presumably because they lack a smooth muscle component they are liable to undergo torsion and this can often result in autoamputation. There is no evidence that isolated juvenile polyps ever undergo malignant change although associated intestinal cancer has been reported in some patients with juvenile polyposis.

In the Peutz-Jeghers' syndrome multiple polyps are present in the gastrointestinal tract, particularly the small intestine, and there is skin pigmentation around the mouth, affecting the lips and buccal mucosa, and sometimes at other sites such as the fingers and toes. However, isolated polyps of the Peutz-Jeghers' type may occur anywhere in the stomach or intestine in individuals who lack the stigmata of the fully developed syndrome. These polyps can reach quite a large size and have a coarsely lobulated surface (Plate 98) not unlike an adenomatous polyp. Histologically, their appearance is characteristic with a tree-like branching core of smooth muscle surmounted by normal mucin-secreting epithelium and lamina propria (Fig. 16.3).

Many of the case reports describing malignant change in Peutz-

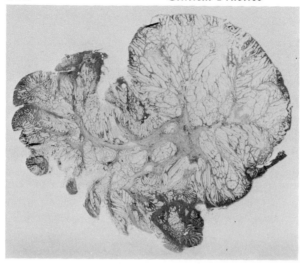

Fig. 16.3 Peutz-Jeghers' polyp. Branching core of smooth muscle derived from the muscularis mucosae and covered by mucus-secreting epithelium. H & E × 3.6.

Jeghers' polyps have misinterpreted the presence of misplaced epithelium in the submucosa and muscle brought about by over-secretion of mucin which becomes trapped between the mucosal folds of the polyp. However, there are authentic cases of gastrointestinal cancer occurring in patients with the Peutz-Jeghers' syndrome and the site of most of the malignancies has been in the stomach and duodenum (Achord and Proctor, 1963; Reid, 1965). Colonic carcinoma has also been described but adenomas were present in addition to the Peutz-Jeghers' polyps in these cases and were more likely to be the source of malignancy. It seems, therefore, that there is a slightly increased risk of cancer in the Peutz-Jeghers' syndrome.

16.2 Inflammatory polyps

In Europe and North America, inflammatory polyps are most frequently encountered in patients with idiopathic inflammatory bowel disease, that is ulcerative colitis and Crohn's disease. They may be single (Plate 131) or multiple (Plate 136), segmental or diffuse and predominate in the colon rather than the rectum. Their formation is related to at least one previous severe attack of colitis and is thought to result from full-thickness ulceration of the mucosa with undermining of surviving epithelium. With healing, these mucosal tags are left projecting into the lumen of the bowel and they can later adhere to the surface mucosa, so forming mucosal 'bridges' (Plates 133–135).

Grossly, they are smooth, shiny, worm-like polyps which may exhibit branching, and with little distinction between stalk and head (Plate 127). Larger polyps may show white patches. On microscopy most consist of variably inflamed mucosa with architectural distortion of the crypts, which may be dilated or cystic. The epithelial cells are often tall, hyperplastic and contain mucin. In some polyps granulation tissue is prominent with little or no glandular component. There is no relationship between inflammatory polyps and the precancerous changes in the bowel which may occur in long-standing ulcerative colitis.

Inflammatory polyps may also occur in ischaemic colitis, following bacillary dysentery and in such parasitic infestations as amoebiasis, schistosomiasis and histoplasmosis when the causative organism may be apparent on microscopic examination (Fig. 16.4).

Polyps composed of normal or hyperplastic lymphoid tissue occur in several situations and whilst not necessarily the result of inflam-

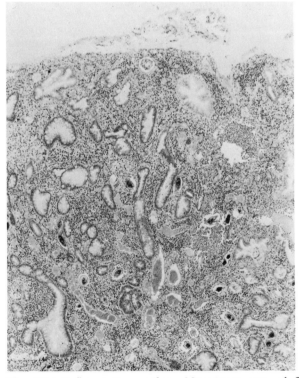

Fig. 16.4 Inflammatory polyp. Numerous ova of *Schistosoma mansoni* are present. H & E × 40.

mation can be conveniently considered under this heading. Minor degrees of lymphoid hyperplasia seen at colonoscopy and most prominent in the rectum is a not uncommon finding in children and is a variation of normal. More exaggerated changes may be familial or occur in patients with immunodeficiency syndromes (Louw, 1968; Shaw and Hennigar, 1974). They have to be differentiated from diffuse malignant lymphomatous polyposis and from familial adenomatous polyposis.

Benign lymphoid polyps (Helwig and Hansen, 1951; Cornes, Wallace and Morson, 1961) are usually solitary, smooth, rounded and sessile lesions up to 1 cm in diameter, although occasionally larger, which are seen, often as an incidental finding, in the lower rectum of adults. Microscopically, they consist of normal lymphoid tissue with prominent follicular differentiation, present mainly in the submucosa and are covered by attentuated mucous membrane (Fig. 16.5). They are harmless, unrelated to malignant lymphomas and probably arise as a response to local inflammation.

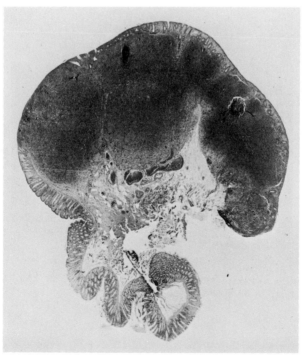

Fig. 16.5 Benign lymphoid polyp of lower rectum. H & E × 10.7.

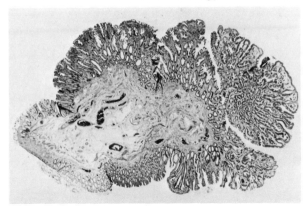

Fig. 16.6 Metaplastic polyp. H & E × 8.4.

16.3 Metaplastic polyps

Metaplastic or hyperplastic polyps are the commonest type of polyp in the large bowel. They are most common in the rectum, more frequent in males and more prevalent with increasing age, being present in 75% of adults over the age of 40. They are usually sessile lesions, the same colour or paler than surrounding mucosa, with a flat convex surface (Plate 66). The majority are small although an occasional polyp may be greater than 1 cm in diameter (Plate 68). Rarely there may be in excess of 50 polyps distributed throughout the bowel so that at endoscopy the appearances suggest familial adenomatous polyposis. Although metaplastic polyps are commonly seen in the neighbourhood of a carcinoma they are harmless lesions with no malignant potential. The histological appearances of this type of polyp are distinctive (Figs. 16.6 and 16.7). Crypts are lengthened and dilated and lined by a serrated epithelium in which there are reduced numbers of goblet cells and an increased proportion of absorptive cells. Cell kinetic studies coupled with electron microscopic observations have shown that cell maturation is normal but that there is a delayed migration of mature cells towards the luminal surface of the mucosa (Kaye, Fenoglio, Pascal and Lane, 1973; Hayashi, Yatani, Apostol and Stemmermann, 1974).

Because of the site of predilection, colonoscopic series of polyps tend to contain a lower proportion of this type of polyp when compared with series of polyps removed at sigmoidoscopy.

16.4 Adenomatous polyps

By far the most important group of polyps are adenomas since these have the potential to undergo malignant change. Leaving aside the

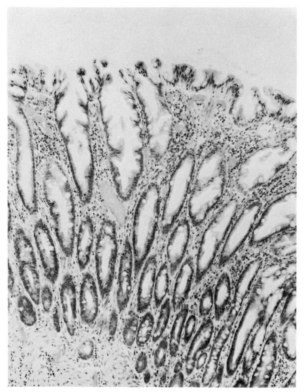

Fig. 16.7 Metaplastic polyp. Higher power showing characteristic serrated epithelium with reduction in goblet cells. H & E × 86.7.

special and uncommon case of malignancy arising in patients with long-standing ulcerative colitis it seems that the majority of, if not all, adenocarcinomas of the colon and rectum arise from adenomas, a process referred to as the adenoma-carcinoma sequence. Studies of the pathology of adenomas have elucidated the factors which make this transformation more likely (Morson, 1978; Morson and Dawson, 1979).

16.4.1 *Prevalence and distribution of adenomas*

Adenomas are common lesions in countries where there is a high incidence of colorectal cancer and their prevalence increases with age. Thus examination of the large bowel at autopsy has shown one or more adenomas to be present in 58% of males and 47% of females over the age of 55 in a series from the USA (Rickert *et al.*, 1979), and in 43% of males and 32% of females in a Norwegian study (Eide and Stalsberg, 1978). In the American series adenomas were more common in the proximal half of the large bowel, whereas the Norwegian data showed that, below the age of 65, adenomas predominated in the distal bowel in both sexes, with a marked shift to the proximal half of the large intestine only in males over 65 years and in females over 75 years. In colonoscopic series, the distribution of adenomas has been predominantly left-sided (Wolff and Shinya, 1973; Gillespie *et al.*, 1979).

16.4.2 *Nomenclature*

The classification proposed by the World Health Organization (Morson and Sobin, 1976) and based on subjective histological appearances subdivides adenomas into tubular, villous and tubulovillous types. It has to be emphasized, however, that these different growth patterns are variants of the same neoplastic process and that the tumours show a common cytology.

Tubular adenomas
The majority of adenomas are of this type and account for 75% of the total in one series (Muto, Bussey and Morson, 1975). Typically they are small, have a lobulated surface and are pedunculated. Histologically, closely packed epithelial tubules are seen which grow and branch horizontally to the muscularis mucosae (Fig. 16.8).

Villous adenomas
By contrast, the typical villous adenoma is large and sessile and has a shaggy or velvety surface composed of numerous frond-like processes. This pattern is present in about 10% of adenomas. Microscopically, finger-like projections of neoplastic epithelium with a core of lamina propria project towards the lumen of the bowel, the epithelium dipping down between the processes to rest on the muscularis mucosae (Fig. 16.9).

Tubulovillous adenomas
This type of adenoma consists of either a mixture of tubular and villous patterns or more commonly has a uniform intermediate appearance with broad and stunted villi overlying epithelial tubules similar to those present in a tubular adenoma (Fig. 16.10).

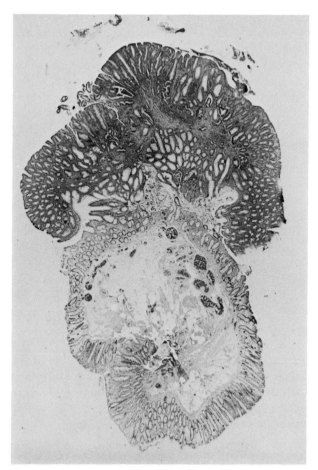

Fig. 16.8 Tubular adenoma. H & E × 15.

16.4.3 *Dysplasia*

All adenomas are composed of neoplastic epithelium in which the component cells contain nuclei which are enlarged, occupying a greater proportion of the cell than normal, more deeply staining (hyperchromatic), and more likely to be undergoing mitosis. Mitoses occur throughout the length of the crypt and are not confined to the basal half as in normal epithelium. Mucus is often markedly reduced although in some villous adenomas and exceptionally in tubular adenomas, it is increased. The term dysplasia is used to describe these changes and on the basis of nuclear changes such as enlargement, pleomorphism, loss of polarity, stratification, and an

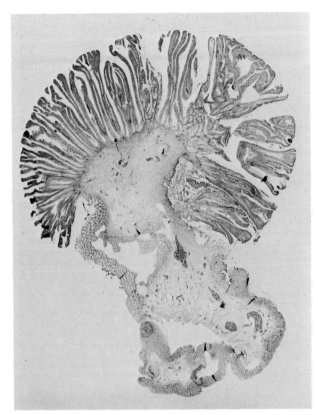

Fig. 16.9 Villous adenoma which in this case is pedunculated. H & E × 5.6.

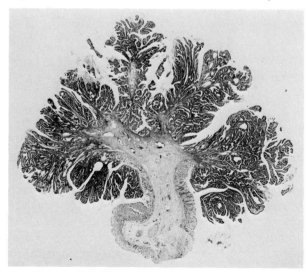

Fig. 16.10 Tubulovillous adenoma. Histological structure intermediate between the typical tubular and typical villous adenoma. H & E × 3.5.

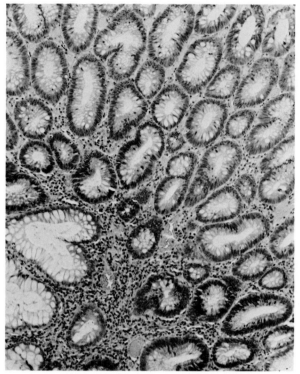

Fig. 16.11 Minor epithelial dysplasia. Nuclear-cytoplasmic ratio is increased and there is a decrease in mucus. Nuclear polarity is maintained. Normal crypts at bottom left. H & E × 107.

increase in the number of mitoses, adenomas may be subjectively graded as showing mild, moderate or severe dysplasia (Figs. 16.11 and 16.12). With severe dysplasia, as well as nuclear abnormalities, irregular budding and a back-to-back arrangement of the glands may be present. An adenoma usually consists of neoplastic tissue showing uniform dysplastic changes but there can be variation in the degree of dysplasia within a tumour. The term carcinoma-in-situ has been used to describe severe dysplasia, and focal carcinoma or focal cancer has been given to an area of severe dysplasia in an adenoma which otherwise shows minor or moderate dysplasia. Both these terms are unsatisfactory and on occasion their use in reports has led to unnecessarily radical surgery. The word cancer or carcinoma to describe neoplastic tissue confined above the muscularis mucosae is inappropriate since in this situation even though the tissue changes

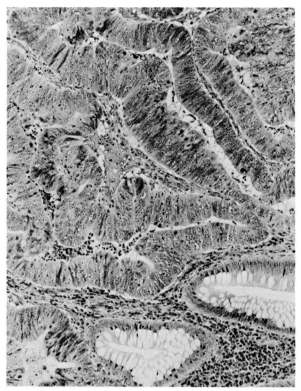

Fig. 16.12 Severe epithelial dysplasia. Nuclear stratification and loss of polarity with frequent mitoses. Total loss of mucus and a back-to-back arrangement of glands. Normal crypts at bottom. H & E × 109.5.

satisfy all the cytological criteria of adenocarcinoma there is no potential for metastasis. This is because in the large bowel no lymphatics are present above this level (Fenoglio, Kaye and Lane, 1973).

16.4.4 *Adenoma-carcinoma sequence*

Much of the evidence for this transition has come from the careful study of lesions removed at operation or at endoscopy. Sometimes it is obvious from macroscopic examination that a tumour is partly benign and partly malignant. When malignant tumours are studied microscopically, a proportion of them will show contiguous benign tissue as well. Thus a grossly obvious carcinoma may have residual adenomatous tissue at its edge. At the other extreme an adenomatous

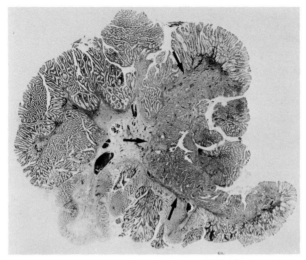

Fig. 16.13 Tubulovillous adenoma with focus of invasive adenocarcinoma (arrowed). H & E × 3.3.

polyp may show a microscopic focus of invasive carcinoma, that is neoplastic tissue deep to the muscularis mucosae (Figs 16.13 and 16.14). The likelihood of finding a benign component is increased the more limited the spread of the malignant tissue through the bowel wall. Thus if spread is limited to the submucosa, 60% of malignant tumours will show benign tumour as well, whereas only 7% will do so when invasion into extramural fat has taken place (Morson, 1966). These results show that, at the least, a majority of large bowel cancers arise from previously benign adenomas and suggest that as cancers spread deeply through the bowel wall they expand also laterally on the mucosal surface and tend to destroy surviving benign tumour (Grinnell and Lane, 1958). If carcinomas of the large bowel arose directly from normal mucosa it would not be uncommon to come across tiny independent carcinomas under 0.5 cm diameter. That this is not the case strongly militates against a *de novo* origin of large bowel cancer.

The fact that carcinomas go through an adenomatous polypoid stage has important implications in terms of detection, prevention and treatment. From the wide disparity between the prevalence of adenomas and carcinomas, however, it is obvious that the vast majority of adenomas do not undergo malignant change and the question arises as to which attributes of adenomas are associated with this malignant transformation.

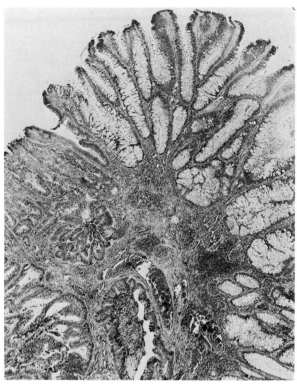

Fig. 16.14 Tubulovillous adenoma. Higher power to show junction of benign and malignant tissue. H & E × 31.

16.4.5 *Malignant potential of adenomas*

From studies of large series of adenomas, three factors, probably interrelated, have been shown to be associated with malignant change. These are increasing size, increasing degrees of epithelial dysplasia, and a villous growth pattern. Thus a series from St. Mark's Hospital (Muto, Bussey and Morson, 1975) showed that 1.3% of 2849 adenomas under 1 cm in diameter contained malignant tissue, whereas adenomas between 1 cm and 2 cm had a malignancy rate of 9.5% and in those greater than 2 cm in diameter the figure rose to 46%. In the same series the malignancy rate for tubular adenomas was approximately 5% but increased to 40% in villous adenomas, with tubulovillous adenomas having an intermediate rate of 22%. Irrespective of the histological growth pattern the malignant potential of adenomas increases with increasing degrees of dysplasia. Thus although it is unusual to find severe epithelial dysplasia in adenomas under 1 cm in size, when it occurs the malignancy rate rises to 27%.

16.4.6 *Life history of the adenoma-carcinoma sequence*

The usual treatment of a polyp when first seen is its removal so that opportunities to follow the transition from adenoma to carcinoma are rare. However, there are two situations where insight into this important area has been gained. The first has been in those few patients who have had a benign tumour but refused operation or who failed to reattend after initial diagnosis and later developed a carcinoma at the same site, and the second in patients with familial adenomatous polyposis. They have shown that adenomas may never develop malignant change and in those that do the sequence evolves over a long period, although it is very variable. Along with studies of metachronous cancer rates and age distribution curves the data suggest that the adenoma-carcinoma sequence is invariably greater than 5 years and averages 10 to 15 years but may even cover a normal life span.

16.4.7 *Malignant adenomas and polypoid carcinomas*

In two large series reporting colonoscopic removal of adenomas (Wolff and Shinya, 1975; Gillespie *et al.*, 1979) the proportion with invasive carcinoma has been 4.5% and 4.8% of the total respectively. In addition, a number of polyps consisted entirely of malignant tissue, so called polypoid carcinomas (Fig. 16.15). In all these cases close liaison between the endoscopist and pathologist is particularly necessary for the future management of the patient. Although there has been no long-term follow-up in patients who have had malignant polyps removed, experience so far suggests that in those lesions where excision is judged to be complete after histological examination (Plate 83) (Figs 16.16 and 16.17), no bowel resection is necessary except in the unusual situation where the malignant tissue is poorly differentiated, when the risk of metastatic spread to local lymph nodes is significantly increased (Morson, 1966). In those cases where malignant tissue extends to the resection margin (Fig. 16.18), which in practice appears to be the case only in a minority of malignant polyps, the policy to be followed depends on such factors as whether the endoscopist considers the lesion was completely removed, and the age and physical condition of the patient. It has been shown that in a considerable proportion of such cases colonic resection fails to show any malignant tumour and this is probably related to the des-

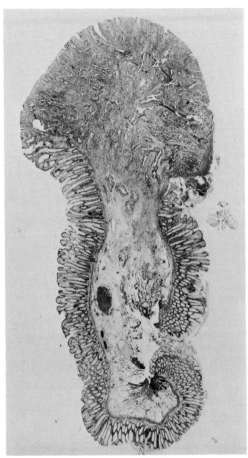

Fig. 16.15 Polypoid carcinoma. The head of this polyp consists entirely of carcinomatous tissue. H & E × 9.

truction of any residual tumour by diathermy at the time of polyp removal (Morson, Bussey and Samoorian, 1977; Gillespie *et al.*, 1979).

16.4.8 *Pseudoinvasion in adenomas*

This refers to the misplacement of benign adenomatous epithelium deep to the muscularis mucosae (Muto, Bussey and Morson, 1973; Greene, 1974). It is important in that it may be misdiagnosed as carcinoma. Histologically, well-circumscribed glandular epithelium and surrounding lamina propria is present in the submucosa, associated

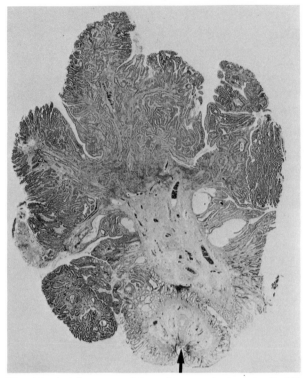

Fig. 16.16 Adenoma with malignant change. Well-differentiated carcinoma is seen arising in the head of a tubulovillous adenoma but is well clear of the line of excision of the polyp (arrowed). H & E × 6.6.

in most cases with the deposition of haemosiderin pigment. The glands, which are frequently dilated, show the same degree of epithelial dysplasia as the epithelium of the head of the adenoma (Figs. 16.19 and 16.20).

This phenomenon is particularly seen in larger tumours with a long stalk and is present most commonly in adenomas of the sigmoid colon, the site of greatest muscular activity in the large bowel. It probably occurs secondary to submucosal haemorrhage related to repeated twisting of the stalk of the adenoma. Follow-up studies have confirmed the benign nature of this condition.

16.4.9 *Multiple adenomas and carcinomas*

One in five patients with neoplastic disease of the large bowel when first seen have more than one tumour, either adenoma or adenocar-

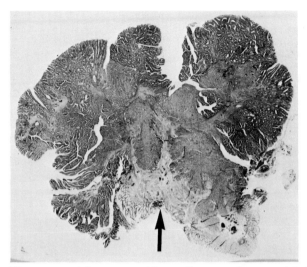

Fig. 16.17 Adenoma with malignant change. Moderately differentiated carcinoma extends close to but stops short of the excision line (arrowed). H & E × 3.6.

cinoma (Muto, Bussey and Morson, 1975). As well as this, 6% of those with a single tumour subsequently present with one or more additional neoplasms of the large bowel. Thus, neoplastic lesions are multiple in at least 25% of patients. In most large series of patients with cancer of the colon or rectum, about 5% will have more than one cancer, either synchronous or metachronous (Heald and Bussey, 1975).

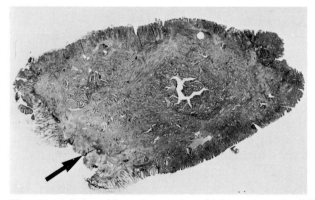

Fig. 16.18 Polypoid carcinoma in which moderately differentiated carcinoma extends to the line of excision as judged by the presence of a diathermy mark (arrowed). H & E × 4.9.

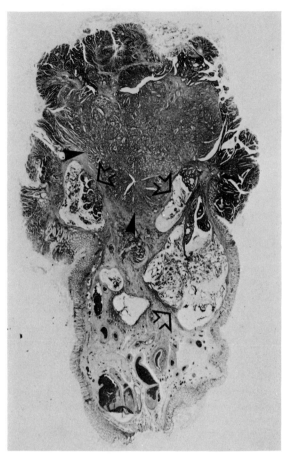

Fig. 16.19 Pseudoinvasion. In this unusual case both true invasion (black arrows) and pseudoinvasion (white arrows) have occurred. H & E × 3.6.

The important clinical implications which follow are that when a single tumour has been discovered in a patient it is essential to examine the whole of the large intestine for other tumours which may be present simultaneously. Because patients who have had one or more tumours removed are at an increased risk of developing further neoplasms such examinations should be repeated regularly. Since the evidence indicates that in general adenomas grow slowly, it would seem that the interval between examinations should be not less than three years and not more than five years, although these limits may have to be modified as more follow-up information becomes available.

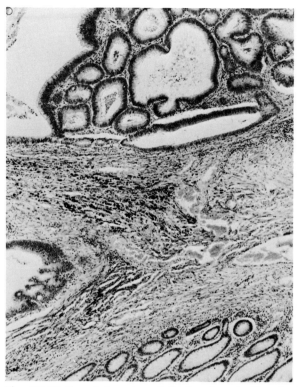

Fig. 16.20 Pseudoinvasion. Misplaced and dilated glandular epithelium in the submucosa with surrounding haemosiderin pigment. H & E × 50.5.

16.5 Other varieties of polyp

A number of polypoid lesions which are occasionally seen will be briefly mentioned

Sometimes what appears to be a discrete lesion at colonoscopy is merely an exaggerated fold or tag of normal mucous membrane. Isolated submucous lipomas, leiomyomas, neuromas, lymphangiomas, and vascular hamartomas can present as polyps endoscopically. Lipomas, which are the commonest of this group, tend to be more frequent in the right colon than in the left colon or rectum. They are mostly found incidentally but when large may give rise to acute or chronic intussusception, when necrosis and haemorrhage of the tumour and its surrounding mucosa may be conspicuous. Lipomas, can often be recognized endoscopically and have a characteristic 'dimpling' sign (Plates 91 and 92). Deposition of excess adi-

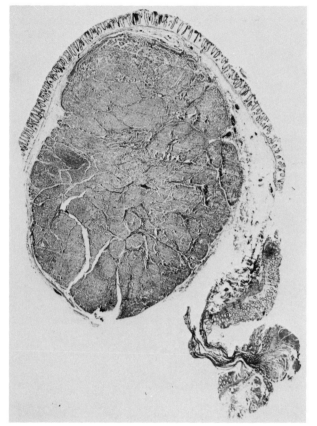

Fig. 16.21 Carcinoid tumour. Local excision of this circumscribed tumour in the rectum is complete. H & E × 10.

pose tissue not infrequently involves the submucosa of the ileocaecal valve (Plate 16), so called lipohyperplasia, and the thickened valve pouts into the caecum and occasionally may become congested and give rise to bleeding.

Carcinoid tumours of the rectum can present as small, hard, submucosal polyps less than 1 cm in diameter and may be discovered accidentally. This type can be treated by local excision, provided that removal is complete (Figs 16.21 and 16.22).

Endometriosis very occasionally gives rise to an ill-defined polypoid mass in the sigmoid colon or rectum. It is covered by intact mucosa. Ulceration only occurs as a complication of biopsy and the histological appearances can easily be mistaken for adenocarcinoma.

In pneumatosis cystoides intestinalis, involvement of the large

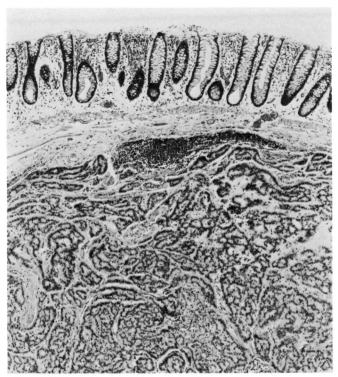

Fig. 16.22 Carcinoid tumour. Characteristic pattern of convoluted and interlacing ribbons of cells. H & E × 56.5.

intestine can give rise to a coarsely polypoid mucosal surface (Plate 187). Histologically, cystic spaces in the submucosa are lined by large macrophages which may be multinucleated (Plate 188). Gas in the cysts appears to be under pressure and a popping sound occurs when they are biopsied at colonoscopy cr sigmoidoscopy.

The Cronkhite–Canada syndrome is a rare form of gastrointestinal polyposis of unknown cause associated with ectodermal changes including alopecia, skin pigmentation and nail atrophy. There is polypoid hypertrophy of the mucosa of the bowel without ulceration (Plate 99). Microscopically, the lamina propria of the mucosa is oedematous and epithelial tubules show cystic dilatation with flattening of the lining epithelium (Plate 100 and Fig. 16.23).

Pseudomembranous colitis results in discrete raised plaques in the large bowel which can often be felt on rectal examination or seen via the sigmoidoscope (Plate 170). However, in some cases the right side of the bowel is affected without rectal involvement and in these the

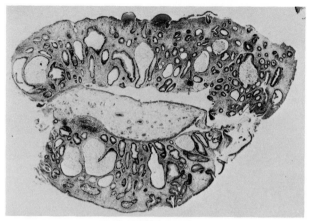

Fig. 16.23 Cronkhite–Canada syndrome. Many glands are dilated and some have ruptured. H & E × 11.5.

diagnosis may be made at colonoscopy (Plate 168) (Tedesco, 1979). Histologically, a focal group of crypts are distended by mucin and polymorphs with loss of the epithelial lining and erosion of the surface (Plate 169). There is an abrupt change to normal adjacent mucosa (Fig. 16.24).

Lastly, and very rarely, heterotopia may occur in the large bowel, nearly always in the rectum and present as a polyp. The commonest

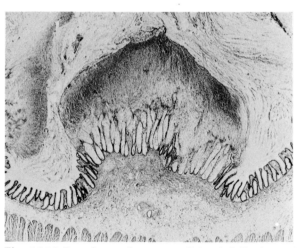

Fig. 16.24 Pseudomembranous colitis. A fully formed plaque composed of a focal group of distended and disrupted crypts with an overlying 'pseudomembrane' of mucin and polymorphs. H & E × 10.4.

tissue is gastric epithelium but pancreatic elements have also been described.

16.6 Summary

In clinical practice most polyps removed at colonoscopy are found to be either inflammatory, hamartomatous, metaplastic or neoplastic on histological examination. The latter is the most important group and consists of adenomas, a small but significant proportion of which have undergone malignant change.

If adenocarcinoma of the large bowel invariably arises via a dysplastic polypoid lesion, the adenoma, then in theory the removal of these precursors would eradicate colorectal cancer. However, because of the wide disparity between the prevalence of adenomas and the incidence of large bowel cancer in high-risk populations, it is obvious that the vast majority of adenomas remain small and do not undergo malignant transformation. In addition, limitations of time, expertise and money as well as the relative risks of the procedure itself necessarily invalidate colonoscopy as a screening procedure. An outstanding problem which remains is to identify the sub-group of people with adenomas who are at most risk of developing malignant change. This notwithstanding, colonoscopy now plays a major role in the detection and removal of polyps and in the examination and follow-up of patients with neoplastic lesions, since this group is known to be at increased risk of having or developing further tumours.

References

Achord, J. L. and Proctor, H. D. (1963), Malignant degeneration and metastasis in Peutz-Jeghers' syndrome. *Archs Intern. Med.*, **111**, 498–502.

Cornes, J. S., Wallace, M. H. and Morson, B. C. (1961), Benign lymphomas of the rectum and anal canal. A study of 100 cases. *J. Path. Bact.*, **82**, 371–82.

Eide, T. J. and Stalsberg, H. (1978), Polyps of the large intestine in northern Norway. *Cancer*, **42**, 2839–48.

Fenoglio, C. M., Kaye, G. I. and Lane, N. (1973), Distribution of human colonic lymphatics in normal, hyperplastic and adenomatous tissue: its relationship to metastasis from small carcinomas in pedunculated adenomas, with two case reports. *Gastroenterology*, **64**, 51–66.

Gillespie, P. E., Chambers, T. J., Chan, K. W., Doronzo, F., Morson, B. C. and Williams, C. B. (1979), Colonic adenomas – a colonoscopy survey. *Gut*, **20**, 240–5.

Greene, F. L. (1974), Epithelial misplacement in adenomatous polyps of the colon and rectum. *Cancer*, **33**, 206–17.

Grinnell, R. S. and Lane, N. (1958), Benign and malignant adenomatous polyps and papillary adenomas of the colon and rectum. An analysis of 1856 tumors in 1335 patients. *Surgery*, **106**, 519–38.

Hayashi, T., Yatani, R., Apostol, J. and Stemmermann, G. N. (1974), Pathogenesis of hyperplastic polyps of the colon: a hypothesis based on ultrastructure and in vitro cell kinetics. *Gastroenterology*, **66**, 347–56.

Heald, R. J. and Bussey, H. J. R. (1975), Clinical experiences at St. Mark's Hospital with multiple synchronous cancers of the colon and rectum. *Dis. Colon Rect.*, **18**, 6–10.

Helwig, E. B. and Hansen, J. (1951), Lymphoid polyps (benign lymphoma) and malignant lymphoma of the rectum and anus. *Surgery Gynec. Obstet.*, **92**, 233–43.

Kaye, G. I., Fenoglio, C. M., Pascal, R. R. and Lane, N. (1973), Comparative electron microscopic features of normal, hyperplastic and adenomatous human colonic epithelium. *Gastroenterology*, **64**, 926–45.

Louw, J. H. (1968), Polypoid lesions of the large bowel in children with particular reference to benign lymphoid polyposis. *J. Pediat. Surg.*, **3**, 195–209.

Morson, B. C. (1966), Factors influencing the prognosis of early cancer of the rectum. *Proc. R. Soc. Med.*, **59**, 607–8.

Morson, B. C. (ed.) (1978), *The Pathogenesis of Colorectal Cancer*. W. B. Saunders, Philadelphia.

Morson, B. C., Bussey, H. J. R. and Samoorian, S. (1977), Policy of local excision for early cancer of the colorectum. *Gut*, **18**, 1045–50.

Morson, B. C. and Dawson, I. M. P. (eds) (1979), *Gastrointestinal Pathology*, 2nd ed, Blackwell, Oxford.

Morson, B. C. in collaboration with Sobin, L. (1976), Histological typing of intestinal tumours. *Int. Histological Classification of Tumours*, No. 15, WHO, Geneva.

Muto, T., Bussey, H. J. R. and Morson, B. C. (1973), Pseudo-carcinomatous invasion in adenomatous polyps of the colon and rectum. *J. Clin. Path.*, **26**, 25–31.

Muto, T., Bussey, H. J. R. and Morson, B. C. (1975), The evolution of cancer of the colon and rectum. *Cancer*, **36**, 2251–70.

Reid, J. D. (1965), Duodenal carcinoma in the Peutz-Jeghers' syndrome. *Cancer*, **18**, 970–7.

Rickert, R. R., Auerbach, O., Garfinkel, L., Hammond, E. C. and Frasca, J. M. (1979), Adenomatous lesions of the large bowel. An autopsy study. *Cancer*, **43**, 1847–57.

Shaw, E. B. and Hennigar, G. R. (1974), Intestinal lymphoid polyposis. *Am. J. Clin. Pathol.*, **61**, 417–22.

Tedesco, F. J. (1979), Antibiotic associated pseudomembranous colitis with negative proctosigmoidoscopy examination. *Gastroenterology*, **77**, 295–7.

Wolff, W. I. and Shinya, H. (1973), A new approach to colonic polyps. *Ann. Surg.*, **178**, 367–78.

Wolff, W. I. and Shinya, H. (1975), Endoscopic polypectomy. Therapeutic and clinicopathologic aspects. *Cancer*, **36**, 683–90.

CHAPTER SEVENTEEN

Colon Cancer

SIDNEY J. WINAWER

Colonoscopy has revolutionized our approach to patients who are at risk for or who have had colorectal cancer (Winawer *et al.*, 1976). Colonoscopy has a clear role in the examination of high-risk groups initially and in their follow-up surveillance; in the diagnosis of patients with positive screening tests; in symptomatic patients suspected of having a neoplastic lesion clinically or on barium enema; and in the follow-up surveillance of patients with a prior adenoma or carcinoma. In addition, a variety of tissue sampling techniques have evolved which can be applied selectively for the clarification of identified lesions. In considering colonoscopy one must now also consider sigmoidoscopy, which recently has developed into a useful examination limited to the distal colon using flexible fibreoptic instruments of varying length. Finally, both colonoscopy and flexible sigmoidoscopy are potential research tools for obtaining samples from the colon in the search for tumour markers and other indicators of malignant or pre-malignant change of the mucosa. Since the current era of colonoscopy is relatively new, in the history of medicine, many of the applications are not yet firmly established and supported by hard data. At this time, a rational approach can be synthesized based on the evidence from clinical trials, personal experience, and known concepts of the natural history of colorectal cancer and its antecedent premalignant lesions both in the normal population as well as in high-risk groups.

17.1 Role of colonoscopy in screening

Although colonoscopy cannot be considered a screening investigation in average-risk patients to be applied on a wide scale, it can be considered as a screening tool in small, select high-risk groups (Kussin, Lipkin and Winawer, 1979). Perhaps it would be even more appropriate to consider the use of colonoscopy in these high-risk groups as a case-finding technique rather than a screening technique in the pure sense, since screening tests should be not only effective, but simple, inexpensive and easy to administer by the medical community to be considered a true screening test. The high-risk groups in which colonoscopy has potential application includes chronic ulcerative colitis, the polyposis inherited colon cancer group, non-polyposis inherited colon cancer, Peutz-Jeghers' syndrome, and patients with a prior adenoma or prior colorectal cancer.

17.1.1 *Ulcerative colitis*

Patients with chronic ulcerative colitis involving the entire colon are at risk for carcinoma approximately seven years after the onset of their ulcerative colitis (Sherlock and Winawer, 1978). Onset of the ulcerative colitis in childhood apparently does not provide any increased risk in addition to the time factor. In such patients, surveillance using colonoscopy should be started approximately seven years after onset and performed either annually or every other year with biopsies for dysplasia and, where cytology is available, lavage cytology. It has not been firmly established as yet whether surveillance every year is more effective than every other year. Most large programmes have given up the barium enema for routine follow-up purposes in this group of patients because of its low yield.

Surveillance can be started later in patients with left-sided ulcerative colitis since the risk appears to increase after approximately fifteen years duration of the disease (Greenstein *et al.*, 1979). The same approach of biopsy for dysplasia and lavage cytology is used in these patients as well. Patients with distal ulcerative colitis involving the distal descending colon or rectosigmoid are at minimal risk of malignant change and it is not clear how often these patients should be put under surveillance, but it is agreed that some surveillance is essential in these patients since they carry at least the same risk as the average population and probably slightly more. In addition, their disease could extend to involve the entire colon which would be missed should they not have any surveillance performed at all. It would be appropriate in this group of patients to reduce the surveillance interval to every other year rather than insist that it be performed annually.

The risk of carcinoma in patients with Crohn's colitis is greater than the general population but not of the order of magnitude as in patients with ulcerative colitis (Lightdale *et al.*, 1975). Their risk has not been firmly established and, in addition, dysplasia has been rarely seen as an indicator of malignancy in these patients. Patients with strictures of the colon with either ulcerative colitis or Crohn's disease can have a carcinoma as the basis for the stricture. Periodic surveillance of both of these groups would detect the development of a stricture, and biopsies and brushings could be obtained for clarification of its nature. The carcinoma in inflammatory bowel disease can be flat (Plate 142) and difficult to detect either by X-ray or visually at colonoscopy: when small they may be detected only by biopsy or cytological techniques.

17.1.2 *Inherited colon cancer*

In the non-polyposis inherited colon cancer groups colonoscopy should be performed periodically to determine whether individuals within a suspect family have been affected. There is increasing evidence from our studies (Lipkin, Sherlock and Winawer, 1978) as well as the studies of Lynch, Lynch and Lynch (1977) that the cancers developing in these groups occur more frequently on the right side of the colon as compared to the left side of the colon, develop from pre-existing adenomas, and develop at a younger age than in the average-risk patient. Given all of these observations, it would be important to use colonoscopy periodically to detect the adenomas especially those on the right side (Fig. 17.1). Sigmoidoscopy would, therefore, be of less value in this group, and faecal occult blood testing with its lower sensitivity for adenomas would also be of limited value in this group as a primary screening investigation.

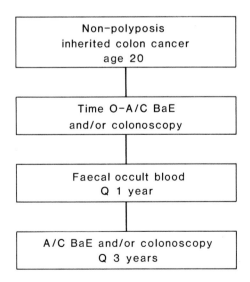

Fig. 17.1 Scheme for inherited colon cancer follow-up.

It may be justifiable, perhaps, in these patients to perform also barium enema initially along with the colonoscopy in an attempt to clear the colon of any existing carcinomas, as well as adenomas, although this approach can be questioned because of the low sensitivity of the barium enema for adenomas and small cancers and the young age of the patients. Once the colon has been cleared of any underlying adenomas or carcinomas, the interval for surveillance can be approximately every three years. This position is extrapolated from the slow doubling time of adenomas in the average-risk population. Although the temporal evolution of new adenomas in this group of patients may not be the same as in the average group of patients, it would seen unreasonable to recolonoscope the patient more frequently especially as they are asymptomatic and their surveillance begins at a very young age, usually in their twenties.

Patients with a family history of polyposis inherited colon cancer of the traditional familial polyposis or Gardner's syndrome (Plate 97) type can have limited flexible sigmoidoscopy to determine whether they are affected, since if they are affected, polyps will be easily visualized in the rectum. This can be done once a year. If affected, recommendations are usually made for sub-total colectomy and periodic follow-up surveillance with flexible sigmoidoscopy. However, if the patients are not psychologically ready for surgery, colonoscopy could be performed in an attempt to keep the colon under surveillance for carcinoma although this is a near impossible task since carcinomas usually evolve from the small adenomas present, and considering the number of adenomas present it would be extremely difficult to keep these patients under effective cancer control with any degree of confidence. Lavage cytology can be added effectively to the endoscopic procedure in this group of patients since we are dealing with a diffuse lesion.

Patients with the Peutz-Jeghers' syndrome (Plate 98) and a history of juvenile polyposis can develop adenomas in adult life anywhere in their colon and, therefore, the type of surveillance just outlined for patients with familial polyposis and Gardner's syndrome may not be applicable to this group (Winawer *et al.*, 1980c). This group of patients probably requires the same type of periodic surveillance with colonoscopy as does the non-polyposis inherited colon cancer group. There is very little data to indicate at what site in the colon adenomas occur in these two groups, but it is our personal observation that they occur commonly above the rectosigmoid. The patients that we have seen with Peutz-Jeghers' syndrome with adenomas in the colon have generally had multiple adenomas rather than a single one.

17.1.3 *Prior neoplasia*

Patients with a prior adenoma or carcinoma of the colon are at high risk for an additional lesion and should, therefore, be kept under surveillance (Winawer *et al.*, 1980c). It is not clear what the metachronous rate or subsequent rate of new adenomas is in the patients who have had a prior adenoma. The reason that data are not firm is because the data on metachronous lesions evolved in the precolonoscopy era before the colon was cleared of all lesions by colonoscopy. In the precolonoscopy era the metachronous rate for new adenomas given an index adenoma at some point in time ranged from 30–50%. There is some information based on the sigmoidoscopy studies which indicate that over a seven year period of time patients having had an adenoma removed from the rectosigmoid during sigmoidoscopy had approximately a 30% frequency of additional new polyps during that period of time. We can extrapolate that figure to the rest of the colon for the purpose of obtaining some reasonable figure although it is clear from a large amount of evidence that neoplastic lesions in the rectosigmoid and the colon do not always behave in the same manner.

We can assume that patients with a prior colorectal cancer have the same metachronous rate as patients with prior adenomas since it is now clearly established that colorectal cancers arise from adenomas and, therefore, these patients would have had an adenoma at some point in the natural history of their colorectal lesion. The metachronous rate for new adenocarcinomas of the colon in patients having had one cancer has ranged from 5–10% in a variety of studies. In the St. Mark's series (Morson, 1976) the patients who had polyps in the resected specimen had a metachronous rate at the higher end of the spectrum. Experience at Memorial Sloan-Kettering Cancer Center with metachronous lesions approaches that of the St. Mark's series. The question of how often to rescreen by colonoscopy patients who have had a prior adenoma or prior colorectal cancer cannot be answered with certainty at this time. A randomized controlled trial has just been initiated with patients in different groups undergoing different intervals of examination to address this issue. However, at the present time considering the slow turnover rate of adenomas that must arise *de novo* and grow to a 1 or 1.5 cm size with a significant premalignant potential, takes about five or more years. A rational approach, therefore, would be to re-examine these patients approximately every three years after the colon has been cleared of all initial polyps and cancer. It has been the experience of most colonos-

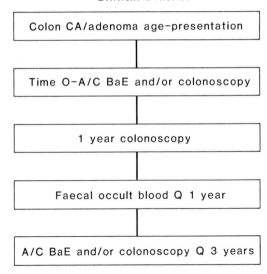

Fig. 17.2 Scheme for the follow-up of a patient with prior cancer or polyps.

copists that it is more difficult to clear the colon of adenomas with certainty if the patient has had several adenomas initially than a single adenoma. It would be reasonable to recolonoscope these patients on an annual basis until the colon has been cleared of all known adenomas before placing the patient on a more extended surveillance programme (Fig. 17.2).

Small adenomas, i.e. those under 5 mm in size, present a special problem. These adenomas are frequently observed and their significance is not clear. It has been previously reported that polyps under 5 mm in size in the rectosigmoid were usually hyperplastic (Plate 66). However, this does not appear to be true above the area of the rectosigmoid. Studies by Waye, Frankel and Braunfeld (1980) and by us (Miller, Kussin and Winawer, 1980) have indicated that a high percentage of these polyps in the rest of the colon, particularly on the right side of the colon, are true adenomas. These can easily be removed by either the diathermy snare technique or the hot biopsy technique (Plate 36). Our approach is to remove polyps of 3 mm in size or more, but to leave the 1 or 2 mm excrescences that are seen in almost every patient. The importance of this approach in cancer control will have to be determined in the future. The two possible reasons for removing these polyps are: (a) as a prevention for their growth into larger adenomas with a premalignant potential, and (b) to determine their histology as an indicator of risk in patients who have no other lesions.

17.2 The role of colonoscopy in diagnosis

17.2.1 *Positive occult blood test*

Asymptomatic patients having a positive faecal occult blood test as well as those with a positive finding on proctosigmoidoscopic examination or barium enema are candidates for colonoscopy. Patients who have a positive faecal occult blood test (Haemoccult) have an approximately 50% probability of having a neoplastic lesion including adenomas (38%) and cancers (12%) (Winawer *et al.*, 1980a). The predictive value of the faecal occult blood test for a neoplastic lesion increases with age. Studies from around the world evaluating the faecal occult blood test for screening have demonstrated that the yield for neoplastic lesions is much higher when colonoscopy is added to the diagnostic work-up in addition to the barium enema (Winawer, Andrews and Miller, 1980d). When single-column barium studies are used, approximately half of the cancers and the majority of adenomas are missed radiologically but detected at colonoscopy. The University of Minnesota controlled trial of screening with faecal occult blood testing has abandoned the use of the single-column barium enema and now uses only colonoscopy in the diagnostic work-up of these patients. In the ongoing controlled trial at the Memorial Sloan-Kettering Cancer Center and Preventive Medicine Institute-Strang Clinic double-contrast barium enemas have been used in addition to colonoscopy in positive screenees. In these patients the barium enema has been highly sensitive for cancers but, as in the University of Minnesota study, the sensitivity for adenomas has been extremely low. The cancers being detected in these controlled trials of screening are to a large extent early cancers of Dukes' A and B stage and smaller in size than the cancers detected in the usual symptomatic population. The false-negativity for the faecal occult blood test is not as yet known, but the false-positivity is about 2%. Even when a lesion is detected by barium enema, colonoscopy is important to search for other lesions as well as obtain a tissue diagnosis or perform polypectomy.

17.2.2 *Positive proctosigmoidoscopy*

In patients having a positive proctosigmoidoscopic examination, colonoscopy is indicated to search for additional lesions. Although the synchronous rate for additional adenomas has been observed to be about 50% with the use of colonoscopy and the synchronous rate for additional cancers in the presence of one cancer has been observed to be between 1.5 and 5%, it is not clear whether this synchronous rate applies to those patients who present with a rectal polyp as compared to a colonic polyp or colonic cancer. This question is now being examined.

A high synchronous rate for additional lesions will undoubtedly be found in the colon in patients who present with rectal lesions, but the exact figure will be forthcoming. In the past, our policy was to obtain a barium enema before doing colonoscopy in patients who have had a rectal polyp detected, but we have given this up because of the extremely low yield of the barium enema for additional synchronous lesions in such patients. We now go directly to colonoscopy in patients who have a rectal polyp of 3 mm in size or greater. At the time of the colonoscopy this lesion is removed and the colon is searched for additional lesions. Should this lesion turn out to be an adenoma, the patient is put under long-term follow-up surveillance, but if it turns out to be a hyperplastic polyp and no other lesions are found at that point in time, no other examinations are performed in this patient for surveillance purposes except for that usually done for the average-risk patients including faecal occult blood testing and sigmoidoscopy.

17.2.3 *Symptomatic patients*

Patients who have symptoms of neoplastic disease are usually worked up with a proctosigmoidoscopic examination first, followed by a barium enema, and then by colonoscopy. If a lesion is found on the proctosigmoidoscopic examination or the barium enema, then of course these patients need a colonoscopy to ascertain the nature of the lesion, to remove it if it is a benign-appearing adenoma, and to obtain tissue sampling if it is a malignant lesion.

When a cancer has been detected by proctosigmoidoscopy or barium enema, the approach will vary regarding colonoscopy depending on the location of the lesion and the nature of the lesion. For small to moderate size polypoid adenocarcinomas anywhere in the colon, colonoscopy can usually be done safely and the lesion passed gently while looking for synchronous lesions. If there is any difficulty, with the colonoscopy requiring considerable manipulation, the procedure is usually terminated. It is more important searching the left colon for a synchronous lesion with an index cancer on the right than it is searching the right colon with an index lesion on the left, because the highest incidence of lesions is found in the left colon, producing a higher yield of synchronous carcinomas in that part of the large bowel. If the lesion is a partially obstructing lesion, we do not like to go past the lesion with the colonoscope. If this lesion is in the proximal colon, then the distal colon can be colonoscoped to clear it of synchronous lesions, but if this obstructing lesion is in the left side or the sigmoid colon, then it is usually unwise to go beyond this lesion and manipulate the colon for fear of perforation. The reason for perforation may be related either to fixation of the bowel caused by the carcinoma or to segmental ischemic colitis that sometimes accompanies a neoplastic lesion with friability and loss of integrity of the bowel wall.

At times it may be wise to omit the first steps of proctosigmoidoscopy and barium enema and proceed directly to colonoscopy. This may be an approach indicated in the patient with moderately severe red rectal bleeding. In patients in whom the rectal bleeding is not quite so severe and there is no clinical urgency, a double-contrast barium enema should precede the colonoscopy. When seeing a patient with rectal bleeding for the first time, a proctosigmoidoscopy in the unprepared bowel should be performed before planning colonoscopy, to be certain that we are not dealing with ulcerative colitis. The activity of the colitis may be such that preparation for colonoscopy should not be performed then but should be deferred until the colitis has been treated and is quiescent.

A double-contrast barium enema should be obtained before colonoscopy whenever possible except in selected circumstances such as the urgent rectal bleeder or a patient with ulcerative colitis under surveillance, in order to provide the most sensitive combination of examinations for neoplasia for each patient. Although the yield of neoplastic lesions is much higher for colonoscopy than it is for the barium enema that is generally performed in a medical community, there is a false-negativity for the colonoscopy, as well. This false-negativity has not been well established for cancers, but we all have had the experience of having missed at least one cancer because of its difficult location. The areas that are potentially difficult for diagnosis are the areas just proximal to the hepatic and splenic flexures and the medial aspect of the ascending colon, especially just proximal to the ileocaecal valve. The false-negativity for adenomas has been established in one study at the University of Wisconsin by Leinicke *et al.* (1977). In their blinded study, colonoscopy was compared to the barium enema and it was shown that colonoscopy had approximately a 6% miss rate for adenomas of 1 cm in size and greater.

17.3 Role of colonoscopy in follow-up surveillance

The rationale and procedure for follow-up of patients after polypectomy or colon cancer resection has been discussed above. In addition to the routine use of colonoscopy in such surveillance, special circumstances require special consideration. If a colostomy has been done temporarily for colorectal cancer, the colon should be examined endoscopically before closure of the colostomy to be absolutely certain that there are no other lesions present in the colon. When following up patients after resection for colon cancer, we routinely biopsy and brush the anastomosis during the surveillance procedures, for the three years following surgery, to detect any anastomotic recurrences. Anastomotic recurrences (Plate 111) are generally uncommon, except for low anterior resections unless the patient has presented under adverse circumstances, such as with obstruction, requiring some compromise of the usual surgical approach. We do brush cytology and biopsies of the anastomosis even if it appears normal (Plates 21 and 22) (Table 17.1). When intra-abdominal recurrences do occur, they usually occur outside of the bowel and involve the bowel secondarily.

In the work-up of a patient with a rising CEA, in addition to the general work-up of the patient, colonoscopy is indicated to look for additional cancers in the colon.

So far the accumulated experience of workers in the field indicate that this approach has not been very productive. In spite of this, however, most physicians feel that colonoscopy is indeed indicated with a rising CEA prior to a second-look operation to be absolutely sure that the colon is clear of new cancers or intraluminal recurrences. Colonoscopy is also useful in the follow-up surveillance of patients who have had radiation. Rectal bleeding that may occur postoperatively in patients who have had both resection and radiation is often secondary to radiation proctitis or radiation colitis, and endoscopic diagnosis of radiation colitis (Plate 166) is helpful as a basis for medical treatment. It is important to be certain that the radiation colitis has become quiescent prior to any contemplation of closure of a colostomy since reanastomosis with restoration of continuity of the bowel can result in a marked worsening of this type of colitis.

Table 17.1 Role of colonoscopy in the follow-up of patients after surgery for cancer

Evaluation of anastomosis
Clear the colon prior to colostomy closure
Evaluation of radiation colitis prior to colostomy closure
Search for synchronous adenomas and cancers
Search for metachronous adenomas and cancers
Evaluation prior to 'CEA-timed second look'

Colonoscopy is not indicated as part of the follow-up of patients who have known residual cancer in the abdomen or distant metastases. In patients who have no known residual disease in the abdomen or metastatic disease, colonoscopy should be considered as part of their routine follow-up after a period of observation has indicated no evidence of recurrence of disease. In patients in whom a polyp has been removed that shows carcinoma (Plates 73 and 74), surgical resection should be considered if the carcinoma appears to be poorly differentiated or has been observed to invade submucosal lymphatics, both of these being unusual, or if the carcinoma has extended down to the line of resection. Under these circumstances a resection should be seriously considered, providing it does not have to be an abdominoperineal resection and the patient is a good risk for surgery. Resection is not indicated for carcinoma-in-situ or for carcinoma that is well differentiated, has not invaded lymphatics, and is well-clear of the line of resection. A large volume of cancer in the polyp often influences our decision (Hertz, 1980). In those patients who have gone to surgery in this setting, only about 5% have demonstrated positive lymph nodes and none have demonstrated distant metastases. The yield of such surgery, therefore, is low and the patient should be managed with a conservative approach.

17.4 Tissue sampling

Adenomas are removed *in toto* and not biopsied unless they appear to be possibly polypoid adenocarcinomas. It has been demonstrated that biopsies of benign-appearing polyps are misleading and do not generally reflect the pathology present (Winawer *et al.*, 1978). Carcinoma detected on biopsy may be in situ or invasive, and carcinoma in the polyp can be easily missed by biopsy of a small portion of the polyp. Exophytic or mass lesions in the colon produce a high yield of positive tissue sampling, and four biopsies are usually sufficient to provide a diagnosis. In flat, infiltrating lesions, such as those seen in inflammatory bowel disease, it is more difficult to obtain a positive tissue diagnosis, and more biopsies from an abnormal area are necessary (Winawer *et al.*, 1978) (Fig. 17.3).

Small polypoid lesions, approximately 5 mm in size or less, can be biopsied with the hot biopsy technique producing a larger size biopsy specimen and fulguration of the remainder. Brush cytology has added to the yield of biopsy and is particularly useful in certain select situations, including strictures, the anastomosis after surgery, and lesions that are difficult to biopsy precisely because of their location. Lavage cytology is now limited to the follow-up surveillance in patients with

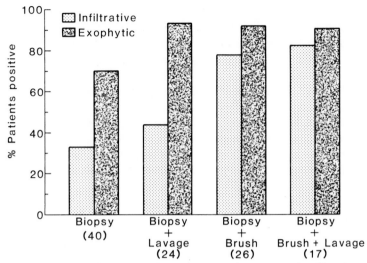

Fig. 17.3 Colonoscopic biopsy and cytology in diagnosis of infiltrative and exophytic cancers. Cytology increases the sensitivity for tissue diagnosis of cancer as compared to biopsy alone. Exophytic or mass-type lesions have a higher yield than the flatter mucosally infiltrating lesions. Lavage cytology adds very little to brush cytology and biopsy and is, therefore, performed only in select situations. (Reprinted with the kind permission of the publishers of Harrison's *Textbook of Medicine*, in press publication of S. J. Winawer and P. Sherlock.)

chronic ulcerative colitis and to other problem situations, such as the patient with a fixed colon and a mass which is difficult to reach or patients with familial polyposis prior to surgery or after surgery with an affected rectal segment.

When biopsies are obtained, a pin or bayonet-type forceps is most useful since the specimen remains on the pin allowing multiple specimens to be obtained with each pass of the biopsy forceps. Graham *et al.* (1980) have developed a valuable technique for increasing the yield of biopsy diagnoses by aspirating the material within the biopsy channel after the biopsy forceps had been removed and collecting this material for cytology. This is especially useful since pieces of the biopsy often come off within the channel on withdrawal of the biopsy forceps. Specimens are placed on gel foam and immediately placed in buffered formalin. When brush cytology is used, we usually use it prior to the biopsy and smear the specimen on several clear glass slides, and immediately place this into a cytology jar, face up, containing 95% alcohol.

When performing lavage cytology, we usually use 200–300 ml of saline, and after aspirating the material back into the trap and with-drawing the colonoscope, we suction into the trap an equal amount of 95% alcohol. The material is then centrifuged and the sediment is smeared on glass slides. Lavage cytology is tedious and time-consuming and, therefore, not done as frequently as before.

There is a significant false-negativity for cytology as there is for biopsy, and the two together have the highest yield. False-positivity can also occur for cytology. This can occur in a setting of considerable inflammation such as active ulcerative colitis, radiation colitis, or in patients on chemotherapy. An experienced cytologist usually has no difficulty distinguishing the false-positive cells from the true-positive cells. False-positives can also occur in patients with polyps having severe atypia or in patients with familial polyposis who have multiple polyps with considerable atypia in many of them. When biopsies are negative and cytology is positive and this becomes a basis for a management decision, we usually ask the cytologist to review the slide again or request another opinion with full clinical information provided so that the cytologist understands the setting in which the material is obtained. If there is any question about the pos-sibility of a false-positivity, we go back and obtain additional mater-ial.

17.5 Sigmoidoscopy: rigid and flexible

Use of the rigid sigmoidoscope has in the past been associated with: a prolonged survival of patients having had a diagnosis of cancer; a reduction in mortality for rectosigmoid cancer in patients screened with sigmoidoscopy; and with a reduction in the expected incidence of rectosigmoid cancer in patients under periodic screening (Winawer *et al.*, 1980c). Sigmoidoscopy, therefore, is a potentially useful approach to the cancer problem. The percentage of neoplastic lesions within the distal 25 cm of colon is 50%, which is a reduction from the older figures and suggests an interruption of the adenoma-adenocarcinoma sequence by identification and removal of antecedent premalignant lesions by this method. The examination procedure with rigid sigmoidoscopy has, however, not been widely accepted by patients or the medical community. There has been a resurgence of interest in sigmoidoscopy with the introduction of flexible instru-ments for this purpose (Winawer *et al.*, 1979). The 60 cm flexible sigmoidoscope has become a popular instrument in the hands of experienced endoscopists, and there have been repeated reports of increased yields when compared to rigid sigmoidoscopy. It is of inter-est that flexible sigmoidoscopy has shown that rigid sigmoidoscopy

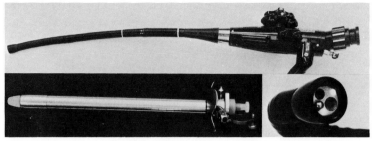

Fig. 17.4 A 30-cm flexible sigmoidoscope. Flexible sigmoidoscopes of varying lengths are available, depending on training, for higher yields of neoplastic lesions and greater patient comfort.

has a false-negativity between 16 and 25 cm, as well as an inability to detect lesions above the 25 cm region (Bohlman *et al.*, 1977). The 60-cm flexible sigmoidoscope however, is an expensive and sophisticated instrument for the trained endoscopist. A 30-cm flexible sigmoidoscope has been introduced for use by the generalist who has no prior endoscopic experience, and our studies to date indicate that this is a feasible instrument for this purpose (Winawer *et al.*, 1980b) (Fig. 17.4). We would expect that some time in the near future 30-cm flexible sigmoidoscopes will totally replace the rigid sigmoidoscope as a primary screening instrument in the hands of the non-endoscopist. It is possible that endoscopists may use this short instrument as well since it provides a comfortable examination for the patient and a consistent insertion by the physician to 30 cm at each examination. The flexible sigmoidoscopes all have facilities for biopsy, brush cytology, photography, and lavage cytology. There is a need to continue the sigmoidoscopy approach for the control of cancer of the colon, since it has been demonstrated that faecal occult blood testing is not a good test for cancer of the rectosigmoid or polyps of the rectosigmoid region, although it appears to be an effective screening test for colorectal cancers above this area. Some combination of faecal occult blood testing, perhaps annually, with flexible sigmoidoscopy perhaps every three years, could provide for the first time a combination of two techniques performed in sequence for the control of colorectal cancer.

17.6 Concluding comments

Dramatic progress has been made in the control of colorectal cancer with the introduction of new technology, including effective colonoscopes, variable length flexible sigmoidoscopes, devices for polypectomy, brush cytology, lavage cytology, and biopsy. The colonoscope may also provide a vehicle for further research into the etiology, screening, and diagnosis of colorectal cancer.

Dye-scattering techniques have been used to enhance biopsy, and lavage has been performed through the colonoscope for assay of tumour markers and other indicators of malignancy and premalignancy. Biopsies have also been obtained to search for proliferative characteristics as an indication of premalignant change, and especially for dysplasia as an indicator of the premalignant change of the colonic mucosa in patients with long-standing ulcerative colitis. The increasing number of physicians being trained in these techniques and the rapid evolution of sophisticated, improved instrumentation has provided an unique opportunity for a dramatic advance in our ability to control cancer of the colon. Hopefully, wide dissemination of new conceptual information and technological advances will provide a greater awareness of these possibilities among the physicians in the general medical community.

Acknowledgement

This work supported in part by Public Health Service Research Grant No. CA-15429 from the National Cancer Institute through the National Large Bowel Cancer Project.

References

Bohlman, T. W., Katon, R. M., Lipschutz, G. R., McCool, M. F., Smith, F. W. and Melnyk, C. S. (1977), Fiberoptic pansigmoidoscopy. An evaluation and comparison with rigid sigmoidoscopy. *Gastroenterology*, **72**, 644–9.

Graham, D. Y., Schwartz, J. T., Cain, G. D. and Gyorkey, F. (1980), Endoscopically directed biopsy of the esophagus and stomach: a controlled study of biopsy number. *Gastrointest. Endosc.*, **26**, 67.

Greenstein, A. J., Sachar, D. B., Smith, H., Pucillo, A., Papatestas, A. E., Kreel, I., Geller, S. A., Janowitz, H. D. and Aufses, A. H., Jr. (1979), Cancer in universal and left-sided ulcerative colitis: factors determining risk. *Gastroenterology*, **77**, 290–4.

Hertz, R. E. L. (1980), The management of adenomas of the large gut. In: *Neoplasms of the Colon, Rectum, and Anus.* (ed. M. W. Stearns Jr.), John Wiley and Sons, Inc., New York, Ch. 5.

Kussin, S. Z., Lipkin, M. and Winawer, S. J. (1979), Inherited colon cancer: clinical implications. *Am. J. Gastroent.* **72**, 448–57.

Leinicke, J. L., Dodds, W. J., Hogan, W. J. and Stewart, E. T. (1977), A comparison of colonoscopy and roentgenography for detecting polypoid lesions of the colon. *Gastrointest. Radiol.*, **2**, 125–8.

Lightdale, C. J., Sternberg, S. S., Posner, G. and Sherlock, P. (1975), Carcinoma complicating Crohn's disease: report of seven cases and review of the literature. *Am. J. Med.*, **59**, 262–8.

Lipkin, M., Sherlock, P. and Winawer, S. J. (1978), Early diagnosis and detection of colorectal cancer in high-risk population groups. In: *Gastrointestinal Tract Cancer* (eds M. Lipkin, R. A. Good and S. B. Day), Plenum Publishing Corp., New York, pp. 241–36.

Lynch, H. T., Lynch, J. and Lynch, P. (1977), Management and control of familial cancer. In: *Progress in Cancer Research and Therapy. Genetics of Human Cancer*, **3**, (eds J. J. Mulvihill, R. W. Miller and J. F. Fraumeni, Jr.), Raven Press, New York City, 235–56.

Miller, C. H., Kussin, S. Z. and Winawer, S. J. (1980), Characteristics of synchronous colonic polyps, (abstract) *Gastrointest. Endosc.*, **26**, 72.

Morson, B. C. (1976), Genesis of colorectal cancer. In: *Clinics in Gastroenterology*, **5**, (eds P. Sherlock and N. Zamcheck), W. B. Saunders Company, Ltd., Philadelphia, pp. 505–25.

Sherlock, P. and Winawer, S. J. (1978), Cancer in inflammatory bowel disease: risk factors and prospects for early detection. In: *Gastrointestinal Tract Cancer* (eds M. Lipkin, R. A. Good and S. B. Day), Plenum Publishing Corp., New York, pp. 479–88.

Waye, J. D., Frankel, A. and Braunfeld, S. A. (1980), The histopathology of small colon polyps (abstract). *Gastrointest. Endosc.*, **26**, 80.

Winawer, S. J. (1973), Colonoscopy as a screening examination. In: *Current Status of Barium Enema and Colonoscopy in Diagnosis of Colonic Disease*. Symposium Proceedings Yale Affiliated Gastroenterology Program/Connecticut Society of Gastrointestinal Endoscopy. (ed. H. M. Spiro and V. A. DeLuca, Jr.), Purdue Frederick Company, Norwalk, Conn., pp. 53–59.

Winawer, S. J., Andrews, M., Flehinger, B., Sherlock, P., Schottenfeld, D. and Miller, D. G. (1980a), Progress report on controlled trial of fecal occult blood testing for the detection of colorectal neoplasia. *Cancer*, **45**, 2959–64.

Winawer, S. J., Andrews, M. and Miller, C. (1980d), Review of screening with fecal occult blood. In: *Colorectal Cancer: Prevention, Epidemiology, and Screening. Progress in Cancer Research*. (eds S. J. Winawer, D. Schottenfeld and P. Sherlock) Raven Press, New York City, Ch. 4.

Winawer, S. J., Cummins, R., Ptak, A. and Andrews, M. (1980b), Feasibility of a 30 cm flexible sigmoidoscopy (FSX 30) by non-endoscopists (abstract), *Gastrointest. Endosc.*, **26**, 80.

Winawer, S. J., Leidner, S. D., Boyle, C. and Kurtz, R. C. (1979), Comparison of flexible sigmoidoscopy with other diagnostic techniques in the diagnosis of rectocolon neoplasia. *Am. J. Dig. Dis.*, (new series) **24**, 277.

Winawer, S. J., Leidner, S. D., Hajdu, S. I. and Sherlock, P. (1978), Colonoscopic biopsy and cytology in the diagnosis of colon cancer. *Cancer*, **42**, 2849–53.

Winawer, S. J., Sherlock, P., Schottenfeld, D. and Miller, D. (1976), Screening for colon cancer. *Gastroenterology*, **70**, 783–9.

Winawer, S. J., Sherlock, P., Schottenfeld, D. and Miller, D. G. (1980c), Screening for colon cancer: an overview. *Cancer*, **25**, 1093–8.

CHAPTER EIGHTEEN

Inflammatory Bowel Disease

ROBIN H. TEAGUE and JEROME D. WAYE

Most patients with inflammatory bowel disease can be adequately investigated and managed using the conventional methods of history, physical examination, sigmoidoscopy and barium enema. A properly performed double contrast barium enema provides a diagnostic record of the whole colon from the rectum to the caecal pole. The double contrast technique is well standardized and can be rapidly carried out by the radiologist with the films available for later inspection and comparison (Bartram, 1977). On the other hand colonoscopy is nearly always more time-consuming to perform than radiology and this is especially true when multiple biopsies are taken or excision diathermy is used. Total colonoscopy may not be uniformly achieved and the depth of intubation as well as the amount of meaningful information obtained may depend greatly on the level of skill of the examiner. It is for these reasons that colonoscopy is considered complementary to the barium enema in the investigation of patients with inflammatory bowel disease.

Colonoscopy does offer some advantages over the barium enema in the ability to see variations in colour of the colon mucosa, visual resolution of tiny lesions, and the means to obtain a tissue diagnosis at any level of the colon. The modern generation of instruments combine differential shaft stiffening, torque stability and 230° distal tip angulation. This means that colonoscopy is now much easier for both the patient and the endoscopist; an important factor when inflammatory bowel disease may render the colon more friable or produce painful fixed loops.

The place of fibresigmoidoscopy in the diagnosis and management of inflammatory bowel disease is not yet established. At the present time, there are few indications for fibresigmoidoscopy in inflammatory bowel disease other than increased patient comfort as compared to the rigid proctosigmoidoscope. The shorter instruments are expensive and there is as yet no evidence that they are any more robust than ordinary colonoscopes.

Table 18.1 The indications for colonoscopy in inflammatory bowel disease

---
Differential diagnosis
Resolution of radiographic abnormalities
  Filling defects
  Strictures
Preoperative and postoperative evaluation in Crohn's disease
Examination of stomas
Screening for premalignant and malignant changes

18.1 Indications for colonoscopy in inflammatory bowel disease

There are only a few fixed indications for colonoscopy in inflammatory bowel disease (Table 18.1) where endoscopy is normally (and properly) the last investigation in the diagnostic armamentarium.

18.1.1 *Differential diagnosis*

The endoscopist may be called on to distinguish, not just between ulcerative colitis and Crohn's disease, but to diagnose a wide range of specific inflammatory conditions of the colon. Whenever colonoscopy is performed in inflammatory bowel disease, the endoscopist must not forget the possibility that a condition other than Crohn's or ulcerative colitis may be present. In many circumstances the intraluminal view is non-diagnostic, and the correct answer is determined by the histopathologist's interpretation of the tiny biopsy specimens provided.

(a) *Infective diarrhoea*
Most of the 'infective diarrhoeas' are self-limiting, and for this reason, rarely come to colonoscopic examination. Acute infection with salmonella, shigella and campylobacter may induce X-ray changes similar to those of early ulcerative colitis. Similar non-specific findings may be seen at colonoscopy and the endoscopic differentiation from ulcerative or Crohn's colitis can be extremely difficult, particularly so in campylobacter colitis.

Shigella and salmonella infections may stimulate large quantities of mucus adherent to a magenta-coloured mucosa. In these cases the surface is less friable than that encountered in ulcerative colitis and histology reveals features of acute inflammation with a cellular infiltrate consisting primarily of polymorphonuclear leucocytes rather than lymphocytes (Day, Mandal and Morson, 1978; Price, Jewkes and Sanderson, 1979).

'*Antibiotic-associated*' *colitis* due to *Clostridia difficile* can be identified endoscopically but involvement is not always uniform and may be confined to the right colon or to the sigmoid colon. A yellow membrane is often present covering most of the mucosal surface (Plate 170) but more commonly small elevated yellow plaques are seen on a moderately inflamed mucosa (Plate 168). Biopsy of the plaques usually produces bleeding and histology shows a polymorphonuclear exudate and the typical 'volcano' lesions of this condition (Plate 169).

Yersinia enterocolitica infection has the appearance of small diffuse ulcerations throughout the colon (Vantrappen *et al.*, 1977).

Tuberculosis can affect any part of the large bowel or terminal ileum, producing appearances indistinguishable from Crohn's disease (Plates 179 and 180) (Bretzholz, Stasser and Kroblanch, 1978; Aoki *et al.*, 1975; Franklin, Mohaptra and Perrillo, 1979). Exuberant inflammatory polyposis commonly follows tuberculosis infections. Minor points which may assist in the differentiation are that in tuberculosis, skip lesions tend to be shorter than those in Crohn's disease; the ulcers may have a rolled edge, and the mucosa is generally less friable. Even at histology the distinction between tuberculosis and Crohn's disease is still difficult to make and although acid-fast staining may show organisms, this is by no means certain (Moshal *et al.*, 1973). A high index of suspicion is required from the clinician, endoscopist and histologist if this potentially treatable disease is not to be misdiagnosed.

Amoebiasis produces an intense inflammatory reaction in the colon with ulcers which may resemble Crohn's disease (Plates 171 and 172) (Crowson and Hines, 1978). Differential points are the very reddened rim of surrounding mucosa in amoebic infestation and the great depth of the ulcers. Positive biopsies can be obtained from any part of the mucosa but the yield is better if the edges of the ulcers are biopsied.

Schistosomiasis is rarely encountered in temperate climates but the colonoscopist may be alerted to the possibility by the presence of inflammatory polyps (Plate 176) especially in a visitor from an endemic area (Nebel *et al.*, 1974). Inflammatory polyps may involve the whole colon but are commonly localized and may also mimic tuberculosis. Calcified polyps containing encysted schistosomes (Plate 173) are a unique feature of schistosomiasis and are readily identified as glistening white nodules.

Endoscopic transmission of *salmonella* has been recorded (Dean, 1977) so that if there is any possibility that a case of infective colitis has been colonoscoped, then the most effective means of instrument cleaning and sterilization should be employed. At the present time this means the use of glutaraldehyde solution or ethylene oxide gas.

Of course, if the colitis is known *in advance* to be infective in origin then colonoscopy is contraindicated but the diagnosis is often in doubt and colonoscopy may then contribute successfully in these situations.

(b) *Specific types of colitis*
An inflammatory reaction of the colon is sometimes observed accompanying diverticular disease. Occasionally the inflammation is confined to the area immediately around the diverticular orifices giving a 'halo' appearance, but more commonly it causes reddening and petechiae on the interhaustral folds in the affected segment (Plate 34). Rarely a confluent inflammation occurs with the thickened folds appearing polypoid. In these circumstances the patient may be experiencing symptoms of 'diverticulitis' and contact bleeding is a feature at endoscopy. The etiology of the colonoscopic findings in diverticular disease is unknown but it may be due to mucosal ischaemia or the trauma of persistent spasm.

Acute ischaemic colitis presents a variable appearance according to the severity of the ischaemic process. Thus, in mild cases only slight oedema with loss of vascular pattern is present but severe cases may reveal the blue/black bowel of incipient gangrene (Plates 160 and 162). Occasionally a pseudomembrane may be present (Plate 163) overlying the ischaemic area which, when removed reveals a reddened, friable mucosa with contact bleeding (Plate 158) (Hunt and Buchanan, 1979). The commonest site for ischaemic colitis is the descending colon just distal to the splenic flexure but it may occur in the sigmoid colon and rectum causing diagnostic confusion. Stricture formation is common (Plate 164) and pseudopolyps may be found (Farinon, 1978). Small ulcers can be seen in the healing phase, but surrounding petechial haemorrhages and biopsies containing haemosiderin, provide a useful diagnostic distinction from Crohn's disease and ulcerative colitis.

Solitary ulcers may be found throughout the colon (Rutter and Riddell, 1975) but the most common site is the rectum (Plate 183). In elderly patients faecal stasis and rectal prolapse are thought to be responsible but in the younger patient self-induced trauma is commonly the cause of the problem. The histological features are unique and allow distinction from other causes of rectal ulceration.

Irradiation colitis is another form of segmental colitis which the colonoscopist may encounter. It is most commonly found in the proximal rectum and distal sigmoid following radiotherapy for cervical carcinoma, but occasionally a mid-sigmoid segment is involved as a result of a fixed redundant loop lying within the irradiated area. Less common sites are the ascending and descending colon following renal irradiation. A symptomatic colitic response of short duration almost always follows radical radiotherapy of the pelvic organs. Symptoms include diarrhoea and tenesmus with the passage of mucus, and occasionally, blood. The endoscopist will rarely be called upon to examine this well recognized and self-limiting phenomenon (Moss and Brand, 1979) which is to a large extent dose- and fractionation-dependent. If, however, the rectum is examined at this stage, an oedematous inflamed mucosa is seen with loss of vascular pattern and multiple small bleeding points. Histology confirms non-specific acute inflammation and mucosal oedema.

A secondary colitis may follow six months to two years after irradiation. This is much less common than the primary reaction and is of obscure etiology, unrelated to the vigour of the initial reaction but occurring at the same site. Endoscopically the appearances are of an acutely haemorrhagic mucosa bleeding spontaneously (Plate 167) and biopsy reveals evidence of chronic inflammation, fibrosis and occasionally haemosiderin granules, suggesting an ischaemic origin. Both the primary and secondary types of irradiation colitis can be followed by the formation of telangiectasias which may present as rectal bleeding, and, when they occur in the right colon, will require differentiation from other forms of acquired angiodysplasia (Rogers and Adler, 1976). This distinction is not usually difficult to make endoscopically as postradiotherapy telangiectasias are diffuse, occur over a wide area, and the surrounding mucosa is atrophic whereas angiodysplastic lesions are usually small (<5 mm), discrete and occur in normal mucosa.

(c) *Irritable bowel syndrome*
Colonoscopy is not normally required to diagnose the irritable bowel syndrome, but as this is a diagnosis usually made by exclusion, the colonoscopist may be asked to give an opinion. The finding of an endoscopically and histologically normal bowel, in a patient who at that time is symptomatic, excludes inflammatory bowel disease of the colon. It is rare for Crohn's disease or ulcerative colitis to heal without any evidence of abnormality. There are no endoscopic features specific to the irritable bowel syndrome. Diffuse or localized spasm may be seen but is common in 'normal' patients and often absent in patients with confirmed irritable bowel syndrome. Melanosis coli resulting from purgative abuse (Plate 27) is often found in irritable bowel syndrome or diverticular disease. In its early stages the non-pigmented lymphoid follicles bear a superficial resemblance to ulceration and the pigmented mucosa appears inflamed. Contact with the

instrument tip or biopsy forceps, however, establishes that there is no friability and the histology is diagnostic.

(d) *Differentiation between ulcerative colitis and Crohn's disease*
The commonest causes of inflammatory bowel disease encountered in clinical practice are Crohn's disease and ulcerative colitis. It is not surprising therefore that the endoscopist is frequently called upon to distinguish between these conditions. On the other hand, it is deluding to imagine that colonoscopy, even with the help of histology, can provide an answer in every case. Endoscopic features which may serve to distinguish the two conditions (Waye, 1977) are listed in Table 18.2. There are exceptions to most of the rules but two may be regarded as absolute. First and most important, in Crohn's disease ulcers of any size may be found in areas of macroscopically and histologically normal mucosa (Plates 144, 146 and 148) (Waye, 1978). This is never seen in ulcerative colitis where ulcers are always accompanied by erythema and loss of vascular pattern in the surrounding mucosa. Secondly, ulcers are never found in the terminal ileum in ulcerative colitis. Backwash ileitis may produce loss of vascular pattern with friability and contact bleeding, but ulcers are always absent.

The typical early change in Crohn's disease is that of aphthous ulcers, each surrounded by a 'halo' of erythema in otherwise normal mucosa (Plate 144) (Morson, 1972; Rickert and Carter, 1977). This is not invariable as some early cases of Crohn's disease show a diffuse granularity and loss of vascular pattern, more typical of ulcerative colitis. The earliest changes of ulcerative colitis are loss of the crisply outlined vascular pattern with intervascular erythema and oedema. These early changes in ulcerative colitis should not be confused with the mucosal oedema produced by irritant enemas such as hypertonic

Table 18.2 Colonoscopic differentiation of inflammatory bowel disease

	Ulcerative colitis	*Crohn's disease*
Early change	Oedema Erythema Loss of vascular pattern	Aphthous ulcers Vascular pattern normal
Moderate change	Granularity Contact bleeding	Linear ulcers Cobblestoning
Late change	Discrete ulcers and pus	Confluent ulcers Contact bleeding

phosphate, or the patchy linear erythema and haemorrhage that results from instrumentation or wash-out procedures.

Progression of ulceration in Crohn's disease produces larger longitudinal ulcers often extending several centimetres along the bowel and causing fissuring (Plate 150). Multiple deep ulcers with intact adjacent mucosa causes one type of 'cobblestoning' appearance. Another type of cobblestoning is associated with granulomatous submucosal involvement giving rise to a bumpy irregularity of the wall covered by normal mucosa (Plates 149 and 152). True cobblestoning is never seen in ulcerative colitis, although some variations of pseudopolyposis may closely resemble it. Rarely Crohn's ulcers may have a deep 'punched out' appearance. These ulcers bleed easily, may perforate, and are almost always associated with a poor prognostic outlook.

Disease progression in ulcerative colitis is accompanied by increased granularity (Plate 115) due to mucosal oedema and multiple small shallow ulcers. Contact bleeding accompanies obvious mucosal inflammation. Later changes are those of larger ulcers which may become confluent but shallow with a mucopurulent yellow exudate. Whenever large deep mucosal ulcers are encountered the examination should be terminated immediately as perforation may be imminent.

Distribution of the inflammatory processes in the colon may give some help in the differential diagnosis. It is unusual for ulcerative colitis to show endoscopic and histological rectal sparing unless topical steroids have been used in treatment. Similarly, right-sided ulcerative colitis, or ulcerative colitis producing skip lesions is not commonly seen. The pattern of involvement of the caecum, ileocaecal valve and terminal ileum may also help in distinguishing these two conditions. Endoscopically it is unusual to see total Crohn's disease of the colon ending abruptly at the ileocaecal valve with a normal terminal ileum. More typically, the valve itself is involved becoming stenosed and rigid with changes of Crohn's disease seen within the terminal ileum. Nodular lymphoid hyperplasia, common in young people, cannot be confused with granulomatous ileitis since the coloration of the bumpy lymphoid nodules is the same as that of surrounding ileal mucosa, and is not friable. Abrupt change to normality at the ileocaecal valve is therefore much more suggestive of ulcerative colitis where the valve is often incompetent and easily intubated.

Other endoscopic features are common to both diseases and are therefore not helpful in the differential diagnosis. Pseudopolyps are an obvious example of this, reflecting the severity of the inflammatory process rather than its etiology (Plates 126, 130 and 136). Mucosal bridges are caused by ulcerations burrowing beneath a strip of normal mucosa which later heals by re-epithelialization of the ulcer bed as well as the under surface of the strip (Plates 134 and 135), thereby producing a mucosal tube. On rare occasions these bridges may cause obstruction to instrument passage but they are common to both Crohn's disease and ulcerative colitis. Healing in both diseases may be associated with absence of haustral folds, strictures, and a reticular pattern of white scars on the mucosa.

Attempts to distinguish between the diseases histologically have proved disappointing despite the use of multiple and target biopsies. There is no doubt however, that multiple biopsies (one or two from each colonic segment – caecum, ascending colon, hepatic flexure, transverse colon, splenic flexure, descending colon, sigmoid and rectum) should always be taken and presented to the histopathologist with a detailed description of the endoscopic findings. Then, if the only histological change is of acute and/or chronic inflammation of varying severity, the pattern of colonic involvement may be mapped out. This information alone may help to distinguish Crohn's disease ('patchy involvement') from ulcerative colitis ('increasing inflammation distally') and a variation of inflammation within an individual biopsy may suggest Crohn's disease.

The finding of granulomas in the biopsy is virtually pathognomonic of Crohn's disease but their presence has been reported in one case of ulcerative colitis (Williams and Waye, 1978). The incidence of granulomas in cases of confirmed Crohn's disease varies according to the literary source. McGovern and Goulston (1968) and Geboes and Van Trappen (1975) and Geboes *et al.* (1978) have found the incidence to be low (<10%) but others (Frühmorgen, 1974; Lux *et al.*, 1978) state that the incidence is higher (25%). This discrepancy may, in part, be due to the type of cases referred for colonoscopy since early cases with aphthoid ulceration tend to have a higher yield of granulomas. The yield is highest when biopsies are taken from the centre of small (<4 mm) ulcers or the edges of large ulcers (Williams and Waye, 1978). In chronic cases with marked mucosal destruction the presence of granulomas is unusual even when the ulcer edges are biopsied.

Other histological features which may help in the diagnosis are microabscesses (twice as common in ulcerative colitis) and other relative factors such as normal goblet cell mucus in a markedly inflamed biopsy, suggesting Crohn's disease (Morson, 1974). In some cases of long-standing Crohn's disease amyloid may be found (Waye, 1977) and this has not been described in biopsies from ulcerative colitis.

It will be obvious from the above description that the distinction between Crohn's disease, ulcerative colitis and other forms of inflammatory bowel disease is not always absolute endoscopically or even histologically. The colonoscopist should, therefore, be aware of the limitations of the investigation and realize that there are only a few pathognomonic features of inflammatory bowel disease. Ulcers in an area of colon that is otherwise grossly normal indicate Crohn's disease as does the presence of cobblestoning.

Even the best double contrast barium enema may underestimate the true extent of inflammatory bowel disease (Teague, Salmon and Read, 1973; Dilawari *et al.*, 1973; Williams, 1975). In addition there are patients whose X-rays are entirely normal but in whom endoscopy plus histology reveals total colitis (Teague, Salmon and Read, 1973; Williams and Teague, 1973).

There are times in the course of inflammatory bowel disease when the clincial progress of the patient may be at variance with the enema report. This may be an indication for colonoscopic examination and the findings may radically alter the treatment regime of that patient. For example, a patient who has radiological proctosigmoiditis which is not responding symptomatically to topical steroid therapy may benefit enormously from the discovery of endoscopic total colitis and a subsequent change to systemic steroids. It is common to find that, when multiple biopsies are taken, the inflammatory process extends beyond the limits visible endoscopically. It is, therefore, mandatory to take multiple biopsies from all levels of the colon in patients with endoscopically subtotal colitis as well as from those patients where there is a high clinical suspicion of organic disease despite a negative endoscopy.

Historically, the histological predictions for malignant and pre-malignant change in ulcerative colitis were developed prior to the advent of colonoscopy and are therefore based on the presence of *radiological* total colitis. Colonoscopic examination has indicated that many cases with radiologically limited colitis do in fact have total colitis, but whether or not these cases have the same malignant risk as X-ray total colitics is not yet known.

18.1.2 *Examination of a radiological filling defect and strictures*

(a) *Radiological filling defects*
In the well-prepared patient with inflammatory bowel disease, in whom retained stool is not a problem, the presence of a filling defect on barium enema indicates pseudopolyps, adenomatous polyps or carcinoma. Pseudopolyps are found in both ulcerative colitis and Crohn's disease (Margulis, 1972). There are several types of

pseudopolyps with the most common resulting from a severe attack of colitis, when small islands of mucosa survive the surrounding destructive inflammation and ulceration. These islands grow more rapidly than the surrounding epithelium and often produce finger-like projections extending 2–3 cm into the lumen (Plate 127). Another theory of pseudopolyp formation is that raging inflammation under-mines a finger-like projection of mucosa, which then projects into the colon lumen when healing occurs. These mucosal tags can exist sur-rounded by histologically normal mucosa and in this situation are the only evidence of the previous extent of inflammation. Other forms of pseudopolyps include granulation tissue polyps (Plates 128 and 129) which are characteristically covered with a white exudate and larger pedunculated polyps composed of epithelialized granulation tissue (Plate 130) (Jalan *et al.*, 1969; Teague and Read, 1975). Inflammatory polyps are usually small and multiple and rarely give rise to diagnos-tic confusion at radiology or endoscopy, but may grow large enough to obstruct the narrowed colitic lumen (Plate 132) (Goldgraber, 1965; Castleman and McNeely, 1972) or cause intussusception (Forde *et al.*, 1978). Large solitary pseudopolyps will require differentiation from carcinoma in chronic total colitics (Plate 131) (Teague and Read, 1975); but because of their histology, biopsies from any portion of the surface will permit the correct diagnosis to be made.

It was originally thought that pseudopolyps were premalignant (Dawson and Pryse-Davies, 1959) but later workers (Edwards and Truelove, 1964; Jalan *et al.*, 1969) proved that they had no malignant potential. It was also thought that there was a negative association between the presence of pseudopolyps and premalignant and malig-nant change (Teague and Read, 1975), but our recent experience sug-gests that these conditions may coexist. When multiple pseudopolyps are present it is obviously impractical to biopsy or remove each polyp but it is wise to biopsy all pseudopolyps exceeding 1 cm in size and all those that are of a different colour from their fellows. Removal or biopsy should also be considered when pseudopolyps show surface irregularity and friability. Endoscopic biopsy is usually sufficient to establish the identity of a pseudopolyp but they can be safely removed using standard electrodiathermy techniques. Discretion must be exercised when the surrounding mucosa is inflamed, or healing may be delayed and serosal burns are more likely. Adenomatous polyps may occur in ulcerative colitis (Teague and Read, 1975) but they are uncommon and may usually be removed by excision diathermy.

The presence of long-standing total ulcerative colitis carries a risk of cancer which is some thirty times greater than that of the normal population (Shearman, 1973; Lennard-Jones *et al.*, 1977). It is widely accepted that cancer arising in colitis has a different genesis from that arising in the 'normal' colon (Counsell and Dukes, 1952; Morson and Pang, 1967; Lennard-Jones *et al.*, 1977). Colon carcinoma usually arises in a neoplastic polyp, spreads to invade the stroma, stalk and finally the colonic wall. In chronic ulcerative colitis dysplastic changes may take place in any part of the colon giving rise to carcinoma-in-situ in some areas (Myrvold, Kock and Ahren, 1974). It follows that the distribution of carcinoma in ulcerative colitis is fairly uniform throughout the colon (Greenstein *et al.*, 1979) and because of its origin it is often flat and plaque-like in appearance (Plate 142). Unfortunately, this is not readily appreciable endoscopically and many colonoscopists have had the experience of performing a biopsy of apparently well healed areas of bowel and receiving the histopathologist's report of severe dysplasia or invasive carcinoma. However, it is worthwhile taking extra biopsies from areas having a pale 'velvety' or villous appearance and from plaques which are raised above the level of the surrounding mucosa (Yardley, Bayless and Diamond, 1979). Large polypoid cancers (Plate 141) may be encountered in ulcerative colitis and these almost certainly reflect an advanced stage of the disease with a poor prognosis (Goldgraber and Kirsner, 1964).

(b) *Strictures*
Most strictures seen in inflammatory bowel disease are benign (Hunt *et al.*, 1975) and are the result of muscle hypertrophy and spasm or fibrosis (Plates 137–139). Fibrotic strictures may also be found in ischaemic and irradiation colitis as well as following amoebic and tuberculous infections. Endoscopic identification of radiologically demonstrated strictures may prove difficult as some are distensible by air insufflation and the spherical aberration produced by modern 'wide angle' optics makes small changes in colonic diameter difficult to appreciate.

The majority of strictures found in inflammatory bowel disease can be successfully negotiated using the standard adult colonoscope (Plate 147) but there are occasions when a paediatric endoscope is required to pass through a tight stricture to inspect the proximal bowel. In every case multiple biopsies should be taken from the edges and lumen of the stricture and these should be supplemented by brush cytology to determine a possible malignant etiology. Malignancy may be suspected endoscopically if the stricture is rigid, has 'shelf-like' edges or is impossible to negotiate with the instrument (Plate 140) (Waye, 1978). Carcinoma complicating ulcerative colitis may be partially submucosal so that negative or inconclusive biopsies are obtained (Crowson, Ferrante and Cathright, 1976). On these occasions referral for surgery may have to be made on the endoscopist's suspicion of malignancy which may be reinforced by the finding of dysplastic change in the proximal or distal epithelium.

18.1.3 *Preoperative and postoperative assessment of Crohn's disease*

In expert hands the double contrast barium enema is capable of demonstrating the presence of small Crohn's aphthous ulcers, especially when magnification spot films are used (Laufer, 1979). Unfortunately, some aphthous ulcers remain undetected even when a technically perfect enema has been carried out (Lennard-Jones *et al.*, 1977). A further problem for the radiologist is to decide whether or not there is active disease in a segment containing pseudopolyps. Most surgeons are unwilling to make an anastomosis through bowel affected by active disease and, for this reason, insist on an accurate preoperative delineation of its extent. As radiology cannot be relied upon to provide accurate information in every case it would seem reasonable to give as many patients as possible the benefit of a colonoscopic assessment which may alter the type of operation planned. When ileocolic fistulae develop in Crohn's disease, it is surgically important to decide whether ileal (as is usually the case) or colonic disease is responsible. A careful endoscopic inspection with multiple biopsies will usually provide an answer in these cases. Inflammatory adhesions consequent upon fistula formation may produce fixed colonic loops making total colonoscopy difficult or impossible. Fortunately it is nearly always possible to reach the site of the fistula and to examine and biopsy the adjacent mucosa.

Postoperative diarrhoea after ileocolic resection for Crohn's disease may be due to choleraic enteropathy (when the terminal ileum has been removed) or to recurrent disease. These cases can present difficulties for the radiologist because of rapid transit through the anastomosis (Fawaz *et al.*, 1976) or because of postoperative distortion of the bowel. Recurrent Crohn's disease will be obvious endoscopically since the colonoscope may almost invariably be passed up to the level of the anastomosis, and beyond to inspect several centimetres of small bowel (Plate 153). If the anastomosis is narrow (Plate 154), the endoscope can be positioned at the stenosed segment providing an opportunity to visualize the area and obtain biopsies.

18.1.4 *Examination of stomas*

Most ileostomies can be intubated with the standard single channel colonoscope but if the stoma is tight its venous drainage becomes obstructed as the instrument is passed through the anterior abdominal wall. It is prudent, therefore, to observe the spout for two or three minutes after intubation and if a dusky blue colour develops then the instrument should be withdrawn and cannulation repeated using the paediatric endoscope. With this proviso it is possible to examine up to 100 cm of the ileal mucosa.

Ileostomy dysfunction may take the form of an increase in effluent possibly with bleeding or mechanical obstruction. If mechanical obstruction takes place in an ileostomy after ulcerative colitis it is important to remember that the original diagnosis may have been wrong and that the obstruction may be due to recurrent Crohn's disease and not to adhesions. In patients whose colectomy was performed for Crohn's disease the presence and extent of recurrence can be visualized and biopsied with the endoscope or, even more important, recurrent disease may be completely ruled out as the etiology for recurrent obstruction. The colonoscopic assessment can be performed in a few minutes after minimal preparation (clear liquid diet for 24 hours) and provides a definitive answer to a problem for which radiology is usually inaccurate or misleading (Fawaz *et al.*, 1976).

In the 'continent' ileostomy pouch of Kock (Kock, 1973) endoscopy may be helpful in both diagnostic and therapeutic roles (Waye *et al.*, 1977). If internal sutures become detached, then kinking of the outflow tract of the pouch may take place. The patient is unable to perform intubation and painful distention of the pouch occurs. The outflow tract can easily be negotiated endoscopically, even when sharply angulated, and the instrument will pass on into the dilated pouch under direct vision. A guidewire may be inserted through the endoscope channel and a catheter passed along this to effect drainage. Alternatively, a rubber tube may be passed along the shaft of the paediatric endoscope to lie proximally in the manner of a colonoscopic stiffening tube. When the pouch has been intubated by the endoscope the lubricated rubber tube is slid down the shaft into the pouch and the endoscope withdrawn. The rubber drain (with plug) may then be left *in situ* for several days or until more definitive measures are carried out.

Incontinence of the Kock ileostomy pouch is a major problem which may benefit from endoscopic assessment and therapy. Continence of the pouch is largely dependent upon a permanently intussuscepted length of ileum at the proximal end of the outflow tract. If the intussuscepted ileum is not fixed in position, then insufficient length protrudes into the pouch to produce the necessary valve effect. This can be determined endoscopically by inverting the endoscope inside the pouch and observing the behaviour of the intussuscepted segment when the instrument is advanced and withdrawn. If it moves freely then it is likely that the securing sutures have given way. This problem may be rectified by injecting a sclerosant at endoscopy to restore a fixed intussusception of appropriate length. Incontinence may also be caused by a fibrous band tethering the intussuscepted segment in a fixed 'skew' position preventing normal function of the valve. This band may be divided using a diathermy snare. Virtually any forward or oblique viewing endoscope can be used and we have also found the paediatric instruments to be helpful (Waye *et al.*, 1977).

18.1.5 *Surveillance for cancer and precancer*

Crohn's disease and subtotal ulcerative colitis carry a slightly higher risk of carcinoma of the colon than that found in the general population (Greenstein *et al.*, 1979). The cancer risk is greatest in patients having total ulcerative colitis for ten years and increases beyond that time. It is thought that the development of frank carcinoma is almost invariably preceded by the appearance of dysplastic cellular changes ('premalignancy') (Morson and Pang, 1967). The presence of dysplasia on biopsy is associated with a high incidence of carcinoma either locally or distally (Morson and Pang, 1967; Lennard-Jones *et al.*, 1974). A high proportion of patients with dysplasia on colonoscopic biopsies will also have dysplasia on sigmoidoscopic biopsies (Riddell, 1976; Nugent *et al.*, 1979) but there are exceptions to this (Evans and Pollack, 1972) and it is now generally agreed that total colonoscopy with multiple biopsies is the best method for detection of early dysplasia. Yardley, Bayless and Diamond (1979) recommend that biopsies be taken at 10-cm intervals throughout the colon so that eight or nine separate levels are investigated and this has also been our practice.

The presence of acute inflammation may cause histological changes closely resembling dysplasia so that if moderate to severe dysplasia is found in association with inflammation, a repeat endoscopy with multiple biopsies is recommended within three to six months for confirmation (Riddell, 1977; Lennard-Jones *et al.*, 1977). If dysplasia is then confirmed the patient should be advised to have a colectomy. If there is no dysplasia at the first endoscopy then the problem of future surveillance arises. The actual interval between the appearance of dysplasia and its progression to carcinoma is not yet known so that a logical time interval between endoscopies is not apparent. Several studies are currently in progress to determine the optimum time interval between colonoscopic examinations (Williams, 1980) but until their results are available it would seem reasonable to carry out colonoscopy with multiple biopsies at yearly intervals and perform interim sigmoidoscopic biopsies every four months. If possible, biopsies from the colitic colon whether taken for surveillance, extent of disease, or for differential diagnosis should be collected from flat, non-inflamed segments of bowel. Although the tendency is to biopsy protruding mounds of tissue such as pseudopolyps, these are not representative of the entire colon. Similarly, one should avoid if possible, taking biopsy specimens for surveillance from areas of inflamed mucosa since the histologic findings of inflammation may be similar to those of dysplasia.

18.2 Contraindications and hazards

The most difficult decision facing the endoscopist is to determine when a patient, recovering from an acute attack of colitis, can be safely endoscoped. Indications must be carefully considered in every patient with inflammatory bowel disease, and no patient should be colonoscoped unless a clearly defined goal has been identified. Each case must be approached individually with the patient's clinical condition as a guide to assessing the proper timing of the procedure. Even when preparation has been completed and the endoscopy begun, the colonoscopist must still decide whether or not the examination may be safely completed.

Fortunately, colonoscopists have been extremely cautious when endoscoping inflammatory bowel disease and reported complications are rare (Teague, Salmon and Read, 1973; Rogers *et al.*, 1975; Smith, 1976). It is obviously very dangerous to attempt colonoscopy in the acute phase of any type of inflammatory bowel disease when the bowel is extremely friable and perforation with the endoscope or proximal perforation due to air insufflation may occur.

Over-inflation and formation of loops on insertion are to be avoided in the friable and non-elastic colon of inflammatory bowel disease and the use of the stiffening overtube is contraindicated. It is possible to perforate the colitic bowel even with the biopsy forceps so that care should be exercised during biopsy procedures and a more gentle technique adopted. Perforation may also result from over-zealous attempts to intubate strictures.

If a sensible approach is used then there are very few unpredictable hazards in the colonoscopy of inflammatory bowel disease.

18.3 Preparation

Bowel preparation for colonoscopy has traditionally utilized a combination of diet, purgation and cleansing enemas, but it is obviously unnecessary and unkind to purge a patient already suffering from diarrhoea. There is also the danger of provoking activity in a recently

Table 18.3 Bowel preparation for colonoscopy in inflammatory bowel disease

	Castor oil	Citrate of magnesia solution	Liquid diet	Enema(s)
Normal	60 ml		24 h	2
Colitis stable		150–300 ml	24–28 h	2
Colitis active			48 h	1

healed colitis by the preparation. This danger may well be over-stated but it seems wise to avoid if possible, an unnecessarily aggressive preparation. Unfortunately, many patients with limited active colitis have faecal stasis in the proximal bowel and these cases will require a full preparation for a meaningful assessment to be obtained. In these circumstances it is sensible to wait for a relatively inactive phase before proceeding with the endoscopy if this is pos-sible. The risk of exacerbating extensive but quiescent colitis by purga-tion appears to be small (Williams and Waye, 1978).

It seems, therefore, that a graded regimen for preparation of colitics should be adopted when a diet, purgation and washout technique is used (Table 18.3). Mannitol 10% has been used as an oral prepara-tion for colonoscopy and may also be employed in patients with inflammatory bowel disease. With this technique, patients with rela-tively inactive colitis can be successfully prepared using 20–30 ml of X-Prep (or similar mild purgation) on the day prior to the examina-tion and then 500 ml of 10% orange or lemon flavoured mannitol orally, at least three hours before colonoscopy. Mannitol characteristi-cally gives a 'wet' preparation but this is more than compensated for by the excellent mucosal cleansing achieved.

When only a limited examination is to be attempted adequate bowel cleansing may be obtained by the use of one or two disposable phosphate enemas. After the enemas have been administered the patient is encouraged to evacuate the bowel and the examination is begun immediately. For examination of ileostomy stomas it is only necessary for the patient to take a 24-hour clear liquid diet and fast overnight.

18.4 Conclusions

Before 1970 endoscopic visualization of the large bowel was limited to its distal 20 cm and unless operation or autopsy supervened then histology was likewise confined. Of all the conditions amenable to colonoscopic diagnosis and therapy, inflammatory bowel disease has proved the most challenging. The indications and limitations are now firmly established and there is no doubt that the technique has proved invaluable for many patients.

References

Aoki, G., Nagasako, K., Nakae, Y., Susuki, H., Endo, M. and Takemoto, T. (1975), The fibercolonoscopic diagnosis of intestinal tuberculosis. *Endoscopy*, **7**, 113.

Bartram, C. I. (1977), Radiology in the current assessment of ulcerative colitis. *Gastrointest. Radiol.*, **1**, 383–92.

Bretholz, A., Strasser, H. and Knoblauch, M. (1978), Endoscopic diagnosis of ileocecal tuberculosis. *Gastrointest. Endosc.*, **24**, 250–1.

Castleman, B. and McNeely, B. U. (1972), Right lower quadrant mass after four-and-one-half years of ulcerative colitis. Case Records of the Massachusetts General Hospital. *New Engl. J. Med.*, **286**, 147–58.

Counsell, P. B. and Dukes, C. E. (1952), The association of chronic ulcerative colitis and carcinoma of the rectum and colon. *Br. J. Surg.*, **39**, 485–95.

Crowson, T. D. and Hines, C. (1978), Amebiasis diagnosed by colonoscopy. *Gastrointest. Endosc.*, **24**, 254–5.

Crowson, T. D., Ferrante, W. F. and Cathright, J. B. Jr. (1976), Colonoscopy: inefficacy for early carcinoma detection in patients with ulcerative colitis. *J. Am. Med. Ass.*, **236**, 2651–2.

Dawson, I. M. P. and Pryse-Davies, J. (1959), The development of cancer of the large intestine in ulcerative colitis. *Br. J. Surg.*, **47**, 113–28.

Day, D. W., Mandal, B. K. and Morson, B. C. (1978) The rectal biopsy appearances in salmonella colitis. *Histopathology*, **2**, 117–31.

Dean, A. G. (1977), Transmission of *Salmonella typhi* by fibreoptic endoscopy. (letter) *Lancet*, **2**, 134.

Dilawari, J. B., Parkinson, C., Riddell, R. H., Loose, H. and Williams, C. B. (1973), Colonoscopy in the investigation of ulcerative colitis. *Gut*, **14**, 426.

Edwards, F. C. and Truelove, S. C. (1964), The course and prognosis of ulcerative colitis. III and IV. *Gut*, **5**, 1–22.

Evans, D. J. and Pollack, D. J. (1972), In-situ and invasive carcinoma of the colon in patients with ulcerative colitis. *Gut*, **13**, 566–70.

Farinon, A. M. (1978), Colonoscopy: a necessary aid in the diagnosis of transient ischaemic colitis. *Endoscopy*, **10**, 112–14.

Fawaz, K. A., Glotzer, D. J., Goldman, H., Dickersin, G. R., Gross, W. and Patterson, J. F. (1976), Ulcerative colitis and Crohn's disease of the colon – a comparison of the long-term post-operative courses. *Gastroenterology*, **71**, 372–8.

Forde, K., Gold, R. P., Holck, S., Goldberg, M. D. and Kiam, P. S. (1978), Giant pseudopolyposis in colitis with colonic intussusception. *Gastroenterology*, **75**, 1142–6.

Franklin, G. O., Mohaptra, M. and Perrillo, R. P. (1979), Colonic tuberculosis diagnosed by colonoscopic biopsy. *Gastroenterology,* **76**, 362–4.

Frühmorgen, P. (1974), Diagnosis of inflammatory disease of the colon by colonoscopy. *Acta Gastroent.,* **37**, 154–8.

Geboes, K., Desmet, V. J., De Wolf-Peters, C. and Van Trappen, G. (1978), The value of endoscopic biopsies in the diagnosis of Crohn's disease. *Am. J. Proctol. Gastroent. Colon Rect. Surg.,* **29**, 21–28.

Geboes, K. and Van Trappen, G. (1975), The value of colonoscopy in the diagnosis of Crohn's disease. *Gastrointest. Endosc.,* **22**, 18–23.

Goldgraber, M. B. (1965), Pseudopolyps in ulcerative colitis. *Dis. Colon Rect.,* **8**, 355–63.

Goldgraber, M. B. and Kirsner, J. B. (1964), Carcinoma of the colon in ulcerative colitis. *Cancer,* **15**, 657–65.

Greenstein, A. J., Sachar, D. B., Pucillo, A., Vassiliades, G., Smith, H., Kreel, I., Geller, S. A., Janowitz, H. D. and Aufses, A. H. (1979), Cancer in universal and left sided ulcerative colitis: clinical and pathological features. *Mt Sinai J. Med.,*

Hunt, R. H. and Buchanan, J. D. (1979), Transient ischaemic colitis – colonoscopy and biopsy in diagnosis. *J. R. Naval Med. Service,* **65**, 15–19.

Hunt, R. H., Teague, R. H., Swarbrick, E. T. and Williams, C. B. (1975), Colonoscopy in the management of colonic strictures. *Br. Med. J.,* **2**, 360–1.

Jalan, K. N., Sircus, W., Walker, R. J., McManns, J. P. A., Prescott, R. J. and Card, I. W. (1969), Psuedopolyposis in ulcerative colitis. *Lancet,* **2**, 555–9.

Kock, N. G. (1973), Continent ileostomy. *Prog. Surg.,* **12**, 180–201.

Laufer, I. (1979), *Double Contrast Gastrointestinal Radiology with Endoscopic Correlation.* W. B. Saunders, Philadelphia.

Lennard-Jones, J. E., Misicwicz, J. J., Parish, J. A., Ritchie, J., Swarbrick, E. T. and Williams, C. B. (1974), Prospective study of outpatients with extensive colitis. *Lancet,* **1**, 1065–7.

Lennard-Jones, J. E., Morson, B. C., Ritchie, J. K., Shove, D. C. and Williams, C. B. (1977), Cancer in colitis – assessment of the individual risk by clinical and histological criteria. *Gastroenterology,* **73**, 1280–9.

Lux, G., Frühmorgen, P., Phillip, J. and Zeus, J. (1978), Diagnosis of inflammatory disease of the colon. *Endoscopy,* **10**, 279–84.

McGovern, V. J. and Goulston, S. J. M. (1968), Crohn's disease of the colon. *Gut,* **9**, 164–76.

Margulis, A. R. (1972), Radiology of ulcerating colitis. *Radiology,* **105**, 251–63.

Morson, B. C. (1972), The early histological lesion of Crohn's disease. *Proc. R. Soc. Med.,* **65**, 71.

Morson, B. C. (1974), The technique and interpretation of rectal biopsies in inflammatory bowel disease. In: *Pathology Annual* (Ed. S. C. Sommers), Appleton-Century Crofts, 209–30.

Morson, B. C. and Pang, L. S. C. (1967), Rectal biopsy as an aid to cancer control in ulcerative colitis. *Gut,* **8**, 423–34.

Moshal, M. G. *et al.* (1973), Colonoscopy: 100 examinations. *S.A. J. Surg.*, **11**, 73–78.

Moss, W. T. and Brand, W. N. (1979), *Radiation Oncology*, C. V. Mosby, St Louis.

Myrvold, H. E., Kock, N. H. and Ahren, C. (1974), Rectal biopsy and pre-cancer in ulcerative colitis. *Gut*, **15**, 301–4.

Nebel, O. T., El-Masry, N. A., Castell, D. O., Farid, Z., Fornes, M. F. and Sparks, H. A. (1974), Schistosomal colonic polyposis: endoscopic and histological characteristics. *Gastrointest. Endosc.*, **20**, 99–101.

Nugent, F. W., Haggit, K. C., Colcher, H. and Kutteruf, G. C. (1979), Malignant potential of chronic ulcerative colitis. Preliminary report. *Gastroenterology*, **76**, 1–5.

Price, A. B., Jewkes, J. and Sanderson, P. J. (1979), Acute diarrhoea Campylobacter colitis and the role of rectal biopsy. *J. Clin. Path.*, **32**, 990–7.

Rickert, R. R. and Carter, H. W. (1977), The gross, light microscopic and scanning electron microscopic appearance of the early lesions in Crohn's disease. *Scann. Electron Microsc.*, **2**, 179–86.

Riddell, R. H. (1976), The pre-carcinomatous phase of ulcerative colitis. In: *Topics in Pathology* (ed. B. C. Morson), Springer-Verlag, Berlin, pp. 197–219.

Riddell, R. H. (1977), Endoscopic recognition of early carcinoma in ulcerative colitis (letter). *J. Am. Med. Ass.*, **237**, 281.

Rogers, B. H. G., Silvis, S. E., Nebel, O. T., Sugawa, C. and Mandelstam, P. (1975), Complications of flexible fiberoptic colonoscopy and polypectomy. *Gastrointest. Endosc.*, **22**, 73–77.

Rogers, B. H. G. and Adler, F. (1976), Haemangiomas of the caecum. *Gastroenterology*, **71**, 1079.

Rutter, K. R. P. and Riddell, R. H. (1975), Solitary ulcer syndrome of the rectum. *Clinics Gastroent.*, **4**, 505–30.

Shearman, D. J. C. (1973), Colonoscopy in ulcerative colitis. *Scand. J. Gastroent.*, **8**, 289–91.

Smith, L. E. (1976), Complications of colonoscopy and polypectomy. *Dis. Colon Rect.*, **19**, 407–12.

Teague, R. H. and Read, A. E. (1975), Polyposis in ulcerative colitis. *Gut*, **16**, 792–5.

Teague, R. H., Salmon, P. R. and Read, A. E. (1973), Fiberoptic examination of the colon – a review of 255 cases. *Gut*, **14**, 139–42.

Vantrappen, G., Agg, H. O., Ponette, E., Geboes, K. and Bertrand, P. (1977), Yersinia enteritis and enterocolitis: gastroenterological aspects. *Gastroenterology*, **72**, 220–7.

Waye, J. D. (1977), The role of colonoscopy in the differential diagnosis of inflammatory bowel disease. *Gastrointest. Endosc.*, **23**, 150–4.

Waye, J. D. (1978), Colitis, cancer and colonoscopy. *Med. Clinics N. Am.*, **62**, 211–24.

Waye, J. D., Kreel, I., Bauer, J. and Gelernt, I. M. (1977), The continent ileostomy: diagnosis and treatment of problems by means of operative fiberoptic endoscopy. *Gastrointest. Endosc.*, **23**, 196–8.

Williams, C. B. (1975), Evaluation of the colonoscopist examination: results of three studies. *Dis. Colon Rect.,* **18**, 365–8.

Williams, C. B. (1980), Personal communication.

Williams, C. B. and Teague, R. H. (1973), 'Colonoscopy'. *Gut,* **14**, 990.

Williams, C. B. and Waye, J. D. (1978), Colonoscopy in inflammatory bowel disease. *Clinics Gastroent.,* **76**, 221–5.

Yardley, J. H., Bayless, T. M. and Diamond, M. P. (1979), Cancer in ulcerative colitis. *Gastroenterology,* **76**, 221–5.

CHAPTER NINETEEN

Diverticular Disease and Strictures

CHRISTOPHER B. WILLIAMS

The dramatic change in colorectal practice made possible by fibreoptic endoscopy is well demonstrated in its application to the management of diverticular disease and strictures of the colon, although the topic is little covered in the literature. The obvious 'plus' of the endoscopist's colour view and tissue specimens is to some extent countered by the 'minus' of technical difficulty in bowel preparation and manoeuvring the instrument in a narrow or rigid area without damage. Most patients coming to colonoscopy with suspicious or undiagnosed strictures do so after one or more preliminary barium enemas and previously would have often progressed directly to surgery. There is, however, every reason for clinicians, radiologists and endoscopists to know about the possibilities and limitations of colonoscopy in the management of strictures. Now that colonoscopy or fibresigmoidoscopy are thought of as 'routine' procedures, the patient may be less likely to suffer unnecessary surgery, but at the hands of an inaccurate endoscopist can still be endangered, inadequately examined or wrongly diagnosed.

19.1. Diverticular disease

Diverticular disease of some degree is so common in the Western world as to be almost a normal finding, especially in old age. Different series have shown 35–50% of subjects over 50 years of age to have diverticula on careful inspection of the colon at post-mortem (Eide and Stalsberg, 1979) although only about 10% will show the muscle hypertrophy which characterizes the more severe degrees of diverticular disease which are difficult to endoscope (Parks, 1968). Whereas diverticula of the left colon are postulated to be 'blow-outs' secondary to intracolonic pressure (Painter *et al.*, 1965) those occurring as an isolated phenomenon in the right colon may represent a different entity (Eide and Stalsberg, 1979), possibly a 'congenital' defect in the colon. Left-sided diverticular disease can be silent but frequently presents with pain, altered bowel habit and other features consistent with functional bowel disorder of the 'spastic colon' variety. True diverticulitis, inferring localized abscess formation in, around or arising from a diverticulum, is relatively uncommon. Perforation and spread of infection are made more likely in such cases by the extremely thin wall of the diverticulum, comprising mucous membrane (and muscularis mucosae) covered by some longitudinal muscle fibres on the antimesenteric side of the bowel; the only other covering is by the peritoneum (Morson, 1979).

Diverticula have been accepted as a cause of bleeding (Rigg and Ewing, 1966) and although present evidence suggests that minor bleeding is frequently due to other pathology such as polyps, massive haemorrhage can result from stercoral ulceration of the vessels associated with the neck of the diverticulum (Meyers *et al.*, 1976). There appears to be no evidence to associate either polyps or cancer directly with the presence of diverticula, except that they are common conditions in the West and therefore likely to occur concurrently (Ponka, Brush and DeWitt Fox, 1959). Furthermore, the combination of circular muscle spasm with hypertrophy and the muscular and mucosal in-foldings resulting from bowel shortening can produce extremely confusing X-ray appearances, which may mimic cancer or conceal polyps; on the other hand the demonstration of a fistulous track or extraluminal barium is clear and valuable evidence of complicated diverticulitis (Nicholas *et al.*, 1972).

Killingback (1965) lucidly summarizes the clinician's dilemma: "Carcinoma is frequently considered as an alternative diagnosis in patients suffering from diverticular disease. The clinical features may be identical, sigmoidoscopy inconclusive and the barium enema difficult to interpret. At laparotomy it may be impossible for the surgeon to be sure of the cause of a large 'inflammatory mass' around the rectosigmoid junction." Something of this dilemma will remain even with fibre-endoscopy because of the sheer numbers of patients involved, some of them aged and frail, others very difficult or impossible to endoscope. The important role of colonoscopy in selected patients is detailed below.

19.2 Colonic strictures

Complete obstruction to retrograde flow of barium occurs in those patients with symptoms suggesting large bowel obstruction. When barium cannot be passed beyond the sigmoid colon, the usual site of this problem, the leading edge of contrast material may fail to show the characteristic changes of either a carcinoma or diverticulitis. Colonos-

Table 19.1 Causes of colonic stricture

Carcinoma	Extracolonic pathology
Spasm	Endometriosis
Pseudostrictures	Pneumatosis coli
Ischaemia	Inflammatory bowel disease
Trauma	Infectious bowel disease
surgical trauma	
Radiation	

copy performed after minimal preparation with a single enema, will invariably provide the diagnosis (Table 19.1). A bulky obstructing cancer can almost always be identified whereas the endoscope will seldom be unable to reach the concentric narrowing of an inflammatory obstruction.

If the commonest form of apparent 'stricture' of the colon is due to diverticular disease with associated muscle hypertrophy, there are numerous other causes to consider. Although *carcinoma* is the most important and certainly the chief cause of anxiety, other strictures are of great diagnostic interest since positive identification often allows conservative management or limited surgery.

Spasm can mimic the 'applecore' effect of a carcinoma on X-ray and failure to distend adequately the colon or to use intravenous spasmolytics (hyoscine-N-butyl-bromide, glucagon) during the filling phase of the barium enema account for a number of radiological errors. *'Pseudo-strictures'* or other inconstant irregularities of colonic outline can be seen in the rare patients with the muscle disturbance of cathartic colon which should not be confused with melanosis coli (Plate 27) which is a clinically unimportant pigmentation of the mucosa secondary to chronic laxative ingestion.

Ischaemic colitis may be of any grade of severity from infarction of the colon to a minor and transient mucosal abnormality with associated muscle spasm (Marston, 1977); the radiologically pathognomonic 'thumb-printing' of submucosal oedema is present only in moderately severe cases. Although the site of ischaemic change is characteristically near the splenic flexure it may occur anywhere in the left colon or the rectum. As the mucosa heals a fibrous stricture may subsequently develop (Plate 165).

Trauma of many aetiologies (including obstetric manipulation) can result in stricturing of the colon, presumably from local ischaemic effects. *Radiation therapy* in particular produces an endarteritis with ischaemia which may cause both mucosal bleeding and subsequent fibrous cicatricial narrowing of the lumen. *Surgical trauma*, including local infection or ischaemia at an anastomosis, may produce bizarre stricturing – an obvious cause of concern when the original resection was performed for cancer. *Extracolonic* or *intramucosal* pathology can also produce unusual appearances of narrowing. Parts of the colon contiguous to other inflamed structures (such as the transverse colon in pancreatitis) may develop marked mucosal oedema and mimic ischaemia or infiltration. Involvement by carcinoma from adjoining organs, intramucosal metastases or foci of lymphosarcoma may all distort or narrow the bowel. *Endometriosis* in the colonic musculature can also produce disturbing appearances. *Pneumatosis coli* (Plate 187) presents less of a problem in diagnosis, since the gas cysts are usually visible in the bowel wall on X-ray.

Inflammatory bowel disease (ulcerative colitis, Crohn's disease, amoebiasis, tuberculosis, schistosomiasis, actinomycosis, lympho-granuloma venereum) can cause strictures either in the active phase of the disease, due to mucosal and submucosal involvement, or in the chronic phase as a result of muscular spasm or fibrosis. The smoothly tapering strictures of ulcerative colitis (Plate 139) usually are a result of muscle thickening or spasm but are sometimes caused by intramucosal carcinoma. Stricturing in Crohn's disease is usually associated with ulceration with inflammation and oedema of the mucosa and submucosa (Plate 147). Inflammatory strictures resolve as the condition of the bowel improves but changes of fibrotic scarring cause permanent damage. In slow-moving infective conditions such as tuberculosis (ileocaecal) or lymphogranuloma venereum (rectosigmoid) stricturing is usually fixed, whereas amoebic strictures treated early can 'melt away' magically.

19.2.1 *Selection of patients*

Each colon stricture has a specific aetiology and the clinician must not only make the diagnosis but also exclude malignancy and judge the activity of the stricturing process and its likelihood of causing clinical problems in the future. It is not difficult to see that on one count or another endoscopy with biopsies is frequently indicated to inform or reassure the doctor, even when the patient is unaware that any problem exists. The presence of continuing symptoms of pain, weight loss, bleeding, etc. merely add urgency for further investigation by endoscopy and clearly the value of endoscopy in the individual patient should be considered in relationship to the whole clinical setting. The history and physical signs taken in conjunction with the X-ray appearances may make endoscopy unnecessary:

(a) an elderly patient with atherosclerotic disease who has an acute onset and spontaneous resolution of abdominal pain and bleeding, with a splenic flexure stricture proximal to diverticular disease can have a check examination by X-ray,

(b) a well patient with proven Crohn's disease and multiple strictures needs no further investigation unless obstructive or other symptoms arise;

(c) a patient with alteration of bowel habit without bleeding and uncomplicated diverticular disease on a good quality aircontrast enema needs no further investigation unless symptoms fail to resolve on suitable treatment.

By contrast, *all* anastomoses after resection for cancer merit endoscopic inspection (rigid or flexible depending on the site of anastomosis). All strictures in chronic ulcerative colitis also need biopsy and all patients with diverticular disease and bleeding should have direct inspection of the bowel. In such high-risk patients the annoyance of repeated bowel preparation and the higher incidence of complications from colonoscopy are more than justified by the extra information gained. In general terms, colonoscopy is indicated if there is any possibility of malignancy, if surgery is in question but not inevitable, or if clinical management may be altered by the results of the procedure. The contraindications to colonoscopy in diverticular disease or strictures are few and apply to any colonoscopy. Examination is avoided if the possibility of perforation is high (acute diverticulitis, severe acute colitis of any cause) or if general medical considerations warrant (recent myocardial infarction, etc.).

19.2.2. *Bowel preparation*

Patients with strictures or diverticular disease need extra thorough bowel preparation. Hypertonic phosphate (Fleet's, Klyx) enemas, effective in evacuating solid stool from the normal distal colon, do not clean diverticular segments or strictures adequately. Even fibresigmoidoscopy or limited colonoscopy will therefore usually require full bowel preparation in these patients. It is essential to clear the bowel proximal to any narrowed area to get a good view without contamination from above during the procedure. In any but the mildest case of diverticular disease, preparation is made difficult because of the functionally abnormal and spastic bowel; additionally there is a tendency for trapped pellets of stool (faecoliths) to be ejected from diverticular pouches during the examination and impact on the instrument tip. Any of the standard regimes for full bowel preparation are acceptable (purge and enema, saline lavage, mannitol, etc.) but it may be useful to administer a stool softening agent or mild aperient for several days beforehand to aid successful evacuation. Patients with obstructive symptoms should be managed with care and the lavage method may be contraindicated in them.

19.2.3 *Medication*

As for the X-ray examination, both the bowel preparation and endo-scopic examination of diverticular disease are made easier and more effective by giving a spasmolytic agent (hyoscine-N-butyl-bromide 40 mg, glucagon 0.5 mg) i.m. or i.v. beforehand. Because the action of these agents is short, it may be necessary to give a further dose to help visualization during withdrawal of the instrument.

Patients with diverticular disease are difficult to examine and col-onoscopy is often painful so that sedation may be needed even for limited examinations, usually with diazepam (Valium) 5–10 mg i.v. and pethidine (Demerol) 25–50 mg i.v. Many patients with inflam-matory strictures can, by contrast, be unexpectedly easy to examine and sedation may be unnecessary. Unless the patient or endoscopist feels strongly one way or the other it may be best to start the procedure without sedation, administering it later if colonoscopy proves more dif-ficult than expected. The usual rules for colonoscopy apply and if sed-ation is used the endoscopist must be proportionately more careful not to employ undue force or to perform manoeuvres which could put the patient at risk because of decreased pain perception.

19.2.4 *Technique and instrumentation*

Diverticular segments and strictures can almost invariably be passed with the correct instrument. Tight strictures may be traversed using small calibre colonoscopes (Rogers, 1981). The combination of acute angulation and fixation of the bowel is usually the limiting factor, caus-ing the distal part of the shaft to loop uncontrollably when propulsive force is applied to coax the instrument tip through the narrowed area. Distal sigmoid colon strictures are therefore easy to examine but proxi-mal lesions or extensive segments of diverticular disease become progressively more difficult. An early study using instruments with limited tip angling reported failure to pass diverticular disease in almost half the cases examined (Dean and Newell, 1973) and later series report failure in 7–26% (Hunt *et al.*, 1975; Sugarbaker *et al.*,

1974; Glerum, Agenant and Tytgat, 1977; Max and Knutson, 1978). The reasons for failure include poor bowel preparation, acute angulation with fixation and 'narrowing'. Poor bowel preparation is presumably remediable with repeat examination if clinically indicated. Many angulations or fixed regions which are apparently impassable with one instrument are actually manageable with another; the very acute tip deflection of the paediatric gastroscope can provide a view around an angle which the longer-bending segment of the adult colonoscope cannot; the more flexible shaft of some paediatric colonoscopes will snake round fixed bends that some stiffer instruments will not. Contrary to popular belief, these thinner instruments are chosen more on the basis of their short tip deflection and shaft flexibility than for their small diameter because the lumen is not significantly narrowed in diverticular disease unless there has been an unusual degree of pericolic inflammation. Although the colon may appear narrowed on barium enema this impression is usually due to muscle spasm and the hypertrophied but distensible circular muscle folds.

Carcinomatous strictures may be impassable with any instrument as the lumen becomes obstructed. It may be technically possible to open a passage using a diathermy loop and in some instances this might be justifiable. Anastomoses are not always passable, but adequate inspection and biopsies may be performed since the 'stricture' is so short in contradistinction to longer strictures where failure to pass through the whole distance means that the examination is non-diagnostic (the taking of biopsies and cytology specimens is discussed later).

In traversing an area of hypertrophic diverticular disease, there are both visual and mechanical problems for any endoscopist. Difficulty with faecoliths has already been mentioned. The thickened circular muscle folds result in greatly exaggerated but shortened haustral segments (Plate 6) in which the ability to see the lumen becomes lost (Fig. 19.1(a)) with the only view being of mucosa in close-up or of a diverticular orifice. The orifice of a diverticulum can very easily be mistaken for the colonic lumen (Plate 31 and Fig. 19.1(b)), potentially a source of disaster and certainly a waste of time. Two principles apply to the endoscopic examination of diverticular disease:

(a) a well-seen and round 'lumen' is *not* the true lumen (Plate 31) which is poorly seen and always distorted (Fig. 19.1(c));
(b) if the instrument is facing a diverticulum it is pointing 90° *away* from the lumen (Fig. 19.1(a)).

Based on these principles, which seem obvious but are usually forgotten by inexperienced endoscopists, the secret of successful intubation through diverticular disease lies in being slow and cautious, con-

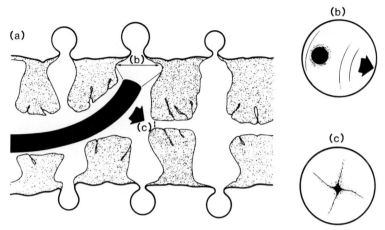

Fig. 19.1 The colonoscope tip impacted in a segment of diverticular disease with (insert b) a diverticulum simulating 'lumen', the true lumen (insert c) being at right angles and distorted by muscular infoldings.

stantly pulling the instrument back to get a view past each successive fold. Because of the prominent muscle hypertrophy, tip movements are restricted and visual judgement must be made with a poor view. It may be necessary to manoeuvre 'blind', and since the instrument tip is usually somewhat hooked, the single most effective movement is to torque or corkscrew the shaft. Providing torqueing movements are made with reasonable gentleness, they are no more stressful to the instrument than attempts at more acute angling with the control knobs. Any manipulation in a fixed segment of colon puts the instrument at some risk and the possibility of cable rupture during a difficult examination must be balanced against its diagnostic benefit to the patient.

At each segment of diverticular disease it may be necessary to pull back a few millimetres and twist or angle the instrument to obtain a partial view of the probable direction of the lumen. Several attempts may be needed to find the right direction and the correct combination of angulation and torque to advance the instrument tip into the lumen. Patience, concentration, determination and 15–20 minutes of time may be required to get through a short segment of severe diverticular disease. The one manoeuvre which is both dangerous and ineffective in diverticular disease is 'slide-by', which the muscular corrugations make completely impossible. Some force may be required to advance the correctly-angled tip past an individual fold following which the shaft is straightened by withdrawal before tackling the next one. This tedious progress, painstakingly repeated through the affected area is eventually rewarded as the instrument passes into the broader lumen of the proximal normal bowel. In most cases the remainder of the examination is easy since the thickened and fixed sigmoid colon 'splints' the colonoscope and keeps it straight during passage to the caecum. If the indication for colonoscopy is strong, the time and trauma involved are clearly worthwhile. Air insufflated during endoscopy is likely to be trapped above the diverticular segment resulting in wind-pain for the patient. There is an advantage in insufflating carbon dioxide throughout colonoscopy, but if the gas is not available at least the proximal bowel should be aspirated before the instrument is withdrawn and insufflation then kept to a minimum thereafter.

These comments relate only to severe diverticular disease; multiple diverticula without fixation or muscle change may confuse the radiologist but present no difficulty to the endoscopist and it is not always obvious how easy or difficult the examination will prove until the instrument is in position.

Simple strictures and stenoses require no change in insertion technique. In the usual fashion (Chapters 8 and 9) the instrument shaft should be straightened if looping interferes with passage. The overtube or splinting device may occasionally be helpful for strictures in the proximal colon; this requires fluoroscopy and should be used with caution since it allows considerable force to be applied directly to the stricture. It is difficult to judge the diameter of a stenotic area with the wide angle lens of the modern endoscopes. If the tip will not pass, it should be withdrawn; a red or haemorrhagic ring of trauma within the stricture caused by impaction of the tip suggests that the instrument is too large and the use of a small-diameter endoscope is indicated. It may be technically easier in some cases to introduce a full-size instrument to the stricture using an overtube and remove the colonoscope leaving the overtube in position as a guide for insertion of the more fragile paediatric instrument. A small diameter fibreoptic bundle may be passed ('mother and baby' scope) through the biopsy channel of a standard size colonoscope. This technique is theoretically possible but does not allow biopsies to be taken (Rogers, 1981). The configuration of impassable strictures can also be demonstrated by the injection of water-soluble contrast medium or barium through the properly positioned endoscope, followed by air insufflation if desired.

It is possible to use mechanical dilators of the Eder-Puestow variety in the colon but no series has been published from which to judge the risk of perforation. As in the oesophagus, a guide-wire must first be passed well above the stricture and then a succession of metal olives of increasing diameter passed over the wire, preferably using fluoroscopic control (Fig. 19.2). In the case of malignant strictures, it is

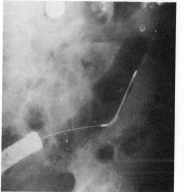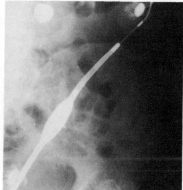

Fig. 19.2 Dilatation of an anastomotic stenosis with Eder–Puestow dilators passed over an endoscopically inserted guide-wire.

theoretically possible after dilatation or endoscopic resection to insert a tube to maintain patency but the prognosis after palliative resection of colonic carcinoma is so good that such procedures are very rarely indicated.

19.2.5 *Biopsy and cytology*

Taking biopsies from colonic strictures and diverticular disease rarely presents any technical problem but it may be difficult to get representative biopsies from all parts of a stricture (especially the proximal end), particularly if the stricture is very narrow. With paediatric instruments, it should be possible to pass through and then retrovert the tip to biopsy the proximal margin, but this is not feasible in the relatively narrow left colon using standard colonoscopes. Because of the problems with biopsy sampling, the use of colonic brushing or washing cytology may be especially useful in tight strictures (Kline and Yum, 1976). Washings for cytology are obtained by injecting saline into or through the strictured area with an endoscopically positioned cannula, then brushing to abrade the inner surface of the stricture with subsequent aspiration into a syringe or via the instrument channel with a bronchial mucus trap placed in the suction line. Cytology performed before biopsy provides specimens with a minimum of red cell contamination. Often, but less desirably, cytology is used as a last resort when the taking of biopsies or passage of the instrument have proved difficult or impossible.

Protuberant areas of possibly abnormal mucosa in diverticular disease or suspicious tissue at the site of an anastomosis are suitable for

snare-loop biopsy, which gives the pathologist a much larger specimen.

19.2.6 *Dangers and complications*

The technical difficulty of colonoscopy in diverticular disease has
already been stressed and the danger of using excessive force during a
difficult examination is obvious. Less obvious is the hidden hazard of
air pressure in causing overt perforation or silent 'pneumoperitoneum'
through thin-walled diverticula. The air pressure generated by some
endoscopic light sources not fitted with safety devices may reach
300–500 mm Hg (Williams *et al.*, 1973, Kozarek *et al.*, 1980). The
bursting pressure of human cadaver colon is around 70–100 mm Hg in
the caecum and 200 mm Hg in the more muscular sigmoid colon
(Quenu, 1882; Wu, 1978; Kozarek *et al.*, 1980) and it may be assumed
that thin-walled diverticula are likely to rupture at similar pressures.
High pressures are rapidly achieved when the instrument tip is in close
contact with the bowel wall, as would occur when the endoscopist
pushes the instrument against a diverticular orifice mistakenly identified
as bowel lumen. These factors presumably account for the immediate
or delayed 'blow-out' perforations reported in diverticular disease
(Sugarbaker and Vineyard, 1973; Meyers and Ghahremani, 1975; Dagradi, Norris and Weingarten, 1978; Taylor, Weakley and Sullivan,
1978) and possibly for the unexplained 'silent' pneumoperitoneum
found in several patients on routine abdominal radiographs performed
after colonoscopy (Glouberman, Craner and Oglenrur, 1976; Ecker,
Goldstein and Hoexter, 1977). In addition there is the possibility of
diverticular disease in the sigmoid colon acting as a non-return valve,
allowing the build-up of high pressures proximally which would
explain the occurrence of lacerations in the right colon when colonoscopy has been limited to the sigmoid region (Kozarek *et al.*, 1980).
Although pneumoperitoneum can usually be managed conservatively
or by needling the abdomen (Jacobsohn and Levy, 1976; Taylor,
Weakley and Sullivan, 1978) these complications are a warning to
insufflate air gently in the presence of diverticular disease, preferably
using rapidly absorbed carbon dioxide. They also warn the manufacturers of the need to fit safety devices.

The presence of signs or symptoms suggesting diverticulitis, when
localized perforation may already have occurred, is a particular contraindication to colonoscopy because of the high likelihood of exacerbating the situation or causing frank perforation (Schwesinger, Levine
and Ramos, 1979).

In addition to these potential dangers of endoscopy is the additional danger of missed diagnosis which should not be forgotten. Once the colonoscope has been successfully passed diagnosis is usually easy but carcinomas have been missed by misinterpretation (Hunt *et al.*, 1975; Forde, 1977) and in tightly strictured areas there is always a danger of inadequate visualization for the inexperienced endoscopist because of reduced tip movement.

19.2.7 *Results of colonoscopy*

There is a relatively small number of studies in the literature on colonscopy in diverticular disease (Dean and Newell, 1973; Sugarbaker *et al.*, 1974; Hunt, 1979, Forde, 1977; Glerum, Agenant and Tytgat, 1977; Max and Knutson, 1978), strictures (Hunt *et al.*, 1975; Rozen, Rajan and Gilat, 1975; Bartnik *et al.*, 1977; Filoche, Delmotte and Pommelet, 1978) or anastomoses (Weill *et al.*, 1974; Gabriellsson, Grandqvist and Ohlson, 1976). All the studies are retrospective analyses of small numbers of differently selected patients, from which some clear principles emerge but no overall calculations are justified.

19.3 Cancer and polyps in diverticular disease

In diverticular disease (Table 19.2) there is a minority of patients in whom unexpected carcinoma or polyps are found, usually in the presence of bleeding. More important perhaps is the ability of colonoscopy to *exclude* the presence of carcinoma with a high degree of confidence in those patients where it is technically successful. The false-positive rate of barium enema in erroneously diagnosing carcinoma is noted by Glerum Agenant and Tytgat (1977) in whose series 12 of 22 patients (55%) with radiologically suspected carcinoma in diverticular disease

Table 19.2 Colonoscopy in diverticular disease

Author	Number of patients	Unsuspected carcinoma present	Failed examination
Dean and Newell (1973)	36	4 (11%)	17 (47%)
Sugarbaker *et al.* (1974)	18	4 (22%)	4 (22%)
Hunt, *et al.* (1975)	39	6 (15≤%)	3 (7%)
Forde (1977)	40	2 (5%)	?
Glerum, Agenant and Tytgat (1977)	30	2 (7%)	3 (10%)
Max and Knutson (1978)	26	2 (8%)	7 (27%)
Hunt (1979)	44	6 (13%)	6 (13%)

were proven normal. In Forde's (1977) series, 11 of 12 (92%) suspected cancers were disproved endoscopically, a rather high figure
which suggests a poor standard of radiology or a high degree of clinical
case selection. All series nonetheless stress radiological inaccuracy in at
least 25% of patients with diverticular disease referred for colonoscopy.
The logical conclusion is that no patient with diverticular disease suspected of cancer on radiological grounds should be operated on without first attempting colonoscopy. A less serious, but initially puzzling,
false-positive result on X-ray results from individual diverticula
simulating polyps; this may be due to simple misinterpretation when
no tangential view has been obtained (the endoscopist identifying only
the neck of the diverticulum concerned) or, understandably, when
barium coats a smooth faecolith projecting from a wide-mouthed
diverticulum. A false-negative inaccuracy of barium enema is demonstrated by the finding of Swarbrick *et al.* (1978) of unexpected carcinoma in four patients (10%) and polyps in nine patients (22%) of 40
patients with diverticular disease and persistent rectal bleeding;
Teague *et al.* (1978) found 20% cancer in their series. Such patients
therefore present an excellent indication for colonoscopy. Even good
air-contrast radiology is difficult to interpret in the presence of diverticula and may miss small to medium-sized polyps. In the presence of
diverticular disease X-ray is so inaccurate that endoscopy is increasingly being requested, posing a problem for the colonoscopist since
these patients are particularly difficult to examine.

In the clinically selected cases included in the series quoted above,
colonoscopy avoided the need for surgery in about half the patients
(Forde, 1977; Glerum, Agenant and Tytgat, 1977) by disproving
cancer or removing polyps. In terms of cost effectiveness, these results
more than justify the extra expense, time taken and discomfort of the
examination, mainly because (for the patient) surgery may be totally
unnecessary and is even more expensive, time-consuming and painful.
Colonoscopy, with the problems inherent in diverticular disease, is the
simplest and most accurate way of reassuring the doctor that all is well
in spite of symptoms, signs and X-rays that mimic cancer.

19.4 Bleeding and inflammation in diverticular disease

Until the concept became accepted of abnormal musculature and functional bowel disorder in diverticular disease, there was a tendency to
ascribe all the symptoms to 'diverticulitis'. Similarly, because occasional patients bleed massively from ulceration of a diverticulum (Plate
60) (Meyers *et al.*, 1976) there has been a mistaken tendency to ascribe
the common lesser degrees of bleeding (Rigg and Ewing, 1966) to the

diverticula as well. The important percentage proven on colonoscopy to be due to polyps and cancer has been mentioned above. In many other patients with persistent minor bleeding the endoscopist will notice reddening and contact bleeding over the mucosal folds in the most severely affected distal segments of diverticular disease, the appearance raising the possibility of chronic inflammatory disease (Plate 34) (ulcerative colitis or Crohn's disease). Crohn's disease has been associated with diverticular disease (Schmidt *et al.*, 1968) although the association may perhaps be no more than chance. Reddened sigmoid folds in diverticular disease are not due to Crohn's disease and neither ulcers nor granulomata are found but biopsies do show these areas to be chronically inflamed: the patchiness of the inflammation is unlike the distribution of ulcerative colitis. On careful inspection, the reddened areas are seen to be remote from the diverticular orifices and situated on the apex of the circular muscle infoldings, the mucosa frequently being redundant as well as red. A plausible explanation of this phenomenon and the bleeding that results from it is that the mucosa is locally traumatized and sometimes prolapsed by the forced passage of faecal contents past the contracted muscle rings. The pathology of biopsies taken from these areas show inflammatory changes analogous to those seen in the early stages of 'solitary ulcer syndrome' of the rectum, where there is also local mucosal prolapse secondary to straining (Rutter and Riddell, 1975).

Acute or massive bleeding makes colonoscopy difficult and the combination of exsanguinating haemorrhage and severe diverticular disease would certainly be impassable. On the other hand, severe bleeding not infrequently originates from diverticula unassociated with muscular changes, particularly on the right side of the colon (Casarella, Kanta and Seaman, 1972) and in such patients colonoscopy in the actively bleeding phase is feasible and likely to be helpful in localization. If the bleeding has stopped, the foulness of melaena stool and the impossibility of aspirating clots make colonoscopy a wretched and inaccurate task. If it must be undertaken it is preferable to use the saline lavage technique (Levy *et al.* 1976) so that any blood washes distally; enemas can reflux blood from the sigmoid colon back into the caecum and even the terminal ileum, which will confuse the issue.

19.5 Strictures and anastomoses

The majority of obvious stricturing carcinomas are not referred for colonoscopy, whereas the more dubious cases are clinically selected for it, so it is gratifying but not surprising that in Rozen, Rajan and Gilat's

(1975) series eight of 10 patients with 'suspected carcinoma', other benign diagnoses were made (ischaemic, inflammatory, irradiation etc.) the patients being spared surgery. Hunt *et al.* (1975) found 31 of 53 (58%) radiologically 'malignant' strictures to be benign. Some of the endoscopically confirmed carcinomatous strictures in this series were referred for surgery on the basis of the visual diagnosis alone, the endoscopic biopsies showing dysplastic tissue but being too small to demonstrate invasion. There was one endoscopically missed carcinoma at the proximal end of an apparently smooth stricture, which reinforces the desirability of using cytology as an adjunct in any narrow area which is not well seen endoscopically, and also of respecting the ability of X-ray to demonstrate all parts of a stricture. Both of these series however, also report examples of colonic spasm radiologically misdiagnosed as malignancy, a result of interpretation of static films without due regard to 'live' fluoroscopic appearances and also to under-use of spasmolytics by some radiologists.

Strictures in chronic ulcerative colitis are a good example of the particular advantage of colonoscopy in being able to inspect fine mucosal detail and to take biopsies. If mucosal biopsies in a colitic stricture show no dysplasia to suggest underlying carcinoma or a precancerous state (Morson and Pang, 1967; Lennard-Jones *et al.*, 1977), and if the outline is smooth on endoscopy and barium enema, the stricture can confidently be considered benign. Hunt, Teague and Swarbrick (1975) found only three of 28 strictures in colitis to show evidence of malignancy by these criteria.

Because of the preponderance of polyps and cancer in the distal colon many anastomoses are within reach of the rigid proctosigmoidoscope. Those that are not (including right hemicolectomy for Crohn's disease) can be examined by colonoscopy. Gabriellson, Grandqvist and Ohlson (1976) confirmed only six of 18 suspected recurrences of cancer. Weill *et al.* (1974) report a small postoperative series, half of whom were considered to have been spared reoperation. They stress in particular, the usefulness of colonoscopic biopsies in differentiating between granulation tissue and recurrent carcinoma, an important point since visually as well as radiologically granulation tissue can look most sinister because of its irregular and friable surface. Radiologically, it may also be very difficult or impossible to diagnose early recurrence of Crohn's disease. Endoscopically, any recurrent ulcers are very obvious and need not be biopsied since the diagnosis will already have been made on the previous operative specimen. Tight stenosis may occur at an anastomosis and be impassable but if so this is an indication for surgery.

Hunt *et al.* (1975) found in their series that the previous (usually radiological) diagnosis was wrong in 52% of 104 patients with strictures and that in a further 50 patients where no diagnosis could be made radiologically, a positive diagnosis was possible with colonoscopy in all but two. They considered that laparotomy was probably avoided in half of their 154 cases.

19.6 Therapeutic colonoscopy

The prime place of colonoscopy in diverticular disease is in diagnosis and clearly it cannot improve the condition. Snare polypectomy in diverticular segments surprisingly may present no particular difficulty and is usually easier than expected because of a tendency to overestimate the size of polyps visually by comparison with the reduced diameter of the bowel. Spasmolytics help in visualization and manoeuvring but even so the resected polyps may be lost between the muscle infoldings; if this happens, a large volume of warm saline solution can be infused through the instrument above the polypectomy site so that the patient evacuates the polyps after withdrawal of the colonoscope.

The use of an endoscopically inserted guide-wire and bougies in dilating strictures (Fig. 19.2) (p. 372) and of electrosurgical loop resection of obstructing carcinomas have been mentioned as rarely-indicated possibilities. It is also feasible to insert a prosthetic tube endoscopically (Den Hartog Jager, Bartelsman and Tytgat, 1979) and this technique can be used *per rectum*, for instance during palliative radiotherapy for recurrent or metastatic carcinoma surrounding the sigmoid colon.

19.7 Conclusion

With patience and a suitable range of colonoscopes most patients with diverticular disease or strictures can be accurately assessed endoscopically. Endoscopy with biopsy or cytology proves considerably more accurate than radiology, particularly in avoiding false-positive diagnoses. Nonetheless, because of its ease and availabilty good radiology is extremely important in delineating strictures and in examining and excluding carcinoma in the majority of patients with diverticular disease. In many patients, out-patient colonoscopy should replace laparotomy and will ensure that those who have surgery really need it. Colonoscopy should be thought of as a possible alternative before considering surgery in any patient with diverticular disease or stricture and may be preferred to repeated radiology as a diagnostic method in selected cases.

References

Bartnik, W. *et al.* (1977), Significance of coloscopy in the diagnosis of colonic stenosis. *Pol. Arch. Med.,* **58**, 415–18.

Casarella, W. J., Kanta, I. E. and Seaman, W. B. (1972), Right-sided colonic diverticula as a cause of acute rectal haemorrhage. *New Engl. J. Med.,* **286**, 450–3.

Dagradi, A. E., Norris, M. E. and Weingarten, Z. G. (1978), Delayed 'blow-out' perforation of sigmoid following diagnostic colonoscopy. *Am. J. Gastroent.,* **70**, 317–20.

Dean, A. C. B. and Newell, J. P. (1973), Colonoscopy in the differential diagnosis of carcinoma from diverticulitis of the sigmoid colon. *Br. J. Surg.,* **60**, 633–5.

Den Hartog Jager, F., Bartelsman, J. and Tytgat, G. N. (1979), Palliative treatment of obstructing eosophagogastric malignancy by endoscopic positioning of a plastic prosthesis. *Gastroenterology,* **75**, 1008–14.

Ecker, M. D., Goldstein, M. and Hoexter, B. (1977), Benign pneumoperitoneum after fibreoptic colonoscopy: a prospective study of 100 patients. *Gastroenterology,* **73**, 226–31.

Eide, T. J. and Stalsberg, H. (1979), Diverticular disease of the large intestine in Northern Norway. *Gut,* **20**, 609–15.

Filoche, B., Delmotte, J. S. and Pommelet, P. (1978), The value of colonoscopy in the etiological diagnosis of sigmoid stenosis. *Lille Med. J.,* **27**, 50–55.

Forde, K. A. (1977), Colonoscopy in complicated diverticular disease. *Gastrointest. Endosc.,* **23**, 192–3.

Gabriellsson, N., Grandqvist, S. and Ohlsen, H. (1976), Recurrent carcinoma of the anastomosis diagnosed by roentgen examination and colonoscopy. *Endoscopy,* **8**, 47–52.

Glerum, J., Agenant, D. and Tytgat, G. N. (1977), Value of coloscopy in the detection of sigmoid malignancy in patients with diverticular disease. *Endoscopy,* **9**, 228–30.

Glouberman, S., Craner, G. E. and Oglenrur, M. (1976), Radiographic survey for extraluminal air following gastrointestinal tract fiberendoscopy. *Gastrointest. Endosc.,* **22**, 165–7.

Hunt, R. H. (1979), The role of colonoscopy in complicated diverticular disease. *Acta Chir. Belg.,* **6**, 349–53.

Hunt, R. H., Teague, R. H., Swarbrick, E. T. and Williams, C. B. (1975), Colonoscopy in the management of colonic strictures. *Br. Med. J.,* **2**, 360–1.

Jacobsohn, W. Z. and Levy, A. (1976), Colonoscopic perforation: its emergency treatment. *Endoscopy,* **8**, 15–17.

Killingback, M. (1965), Current aspects of the diagnosis and treatment of diverticulosis and diverticulitis of the sigmoid colon. *Postgrad. Bull. Sydney,* **20(12)**, 349–57.

Kline, T. S. and Yum, K. K. (1976), Fibreoptic colonoscopy and cytology. *Cancer,* **37**, 2553–6.

Kozarek, R. A., Earnest, D. L., Silverstein, M. E. and Smith, R. G. (1980), Air-pressure induced colon injury during diagnostic colonoscopy. *Gastroenterology,* **78**, 7–14.

Lennard-Jones, J. E., Morson, B. C., Ritchie, J. K., Shove, D. C. and Williams, C. B. (1977), Cancer in colitis – assessment of the individual risk by clinical and histological criteria. *Gastroenterology,* **73**, 1280–9.

Levy, A. G. *et al.* (1976), Saline lavage: a rapid, effective, and acceptable method for cleansing the gastrointestinal track. *Gastroenterology,* **70**, 157–61.

Marston, A. (1977), *Intestinal Ischaemia,* Edward Arnold, London.

Max, M. H. and Knutson, C. O. (1978), Colonoscopy in patients with inflammatory colonic strictures. *Surgery,* **84**, 551–6.

Meyers, M. A. and Ghahreman, G. G. (1975), Complications of fibreoptic endoscopy: colonoscopy. *Radiology,* **115**, 301–7.

Meyers, M. A., Alonso, D. R., Gray, G. F. and Baer, J. E. (1976), Pathogenesis of bleeding colonic diverticulosis. *Gastroenterology,* **71**, 577–83.

Morson, B. C. and Pang, L. S. C. (1967), Rectal biopsy as an aid to cancer control in ulcerative colitis. *Gut,* **8**, 423–34.

Morson, B. C. (1979), Diverticular disease of the colon. *Acta Chir. Belg.,* **6**, 369–76.

Nicholas, G. G., Miller, W. T., Fitts, W. T. and Tondreau, R. L. (1972), Diagnosis of diverticulitis of the colon: role of the barium enema in defining pericolic inflammation. *Ann. Surg.,* **176**, 205–9.

Painter, N. S., Truelove, S. C., Ardran, G. M. and Tuckey, M. (1965), Segmentation and the localisation of intraluminal pressures in the human colon, with special reference to the pathogenesis of colonic diverticula. *Gastroenterology,* **49**, 169–73.

Parks, T. G. (1968), Post-mortem studies on the colon with special reference to diverticular disease. *Proc. R. Soc. Med.,* **61**, 932–4.

Ponka, J. L., Brush, B. E. and DeWitt Fox, J. (1960), Differential diagnosis of carcinoma of the sigmoid and diverticulitis; evaluation of aids. *J. Am. Med. Ass.,* **172**, 515–9.

Quenu, P. E. (1882), Des ruptures spontanees du rectum. *Rev. Chirurg.,* **2**, 173–88.

Rigg, B. M. and Ewing, M. R. (1966), Current attitudes on diverticulitis with particular reference to colonic bleeding. *Archs Surg.,* **92**, 321–32.

Rogers, B. H. G., Cot, C., Meiri, S. and Epstein, M. (1981), Endoscopic extender for flexible fiberoptic colonoscopes (abstract), *Gastrointest. Endosc.,* **27**, 26–27.

Rozen, P., Rajan, J. and Gilat, T. (1975), Colonoscopy in the differential diagnosis of colonic strictures. *Dis. Colon Rect.,* **18**, 425–9.

Rutter, K. R. P. and Riddell, R. H. H. (1975), The solitary ulcer syndrome of the rectum. *Clinics Gastronent.,* **4(3)**, 505–30.

Schmidt, G. T., Lennard-Jones, J. E., Morson, B. C. and Young, A. C. (1968), Crohn's disease of the colon and its distinction from diverticulitis. *Gut,* **9**, 7–16.

Schwesinger, W. H., Levine, B. A. and Ramos, R. (1979), Complications in colonoscopy. *Surgery Gynec. Obstet.,* **148**, 270–81.

Sugarbaker, P. H. and Vineyard, G. C. (1973), Fiberoptic colonoscopy – a new look at old problems. *Am. J. Surg.,* **125**, 429–31.

Sugarbaker, P. H., Vineyard, G. C., Lewick, A. M., Pinkus, G. S. and

Warhol, M. J. (1974), Colonoscopy in the management of disease of the colon and rectum. *Surgery Gynec. Obstet.,* **139**, 341–9.

Swarbrick, E. T., Fevre, D. I., Hunt, R. H., Thomas, B. M. and Williams, C. B. (1978), Colonoscopy for unexplained rectal bleeding, *Brit. Med. J.,* **2**, 1685–87.

Taylor, R., Weakley, F. L. and Sullivan, B. H. (1978), Non-operative management of colonoscopic perforation with pneumoperitoneum. *Gastrointest. Endosc.,* **24**, 124–5.

Teague, R. H., Thornton, J. R., Manning, A. P., Salmon, P. R. and Read, A. E. (1978), Colonoscopy for investigation of unexplained rectal bleeding *Lancet,* **1**, 1350–1.

Weill, J. P., Kerschen, A., Meknini, B. and Monath, C. (1974), Interêt de la coloscopie dans l'étude des anastamoses après colectomie. *Ann. Gastroent. Hepat.,* **10**, 491–5.

Williams, C. B., Lane, R., Sakai, Y. and Hanwell, A. (1973), Air pressure: a hazard during colonoscopy. *Lancet,* **2**, 729.

Wu, T. K. (1978), Occult injuries during colonoscopy. Measurement of forces required to injure the colon and report of cases. *Gastrointest. Endosc.,* **24**, 236–8.

CHAPTER TWENTY

Paediatric Colonoscopy

ANGELITA HABR-GAMA

Colonoscopy has become an established procedure for the diagnosis, evaluation and treatment of many colonic disorders in adults. Despite this important advance, experience of colonoscopy in children is still limited. In a review of the literature up to the middle of 1979, no more than 500 colonoscopies in children had been reported. In spite of this, colonoscopy should be considered a valuable diagnostic and therapeutic procedure in several conditions affecting the paediatric age group. Among these conditions, the most important application for colonoscopy is in the child with rectal bleeding. With improvements in both the instrumentation and the technique of fibreoptic colonoscopy, it is now possible not only to diagnose colon polyps, but also simultaneously to provide definitive therapy.

Most polyps visualized during colonoscopy can be completely removed by diathermy, avoiding the risks and inconveniences of surgery. Accumulated experience has shown that morbidity, mortality and cost are significantly lower than those associated with polypectomy through laparotomy. In children, surgery is only justified when an experienced endoscopist determines that the polyp is too large to be removed safely or when endoscopic resection is prevented by some technical difficulty. Besides polyps, an increasing number of vascular lesions of the colon have been detected by colonoscopy, making a correct diagnosis possible and sometimes avoiding an unnecessary operation. Furthermore, colonoscopy has become an essential aid for the accurate diagnosis and follow-up of inflammatory bowel diseases in infants and children.

Despite the diagnostic potential of colonoscopy, the indications for this technique must be carefully considered. The technique carries some risk and must be performed only by an experienced endoscopist. The co-operative role between paediatrician and endoscopist cannot be overemphasized.

20.1 Indications

The main indications for colonoscopy in infants and children are:
   Unexplained rectal bleeding;
   Unexplained diarrhoea/mucopus/blood;
   Doubtful radiological findings or colonic strictures;
   In selected patients with inflammatory bowel;
   Therapeutic endoscopy for removal of colonic polyps.

20.2 Instruments

Most colonoscopies in children so far reported have been performed with adult instruments. Some endoscopists (Lux *et al.*, 1976) have reported the use of a paediatric small-calibre upper intestinal fibrescope (GIF-P2 Olympus, F7-ACMI) for children less than six years old, while we have used the standard colonoscopes (Habr-Gama *et al.*, 1977). With good technique, patience and experience, the adult instruments can be safely used, although a light general anaesthesia may be helpful in selected cases during examination in smaller children.

Colonoscopes specifically designed for children are not yet widely available. However, prototypes are under trial with good preliminary results reported. These instruments have excellent flexibility, and the tip can be deflected in four directions. They are equipped with air, water, suction, biopsy channels and lens-washing systems similar to those for adult use. These paediatric models are easier to handle and cause less discomfort to the patient due to their greater flexibility, shorter bending section and smaller diameter. With appropriate instruments colonoscopy may be performed routinely in infants and children without general anaesthesia. However, the thinner upper gastrointestinal instruments present some disadvantages, such as: the colon must be perfectly clean to prevent faecal blocking of the narrower suction channel; the lens-washing system is weak; and the biopsy channel is narrow resulting in small biopsy specimens which do not allow satisfactory histological studies. Since the optical bundle of these paediatric models is about four times smaller than that of the standard fibrescopes, the optical definition and the quality of endoscopic photographs is reduced (Cadranel *et al.*, 1977; Cremer *et al.*, 1974; Rodesch *et al.*, 1976). The newer purpose-built paediatric colonoscopes avoid some of these problems, particularly the small biopsy channel.

20.3 Technique

20.3.1 *Bowel preparation*

A liquid diet is recommended for 48 hours prior to the procedure. We have found that children have an excellent tolerance for this. Laxatives must be prescribed unless there is diarrhoea. Sodium sulphate 0.3 g/kg is given in a single dose in the afternoon preceding the day of colonoscopy. In the very young or in the presence of diarrhoea, bisacodyl suppositories (5–10 mg) may replace the use of laxatives. In older children, or when clear liquid faecal effluent is not induced by cathartics, mechanical bowel cleansing with saline wash-outs must be carried out until the water returns clean. Since intestinal transit time is rapid in the child, enemas should be given about 1–2 hours before colonoscopy. If the patient already has diarrhoea, a single large-volume saline enema should be sufficient. The preparation described above is adequate in more than 90% of cases (Habr-Gama *et al.*, 1980).

Attempts to avoid the need for enemas in children have stimulated interest in bowel preparation by the oral ingestion of a hypertonic solution of 10% mannitol. The principle of this technique is to present an osmotic load to the small intestine promoting the rapid transport of a large fluid volume, resulting in the elimination of clear watery waste. The solution of 10% mannitol is given in a calculated volume and frequency. In adults, good cleansing for colonoscopy may be achieved by giving 150 ml of 10% mannitol every 15 min until a total volume of 0.5–1.0 l is ingested. In children, half of this dosage is usually necessary. Nausea and vomiting may occur in some patients, but the incidence may be reduced by an injection of metoclopramide before drinking begins. In adults, the mannitol load may be better tolerated than the standard preparation, since diet, laxatives and enemas are not necessary. Despite the sweet taste of the solution, some children do not accept all the volume required. Bowel preparation with mannitol must be further evaluated in children to determine its efficacy.

20.3.2 *Technique of colonoscopy*

Colonoscopy in children should be performed early in the morning to prevent a prolonged period of fasting. Light general inhalatory anaesthesia may be valuable for performing the examination in very young children. Some infants may tolerate total endoscopy with any medication, but others may be quite restless, rendering attempts to intubate without anaesthesia too risky and traumatic. In co-operative older children, colonoscopy may be performed under sedation provided by the intravenous injection of meperidine/pethidine 1 mg/kg and diazepam 0.04–0.2 mg/kg (maximum 5 mg) administered just before the examination.

Colonoscopy can be safely performed in children without fluoroscopy; this should only be used when some difficulty arises or to confirm the position of the tip of the instrument. Determination of the depth of intubation of the colonoscope follows the same principles as that described for adults (Nagasako and Tatemoto, 1973; Waye, 1975; Williams and Teague, 1973), using the internal characteristic landmarks of the colon, the palpation of the tip of the instrument and transillumination of the light of the colonoscope on the abdominal wall, which in children is easier to observe than in adults.

The position of the child may be similar to adults using the left lateral decubitus position, but we prefer to conduct the examination with the child lying supine. The supine position permits manual compression and manipulation of the colonoscope through the abdominal wall by an assistant. Abdominal pressure is important to prevent over-distension and torsion of the sigmoid loop by the instrument. Since the patient is sedated, suction of air must be repeated continuously to avoid over-inflation.

Advancing the instrument in children should be done gently and as with adults only when the lumen of the bowel is in view. The sigmoid colon is commonly redundant in small children, causing occasional difficulty with its intubation. Introduction may be facilitated by frequent efforts to straighten the sigmoid by a combination of hooking, jiggling and withdrawal of the instrument. Changing the patient's position and repeating manual compression on the abdomen may also help progression of the instrument. Total colonoscopy to the caecum should be attempted, even when pathology is found in the left side of the colon; this is particularly important in patients with polyps, since about 25% of them may have more than one lesion (Habr-Gama *et al.*, 1980). The reasons for incomplete colonoscopy include an organic bowel stenosis or problems encountered during the procedure, but should not include the colonoscopist's lack of expertise. The endoscopist's skill, experience and patience for paediatric colonoscopy must be emphasized. General anaesthesia, the relative stiffness of various instruments, and the thinness of the bowel wall in children all increase the risks. However, total colonoscopy becomes easier and faster in children if the endoscopist has accumulated sufficient experience with adult patients.

20.3.3 *Technique of polypectomy*

Polypectomy in children is performed using the same technique as applied in adults. The bowel preparation must be good; the colonoscope must be correctly introduced and straightened; the polyp must be well positioned in the lumen; after lassoing the polyp head, the snare loop must be placed on the pedicle at a distance away from the bowel wall. Coagulation current is applied as the snare is gradually closed until the pedicle has been thoroughly coagulated in order to avoid premature mechanical cutting of the pedicle with consequent bleeding. In children, this technical detail is important, since the stalk of the polyp is usually slender. Because of the previously mentioned thinness of the bowel wall, the intensity of coagulation current should be low and cutting current is not needed unless the pedicle is thick.

When more than one polyp is encountered, all should be removed, starting with the most proximal one, thus avoiding repeated trauma by passage of the colonoscope over recently cauterized polypectomy sites.

Once the polyps have been snared and resected, they must be retrieved for histological investigation. Retrieval may be accomplished by suction onto the tip of the colonoscope, by resnaring the polyp, by the use of special grasping forceps, or rarely by means of subsequent enemas.

20.4 Complications

Complications of colonoscopy in children may be related to medication or anaesthesia, to the introduction of the instrument, or to polypectomy procedures.

In adults, complications occur with diagnostic colonoscopy in about 1.3%, and with polypectomy in about 2.4% of patients. Considering the difficulties in performing the examination in the young age group, and the fact that the instruments in general use to date are not especially designed for endoscopy in children, a higher morbidity should be expected. About 430 diagnostic colonoscopies and 100 polypectomies in children have been reported in the literature (see authors' reference section). No reported complication was related to introduction of the instrument but four perforations occurred during polypectomy (4%) (Gans, Ament and Cristie, 1975; Habr-Gama *et al.*, 1980; Holgersen, Mossberg and Miller, 1978). There have been no cases of severe bleeding, and no mortality. An immediate laparotomy is mandatory when the bowel is perforated. The perforation may be sutured, or the affected segment may be resected with a primary anastomosis, without colostomy, according to the size of the lesion and the condition of the bowel wall. The prognosis of the patient is usually good, since the colon is clean, and there is little time for the development of peritonitis.

20.5 General considerations about common colonic conditions in children and their relation to colonoscopy

20.5.1 *Rectal bleeding*

Rectal bleeding is a common complaint in infants and children. Often, the exact cause of rectal bleeding remains obscure after all the conventional diagnostic techniques have been used. It is well known that children with minimal to moderate amounts of rectal bleeding may have a self-limiting course with no recurrence of bleeding. However, if rectal bleeding is persistent or recurrent or severe enough to produce anaemia, colonoscopy is indicated. In a significant number of patients, this examination may disclose unsuspected pathology such as polyps, vascular lesions, infections, or inflammatory bowel disease.

Polyps are the commonest cause of moderate bleeding in paediatric patients. Severe bleeding rarely occurs. Ulcerative or granulomatous colitis and parasitic and bacterial diseases may also be associated with moderate bleeding, but more often these diseases are associated with a variable degree of abdominal pain and diarrhoea with or without the passage of mucus.

Large bowel polyps are frequent in childhood. Almost all polyps in children are hamartomatous lesions (Plate 88) without malignant potential and designated juvenile polyps. However, sporadic cases of solitary adenomas have been reported (Lowu, 1968). Of all solitary polyps resected by colonoscopy in children, only one has been reported to be of the mixed type – juvenile and adenomatous (Liebman, 1977). Schistosomal polyps have also been described in endemic areas (Plates 174 and 176) (Habr-Gama *et al.*, 1977).

Juvenile polyps may occur throughout the whole colon, but they are more common in the distal part, often within reach of the rectosigmoidoscope and about 20% are beyond this area (Roth and Helwig, 1963). They may be single or, if multiple, may represent a form of the well-known juvenile polyposis syndrome. They may be sessile but more often are pedunculated. Their stalks are usually slender, and the size ranges from a few millimetres to several centimetres in diameter. They are usually smooth in contour, with the surface being red and often haemorrhagic as a result of infarction. Gross anatomic findings may be misleading, since such juvenile polyps may be macroscopically indistinguishable from an adenoma. The combination of a large polyp with a narrow stalk accounts for the well-recognized propensity for autoamputation of these polyps, leading to the endoscopic finding of a stalk without a polyp head.

Juvenile polyposis is a rare condition and the polyps of this syndrome may occur anywhere in the gastrointestinal tract, but they are more common in the large bowel and are often limited to this region (Bussey, Veale and Morson, 1978; Veale, McColl and Bussey, 1966). Bleeding causing severe anaemia with malnutrition and physical retardation are the main symptoms. About 20% of patients with juvenile polyposis have other congenital defects, such as heart lesions, bowel malrotation, Meckel's diverticulum and an anomalous cephalic bone structure with a large and abnormally shaped head (Bussey, Veale and Morson, 1978).

Although juvenile polyposis is usually considered to have no malignant potential, this concept is under revision. Most tumours in juvenile polyposis have the same characteristic structure as the isolated juvenile polyps found in children, but some may contain atypical epithelial changes indistinguishable from the mild or moderate dysplasia seen in adenomas. According to Bussey (Bussey, Veale and Morson, 1978) there is no reason why these polyps should not have a neoplastic potential at least as great as that of the tissues from which they arise.

If the mucosa of the large intestine is prone to produce one type of neoplastic growth, it is not surprising if other neoplasms, such as adenomas or carcinomas, occurred in association with juvenile polyposis. Associated intestinal cancer has been observed in some patients with juvenile polyposis, as well as in other family members. Juvenile polyposis is now considered a biologic marker of neoplasia for the patient and his family. An apparent association has been reported between adenomatous polyposis coli and juvenile polyposis in different members of the same family. This association is in accordance with the hypothesis that hamartomas and adenomas could represent different phenotype expressions of the same genetic pattern (Habr-Gama *et al.*, 1980). In adenomatous polyposis, polyps do not usually appear until after the age of 10 years (Morson and Dawson, 1974). However, sporadic cases of familial polyposis have been reported before the age of 10 years. The premalignant character of this disease is well established, and all adolescents with familial polyposis must be submitted to colectomy before malignant changes occur.

Taking into account these concepts of polyps and polyposis in the paediatric age group, a general management programme may be adopted. All rectal polyps should be resected and examined. To increase the yield of pathology in individual patients, children with polyps occurring within the range of rectosigmoidoscopic examination should have a double-contrast barium enema to search for other polyps which may occur in about 25% of patients. Colonic polyps discovered on X-ray should be removed at colonoscopy if bleeding is persistent, recurrent or severe enough to produce anaemia. However, the mere presence of a polyp on X-ray does not require its removal. Most parents are worried about any visible degree of rectal bleeding in their children, and, they must therefore be informed that the great majority of polyps in this age group are benign, and that haemorrhage may only be occasional or may never recur. When a single juvenile polyp is resected, any follow-up of the child is unnecessary unless symptoms recur. If the polyp is an adenoma, follow-up is mandatory. When more than one polyp is resected, all of them must be examined, since the coexistence of adenomas and juvenile polyps may rarely occur. Children with multiple polyps should be examined periodically thereafter, searching for the development of polyposis and possible malignancy. Although cancer of the colon is rare in children, it may occur and is more often associated with adenomas or familial polyposis.

A Meckel's diverticulum or a vascular abnormality of the colon may be the cause of acute severe or chronic rectal bleeding in children. Vascular lesions are often beyond the reach of sigmoidoscopy, and their diagnosis may be difficult either by radiological techniques or by laparotomy. The location of the bleeding site in the colon is so common that children with significant rectal bleeding and with negative barium enema and proctosigmoidoscopic examinations should be submitted to colonoscopy before the performance of small bowel X-ray, arteriography or laparotomy. A negative total colonoscopy diminishes the possibility of colonic disease, thus making the diagnosis of small bowel disease and even an abdominal surgical exploration easier (Holgersen, Mossberg and Miller, 1978). About thirteen cases of vascular lesions in children have been reported during colonoscopic examinations (Fisher, Harrison and Adkins, 1979; Rodesch *et al.*, 1976; Skovgaard and Sorensen, 1976; Soehendra, 1979). Electrocoagulation or photocoagulation by laser have been employed for treatment of some vascular lesions in adults (Frühmorgen, Zens and Demling, 1975), and this method may soon be used for children.

20.5.2 *Lymphoid hyperplasia*

Spherical nodules of lymphoid tissue which vary from 0.6–3 mm occur throughout the intestinal tract, and those in the ileum are referred to as Peyer's patches (Capitanio and Kirkpatrick, 1970). Lymphoid follicles are numerous and prominent in children, and under certain circumstances hyperplasia may occur. When identified, it is a benign condition which does not undergo malignant transformation. However, it may be misdiagnosed as multiple polyposis with resultant unnecessary surgery. In recent years, lymphoid hyperplasia of the colon has been proposed as a cause of symptoms in children characterized by vague recurrent abdominal pain, diarrhoea and rectal bleeding.

The aetiology of lymphoid hyperplasia is not known. Infection, allergy and dysgammaglobulinaemia have been pointed out as possible aetiologic factors. Most probably, lymphoid hyperplasia represents the normal response of lymphoid tissue in children to a variety of stimuli.

Barium enema X-rays must be performed with excellent double contrast coating of the mucosa in order to demonstrate the umbilicated polyps characteristic of the disease. The nodularity is best delineated if maximum dilatation of the colon has not been obtained (Franken, 1970). Colonoscopy and biopsy of the submucosa are indicated to confirm the clinical and radiological suspicion of lymphoid hyperplasia before any kind of treatment is undertaken (Habr-Gama *et al.*, 1980).

20.5.3 *Ulcerative colitis*

Ulcerative colitis has been found in infants aged 2–3 months, but symptoms usually show up later in life, commonly between 8–15 years of age. In general, the clinical picture in children is the same as in adults. Anorexia, diarrhoea with loss of mucus or blood in the stools; fever, abdominal pain, and extracolonic symptoms may occur. Retardation of growth occurs in a significant percentage of patients and is inversely proportional to the age of onset of the disease. The endoscopic appearance, histology, bowel X-ray, course of the disease, complications, and response to treatment are similar to ulcerative colitis in the adult. However, in young patients, the severe forms with total colon involvement and the association with later carcinoma are more frequently seen.

Endoscopic findings in the early stage include hyperaemia (Plate 116), loss of the normal vascular pattern (Plate 117), mucosal friability, granularity (Plate 115), oedema and shallow small ulcerations or erosions. Later changes include a coarsely granular appearance, deeper mucosal ulcerations, pseudopolyps, shortening and loss of haustrations and mucosal bridging (Waye, 1977).

Children with diarrhoea and negative stool examination for bacteria or parasites and those with negative or doubtful barium enemas should be colonoscoped. An increasing number of cases of inflammatory bowel disease have been diagnosed with the help of colonoscopy and appropriate treatment instituted. About one-third of children investigated by colonoscopy for clinical symptoms and a negative barium enema will be found to have inflammatory bowel disease (see author's reference section). Besides its use for diagnosis of ulcerative colitis, colonoscopy is a valuable method of follow-up in children with long-standing colitis, thus avoiding excessive exposure to X-ray.

20.5.4 *Crohn's disease of the colon*

The incidence of Crohn's disease is apparently increasing. Although no statistics provide a true picture of its prevalence in children, many reports have been published in the last decade describing new cases of the disease in this age group (Guttman, 1974; Lux *et al.*, 1976; Gryboski and Spiro, 1978; Soehendra, 1979). Although the greatest prevalence in most series occurs in children over 10 years of age, recent publications have described a growing number of cases under the age of 10 (Guttman, 1974; Holgersen, Mossberg and Miller, 1978; Lux *et al.*, 1976).

Clinical manifestations of Crohn's disease in children are often subtle and non-specific and a long duration of disease before diagnosis is common. Abdominal pain, diarrhoea, rectal bleeding, anal abscess or fistula are the most prominent gastrointestinal complaints. Fever, anorexia, weight loss, unexplained anaemia, hypoalbuminaemia growth retardation, and arthralgia are the commonest extraintestinal manifestations. In some children, these problems are more prominent than the intestinal symptoms, which may be so mild that complete investigation of the gastrointestinal tract is not performed.

Proctosigmoidoscopy, barium enema and small bowel series are the most useful diagnostic investigations. However, when the disease does not affect the rectum, or when X-rays are negative, colonoscopy should be requested.

Although the specimens taken by endoscopic biopsies are often small and non-specific (Waye, 1977), they may aid in the differentiation between ulcerative colitis and Crohn's disease by finding granulomas (Frühmorgen, 1974; Geboes and Vantrappen, 1975).

Endoscopic features of Crohn's disease in the earliest phase include limited areas of hyperaemia, oedema with clear skip areas, and 'aphthoid' ulcerations (Plate 144) with sharply defined craters and thin bright red edges. In more advanced stages of the disease, deep serpiginous transverse ulceration and a 'cobblestone' appearance (Plate 152) are characteristic. Friability is rarely seen, and the occurrence of ulcers with adjacent normal mucosa and a normal vascular pattern are common (Plate 148).

In the literature, colonoscopy has been performed in about 40 children to confirm or to diagnose colonic Crohn's disease (Burdeski, Lucking and Siefert, 1975; Cadranel *et al.*, 1977; Cremer *et al.*, 1974; Habr-Gama *et al.*, 1980; Liebman, 1977; Lux *et al.*, 1976). In some children, the intubation of the colonoscope through the ileocaecal valve, permitting a view of the ileum, has contributed to the diagnosis of small bowel Crohn's disease.

20.6 Colonoscopy and radiology of the colon in the paediatric age group

Large neoplastic lesions or advanced colonic inflammatory diseases are easily identifiable either by radiological or endoscopic procedures. The accuracy of information obtained through colonoscopy or radiology depends to a large extent on two factors: good colon preparation, and the enthusiasm of the examiner.

Barium enema studies allow a precise evaluation of the diameter of a segment of colon and an indirect measurement of the degree of scarring of the colon wall as a whole.

Colonoscopy provides accurate information about the state of the colon's mucosal surface. Endoscopy has a splendid capacity to detect minute mucosal processes and affords a unique view of the submucosal vascular pattern (Plate 3).

Usually, there is no difficulty in preparing the colon for examination, but the ability of the examiner to demonstrate a lesion may be hindered by an uncooperative patient. Colonoscopy in the sedated paediatric patient allows the examiner to perform a careful and complete study of the colon with the collaboration of the passive patient. On the other hand, a good colon X-ray may be difficult in the awake and restless child. The radiographic demonstration of minute lesions requires a careful air/barium double contrast technique, for the ordinary barium enema fails when fine detail is sought. In paediatric patients, a good double contrast barium X-ray is considerably more difficult to achieve than an ordinary barium enema.

The differences between the information obtained from a barium enema and colonoscopy must be considered in the light of the diagnostic possibilities in the age group studied. The major pathology will be in the discovery of polyps, lymphoid hyperplasia, vascular abnormality, or inflammatory bowel disease. Another major diagnostic problem lies in the ability to conclude that the colon is or is not normal.

Positive radiological images may or may not represent actual pathology, since a defect in the barium column may actually be caused by the presence of stool. On the other hand, at colonoscopy, there are no false-positive results, but some lesions may be missed by the endoscopist giving a false-negative impression. The comparison of endoscopic and radiological results suggests that more pathology is missed by the barium enema when compared with the high accuracy of colonoscopy.

With lymphoid hyperplasia, errors in diagnostic precision are common. A barium enema of excellent quality is required to demonstrate with accuracy the presence of disease. However, the endoscopic view of the submucosal nodules is unmistakable and biopsy is helpful.

Barium enema is usually normal with vascular abnormalities of the colon. Although colonoscopy may detect vascular abnormalities in patients examined for a history of blood loss, it is not always possible to implicate them as the source of bleeding. Only seldom will the endoscopist have the opportunity to observe actual bleeding from these lesions.

In the early stages or in mild forms of inflammatory bowel disease, when the lesions are exclusively or predominantly confined to the mucosal layer, barium enema studies may fail to demonstrate the presence of disease. This possibility is greater when the abnormality is localized, as in Crohn's disease. In some cases, colonoscopy is helpful for judging the extent of the disease and the detection of mild lesions in a region previously considered normal by radiological criteria may provide assistance in the selection of therapy. In addition to visual data, colonoscopy may also provide a tissue biopsy specimen for histologic study.

Although the endoscopic information is more direct than the radiological data, comparison of the two methods does not prove the superiority of endoscopy. The basic nature of the methods are quite dissimilar, and they should be used in different stages of investigation.

Prior to colonoscopy, a barium enema should be performed in order to obtain a total view of the bowel, its configuration, dimensions, to localize segments of greatest interest, and to delineate strictured areas (Hunt *et al.*, 1975). When there is a stenotic segment that

cannot be intubated with the colonoscope, the segment proximal to
the stenosis can only by seen by radiological studies. Colonoscopy
without a barium enema must be performed very judiciously, if ever.

20.7 Author's experience of paediatric colonoscopy

In our early experience of 70 paediatric colonoscopic examinations, 63
have been performed in infants and children between 4 months and
16 years of age.

The examination was performed under general anaesthesia in 52
patients and under sedation in 11 children older than 7 years. The
instruments used were the same as for adult colonoscopy.

Colonoscopy was not successfully performed in two children with
extremely redundant sigmoid colons and in one of them, a polyp in
the transverse colon could not be endoscopically resected.

There were no complications due to medication or anaesthesia or to
the actual performance of colonoscopy. One complication during a
polypectomy occurred from excessive use of coagulation current, with
subsequent perforation of the sigmoid colon. Following immediate
resection of the affected bowel segment, the child made an uneventful recovery.

The main indications and results of the examinations are presented
in Figs. 20.1.

In the 42 children with rectal bleeding (Fig. 20.1(a)) polyps were by
far the most common pathology found: 59 polyps were found in 32
children, seven of them having more than one polyp (21.8%). Two
children, a brother and a sister had polyposis, one of the juvenile
type (5 years old) and the other (11 years old) of the familial
adenomatous type. In this series 59 therapeutic polypectomies were
performed for single or multiple polyps, and two diagnostic
polypectomies were performed in the two children with polyposis.
Forty-seven polyps (77%) were located in the left colon. Excluding 13
schistosomal polyps found in one child, and the adenomatous polyp
in the child with polyposis, all the other polyps were histologically
of the juvenile type.

There was a poor correlation between radiologic and endoscopic
findings in the children with rectal bleeding. In 11 children with significant rectal bleeding and with normal X-ray findings, polyps were
found in seven during colonoscopy; five of the 23 patients with
radiological diagnosis of a single polyp were found on endoscopy to
have further undetected lesions. One patient with the radiological
diagnosis of three polyps was found to have mutiple colonic polyps.

Based on these findings, colonoscopy was performed in seven small

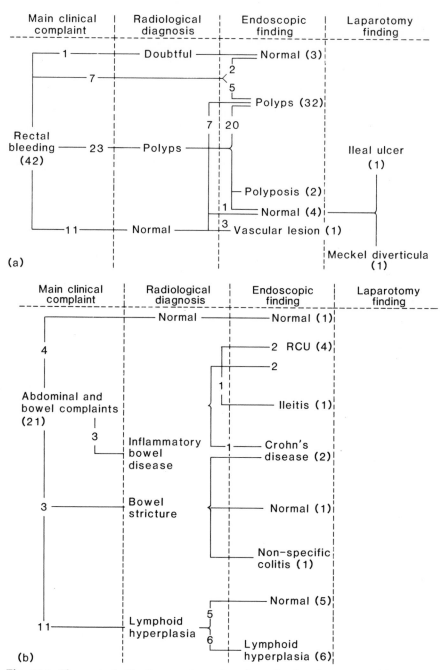

Fig. 20.1 The main indications and results of paediatric colonoscopy (a) rectal bleeding, and (b) abdominal and bowel complaints in the author's hospital.

children without prior X-ray studies of the colon, since bleeding was significant and high-quality bowel X-rays were not available in the hospital where the infants were admitted. Polyps were detected in five of these children, and in two endoscopic examinations were normal. However, in our series, there were very few false-positive diagnoses of polyps by X-ray.

In one child with recurrent bleeding, an area of vascular abnormality was found in the ascending colon. She has not yet been treated and continues to have intermittent bleeding.

In seven out of the 42 children with rectal haemorrhage, colonoscopy was normal (16.6%). Two of them were submitted to laparotomy and a Meckel's diverticulum in one child and an ileal ulcer in the other were found to be the source of bleeding. In two children, rectal bleeding ceased spontaneously. One child with a radiological suspicion of intestinal duplication died of complications secondary to malnutrition and two other children were lost to follow-up.

Twenty-one children were examined because of unexplained abdominal and bowel complaints (Fig. 20.1(b)): 11 had bowel X-rays with suspicion of lymphoid hyperplasia; colonoscopy confirmed this diagnosis in six cases and was normal in five. Ten children were colonoscoped with the clinical suspicion of inflammatory bowel disease: in four patients, X-rays were normal, and yet mild ulcerative colitis was found in two by colonoscopy. In another child, intubation of the ileocaecal valve disclosed the presence of small bowel inflammation and biopsy showed mild non-specific ileitis. A radiographic study of the small bowel, performed some hours later, demonstrated mucosal irregularity reported as lymphoid hyperplasia of the terminal ileum. The clinical course of this child, with recurrent periods of diarrhoea, rectal bleeding, and abdominal pain, is suggestive of the diagnosis of Crohn's ileitis.

In three children with clinical signs and typical radiological findings of inflammatory disease, colonoscopy and biopsy confirmed the diagnosis of ulcerative colitis in two, and the diagnosis of Crohn's disease in one. Granulomas were not found on the histological studies, but all the symptoms, signs and the evolution of the disease with deterioration of the general state and the development of fistulae were typical of Crohn's disease.

Three children were colonoscoped to clarify the nature of radiological bowel strictures. In one of these children with two areas of stricture, one in the sigmoid colon and the other at the splenic flexure, oedema, thickened interhaustral septa and many serpiginous ulcerations surrounded by a narrow rim of erythema were seen in the descending colon. Although the colonoscope could not pass the second stricture, several biopsies were suggestive of Crohn's disease. In the second child with a single stenosis at the rectosigmoid junction, the colonoscope easily passed through it, and only a mild degree of inflammation was seen in the narrow segment. The biopsies disclosed a non-specific inflammatory process. In the third child with a radiological suspicion of stenosis at the hepatic flexure, colonoscopy to the caecum was normal.

In our series a good correlation was observed between the radiological and endoscopic findings for the diagnosis of inflammatory bowel disease in children and for the evaluation of strictures, colonoscopy is extremely valuable to confirm their presence and determine their nature.

20.8 Conclusion

Although the published reports of paediatric colonoscopy are so far limited, experience is now growing rapidly and with the development of specialized paediatric colonoscopes and growing expertise both diagnostic and therapeutic colonoscopy are going to make a significant contribution to the practice of paediatric gastroenterology.

References

Burdeski, M., Lucking, Th. and Siefert, E. (1975), Uber die bedeutung der Coloskopie in der beurteilung von dickdarmerkrankungen in kindesalter. *Wscht. Kinderheilk.*, **123**, 434–5.

Bussey, H. J., Veale, A. M. O. and Morson, B. C. (1978), Genetics of gastrointestinal polyposis. *Gastroenterology*, **74**, 1325–30.

Cadranel, S., Rodesch, P., Peeters, J. P. and Cremer, M. (1977), Fiberendoscopy of the gastrointestinal tract in children. *Am. J. Dis. Child.*, **131**, 41–45.

Capitanio, M. A. and Kirkpatrick, J. A. (1970), Lymphoid hyperplasia of the colon in children. *Radiology*, **94**, 323–7.

Cremer, M. Peeters, J. P., Emonts, P., Rodesch, P. and Cadranel, S. (1974), Fiberendoscopy of the gastrointestinal tract in children. Experience with newly designed fiberscopes. *Endoscopy*, **6**, 186–9.

Fisher, S. E., Harrison, M. and Adkins, J. C. (1979), Colonoscopic diagnosis of vascular anomalies in children. *Clin. Pediat.*, **18**, 299–303.

Franken, E. A. (1970), Lymphoid hyperplasia of the colon. *Radiology*, **94**, 329–34.

Frühmorgen, P. (1974), Diagnosis of inflammatory disease of the colon by colonoscopy. *Acta Gastroent. Belg.*, **37**, 154.

Frühmorgen, P., Zens, J. and Demling, L. (1975), New aspects of therapeutic coloscopy. *Endoscopy*, **7**, 59–63.

Gans, S. L., Ament, M. and Cristie, D. L. (1975), Pediatric endoscopy with flexible fiberscopes. *J. Pediat. Surg.*, **10**, 375–80.

Geboes, K. and Vantrappen, G. (1975), The value of colonoscopy in the diagnosis of Crohn's disease. *Gastrointest. Endosc.*, **22**, 18–23.

Geenen, J. E., Schmitt, M. C. Jr and Hogan, W. J. (1974), Complications of colonoscopy. *Gastroenterology*, **66**, 812.

Gleason, W. A. Jr., Goldstein, P. D. and Shotz, B. A. (1975), Colonoscopic removal of juvenile polyps. *J. Pediat. Surg.*, **10**, 519–21.

Gryboski, J. J. and Spiro, H. M. (1978), Prognosis in children with Crohn's disease. *Gastroenterology*, **74**, 807–17.

Guttman, F. J. (1974), Granulomatous enterocolitis in childhood and adolescence. *J. Pediat. Surg.*, **9**, 115–21.

Habr-Gama, A., Gama-Rodrigues, J. J., Alves, P. R. A. and Verane, E. (1977), Colonoscopic polypectomy. *Am. J. Gastroent.*, **68**, 535–41.

Habr-Gama, A., Alves, P. R. A., Gama-Rodrigues, J. J., Teixeira, M. G. and Barbieri, D. (1980), Pediatric colonoscopy. *Dis. Colon Rect.*, **22**, 530–5.

Holgersen, L. O., Mossberg, S. M. and Miller, R. E. (1978), Colonoscopic for rectal bleeding in childhood. *J. Pediat. Surg.*, **13**, 83–85.

Hunt, R. H., Teague, R. H., Swarbrick, E. T. and Williams, C. B. (1975), Colonoscopy in management of colonic strictures. *Br. Med. J.*, **3**, 360.

Liebman, W. M. (1977), Fiberoptic endoscopy of the gastrointestinal tract in infants and children. Fiberoptic colonoscopy and polypectomy in 15 children. *Am. J. Gastroent.*, **68**, 452–5.

Lowu, J. H. (1968), Polypoid lesion of the large bowel in children with particular reference to benign lymphoid polyposis. *J. Pediat. Surg.*, **3**, 195–209.

Lux, G. Rosch, W., Phillip, J. and Fruhmorgen, P. (1976), Gastrointestinal fiberoptic endoscopy in pediatric patients and juveniles. *Endoscopy*, **10**, 158–63.

Morson, B. C. and Dawson, I. M. P. (1974), In: *Gastrointestinal Pathology*, Blackwell Scientific, Oxford.

Nagasako, K. and Tatemoto, T. (1973), Endoscopy of the ileocecal area. *Gastroenterology*, **65**, 403.

Nelson, E. W., Rodges, B. M. and Zawatzky, L. (1977), Endoscopic appearance of auto-amputated polyps in juvenile polyposis coli. *J. Pediat. Sur.*, **12**, 773–6.

Rodesch, P., Cadranel, S., Peeters, J. P. and Cremer, M. (1976), Colonic endoscopy in children. *Acta Pediat. Belg.*, **29**, 181–4.

Roth, S. I. and Helwig, E. B. (1963), Juvenile polyps of the colon and rectum. *Cancer*, **16**, 468–79.

Skovgaard, S. and Sorensen, F. H. (1976), Bleeding hemangioma of the colon diagnosed by coloscopy. *J. Pediat. Surg.*, **11**, 83–4.

Smith, G. E. (1974), Endoscopic removal of recurrent juvenile polyps in a 6 years old. *Gastroenterology*, **66**, 815.

Soehendra, N. (1979), Colonoscopy in children. *Proctology*, **1**, 8–14.

Stillman, A. E., Long, Paul and Komar, N. N. (1976), Arteriographic demonstration and colonoscopic removal of a bleeding juvenile polyps. *J. Pediat.*, **88**, 445–6.

Surikova, O. A. (1979), Colonoscopy in children. *Vopr. Okhr. Makrin. Det.* **24**, 39–42.

Veale, A. M. D., McColl, I. and Bussey, H. J. R. (1966), Juvenile polyposis coli. *J. Med. Genet.*, **3**, 5–16.

Waye, J. D. (1975), Colonoscopy: a clinical view. *M. Sinai J. Med.*, **42**, 1–34.

Waye, J. D. (1977), The role of colonoscopy in the differential diagnosis of inflammatory bowel disease. *Gastrointest. Endosc.*, **23**, 150–4.

Williams, C. and Teague, R. (1973), Progress report: colonoscopy. *Gut*, **14**, 990–1003.

Williams, C. B., Hunt, R. H., Loose, H., Riddell, R. H., Sakai, Y. and Swarbrick, E. T. (1974), Colonoscopy in the management of colon polyps. *Br. J. Surg.*, **61**, 673–82.

Willital, G. H. (1978), Significance of pediatric endoscopy. *Endoscopy*, **10**, 153–7.

PART THREE

Colour Atlas of Colonoscopy

Introduction

This atlas is intended to be primarily a collection of slides of the endoscopic appearances of the normal and diseased colon. Where appropriate, histological slides have been included to amplify the pathology, but no attempt has been made to be comprehensive in this respect, and a more detailed discussion will be found in Chapter 16.

The illustrations have been obtained from the extensive slide collections of the editors, supplemented by the authors of this book. The atlas essentially follows the outline of the book and is extensively referred to in the text. The first section (Plates 1–29) demonstrates the normal colon and the intraluminal landmarks, knowledge of which helps the endoscopist to localize the tip of the instrument at any site within the colon. Photographs of diverticular disease, an extremely common entity, are placed at the end of the normal findings (Plates 30–35) to point out the spectrum of abnormalities encountered in this ubiquitous condition. This is followed by a section illustrating the correct techniques of snare placement for polypectomy procedures (Plates 37–46), and photographs demonstrating the need to tighten the snare loop around the base of the polyp prior to the application of current. The technique of hot-biopsy polypectomy is also shown.

Rectal bleeding is frequently an indication for colonoscopy, and a variety of the causes seen endoscopically are illustrated in the next section (Plates 46–64), including the spectrum of vascular abnormalities.

The section on polypoid lesions (Plates 65–100) emphasizes the difficulties in the visual recognition of individual types of polyps, since most have a similar appearance even to the trained observer. Flat lesions are usually villous tumours, but some villous adenomas are pedunculated and indistinguishable from tubular adenomas. The only certain way to differentiate between the various histological types of polyps is to remove them *in toto* and submit the entire specimen to examination by the histopathologist.

The section on cancer of the colon (Plates 101–114) shows many typical intraluminal tumours – fungating, ulcerated and obstructing – which can almost always be immediately recognized as malignant.

However, some polyps may harbour invasive carcinoma, and yet have a benign appearance with a regular surface configuration. The endoscopic characteristics of carcinoma are those of a mass lesion with an irregular nodular and friable mucosal surface. Biopsy of the edges of such tumours usually provides histological confirmation of the visual endoscopic diagnosis of cancer, but a number of biopsies should always be taken because contiguous benign and malignant tissue can often occur in colon cancer.

Inflammatory bowel disease is comprehensively covered (Plates 115–180), since this presents a special challenge to the endoscopist. In ulcerative colitis (Plates 115–142), the colonoscopist's visual impression is most important in the differential diagnosis, because biopsies are usually non-specific. These pictures also provide the endoscopist with the opportunity to compare different disease entities, such as the similarities between the cobble-stoning of tuberculosis, that of Crohn's disease and of pseudopolyps. The polyps of schisto-somiasis may resemble adenomatous or inflammatory polyps.

The final portion of the atlas (Plates 181–188) demonstrates less common colonoscopic findings, such as ischaemia, radiation changes in the bowel wall, infections and pneumatosis coli.

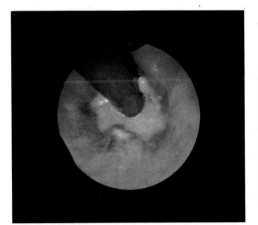

Plate 1 U-turn inversion of the colonoscope in the rectum showing the dentate line, anal papillae and dark bluish internal haemorrhoids.

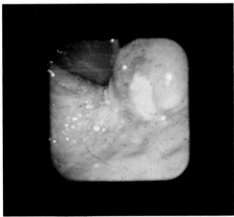

Plate 2 An ulcerated haemorrhoid in the rectum observed by inversion of the colonoscope, seen in the left upper part of the picture.

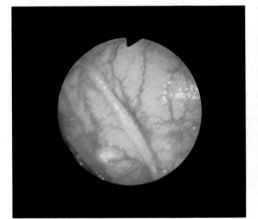

Plate 3 The normal healthy vascular pattern of the colon.

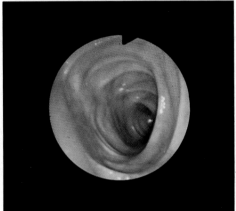

Plate 4 The normal descending colon.

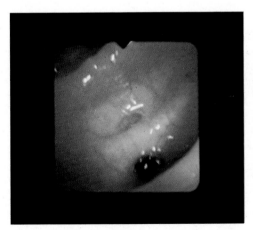

Plate 5 The arcuate highlights and folds which indicate that the lumen is to the top left.

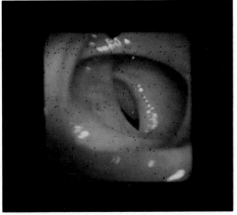

Plate 6 Circular muscle hypertrophy in the sigmoid colon.

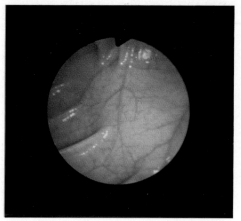

Plate 7 The characteristic 'blue' coloured impression of the spleen often seen at the splenic flexure.

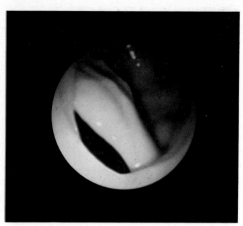

Plate 8 The gatelike fold commonly seen just below the splenic flexure.

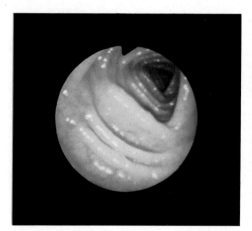

Plate 9 The transverse colon showing the typical triangular folds.

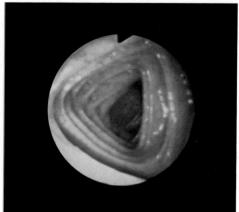

Plate 10 The characteristic triangular appearance of the transverse colon.

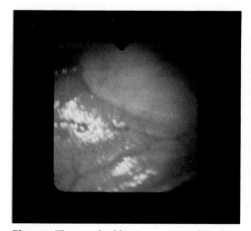

Plate 11 The angular blue impression of the liver seen at the hepatic flexure.

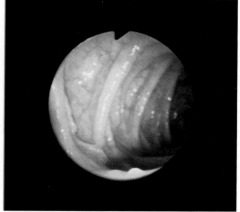

Plate 12 The ascending colon showing the characteristic incomplete arcuate folds.

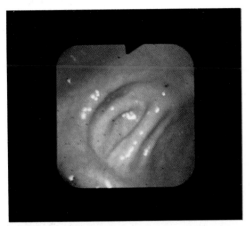

Plate 13 The appendix orifice seen with a pool of ileal fluid and prominent caecal folds.

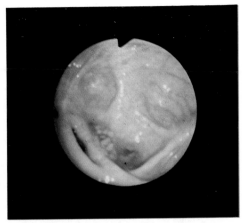

Plate 14 The normal caecum showing the ileocaecal valve.

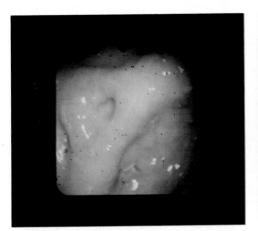

Plate 15 The orifice of the appendix seen at the junction of the taenia coli at the pole of the caecum.

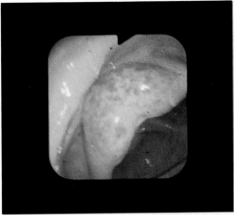

Plate 16 The appearance of a lipomatous ileocaecal valve.

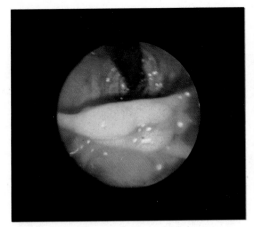

Plate 17 The ileocaecal valve which has a downward aspect can be seen on inversion of the colonoscope in the caecum.

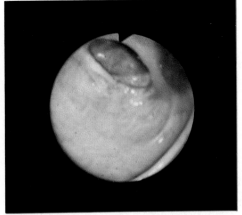

Plate 18 Flattening of the arcuate fold indicating the superior lip of the ileocaecal valve.

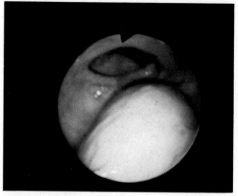

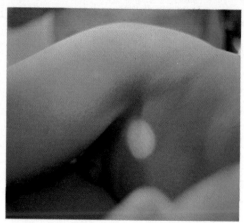

Plate 19 The same patient as in Plate 18, demonstrating identation of the caecum by finger palpation in the right iliac fossa just below the point of transillumination (see Plate 20).

Plate 20 The same patient as in Plate 18 in the left lateral position.

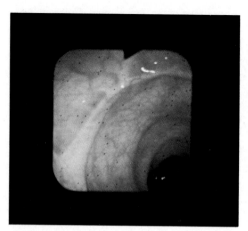

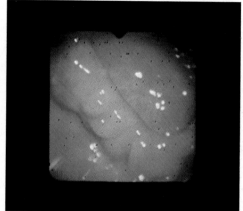

Plate 21 The smooth curvilinear appearance of a healed anastomosis in the sigmoid colon.

Plate 22 The nodularity often seen at a healthy colonic anastomosis.

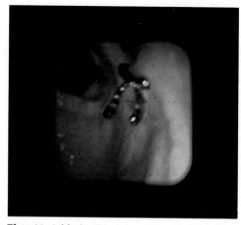

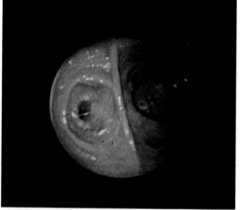

Plate 23 A black silk suture at the site of a colonic anastomosis.

Plate 24 A healthy ileo-colic anastomosis following right hemicolectomy. The ileum is on the left, the blind pole of the colon on the right.

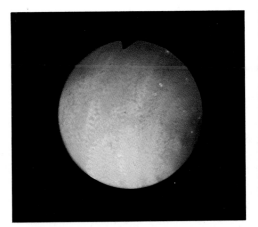

Plate 25 The normal terminal ileum.

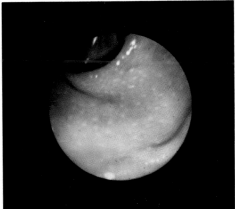

Plate 26 The mottled effect of early melanosis coli.

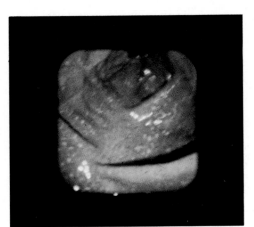

Plate 27 Prominent changes of melanosis coli seen throughout the colon.

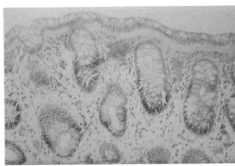

Plate 28 Groups of intramucosal pigment laden macrophages in a biopsy from melanosis coli.

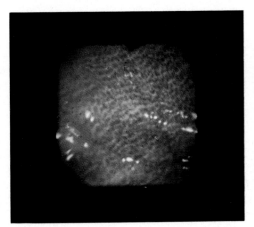

Plate 29 The angular impression created by the liver at the hepatic flexure seen in a case of melanosis coli.

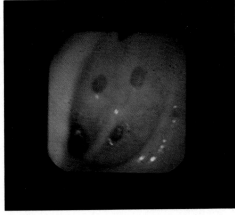

Plate 30 Orifices of diverticula in the sigmoid colon.

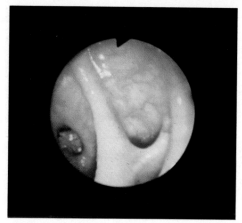

Plate 31 Large diverticular orifices which may easily be confused with the colonic lumen.

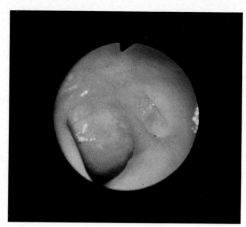

Plate 32 An inverted diverticulum.

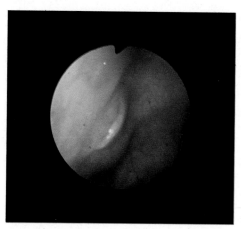

Plate 33 An inverted diverticulum in the sigmoid colon.

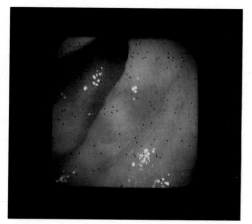

Plate 34 Reddened folds associated with diverticular disease in the sigmoid colon.

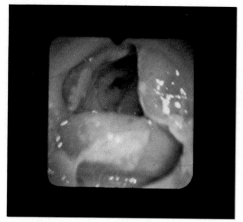

Plate 35 Acute diverticulitis with mucopus and oedema. Acute diverticulitis is generally a contra-indication to colonoscopy.

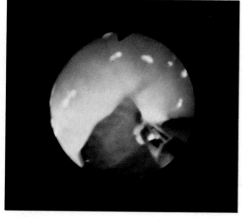

Plate 36 Hot biopsy being taken of a small adenoma.

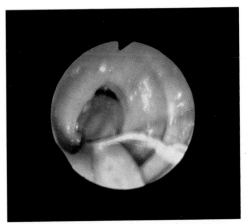

Plate 37 Snare approach. The polypectomy snare is being placed around the polyp stalk after encircling the polyp head.

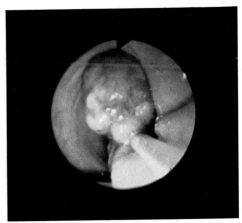

Plate 38 Snare placement. Placing the polypectomy snare at the junction of the polyp head and the pedicle.

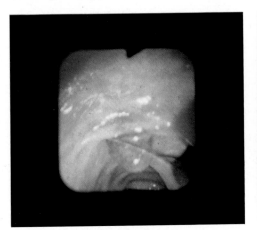

Plate 39 Removal of a small sessile polyp. Placing the polypectomy snare.

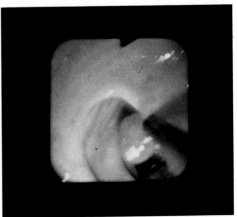

Plate 40 Removal of a small sessile polyp. 'Tenting' the polyp away from the wall to form a pseudo-pedicle.

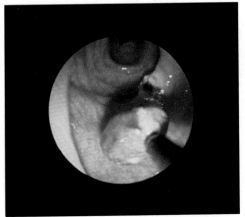

Plate 41 A small polyp being retrieved within the polypectomy snare. The polypectomy site can also be seen.

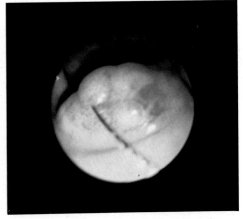

Plate 42 Piecemeal polypectomy. Placing the polypectomy snare over a portion of a broad-based adenoma.

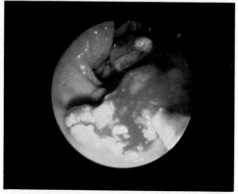

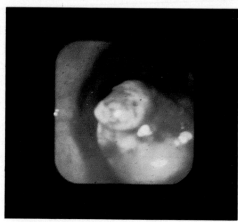

Plate 43 Piecemeal polypectomy. Removal of remaining tissue by diathermy snare. The already resected portion of the lesion may be seen beyond the polyp base.

Plate 44 Bleeding after polypectomy. A bleeding polyp pedicle.

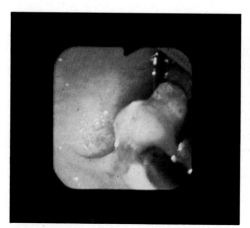

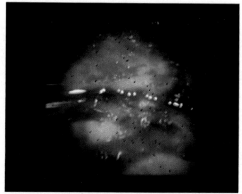

Plate 46 Angiodysplasia in the caecum. Solid stool is present and emphasizes the importance of meticulous bowel cleansing when searching for vascular abnormalities.

Plate 45 Bleeding after polypectomy. The pedicle is grasped and held within the diathermy snare but current is not applied.

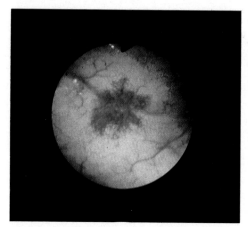

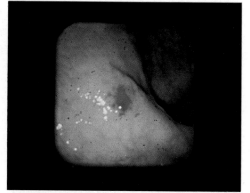

Plate 48 An angiodysplasia lesion on the superior fold of the ileocaecal valve showing the typical foot processes of the dilated superficial mucosal capillaries.

Plate 47 An unusually prominent vascular lesion in a patient with Osler–Rendu–Weber syndrome.

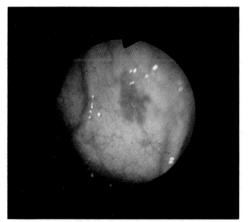

Plate 49 Angiodysplasia in the right colon showing a typical cherry red lesion.

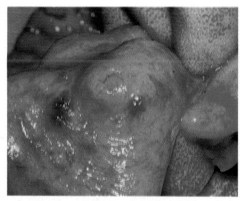

Plate 50 Angiodysplasia of the caecum diagnosed at colonoscopy and seen on the operation specimen (by courtesy of Mr F. I. Tovey).

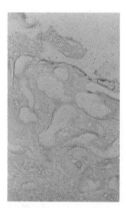

Plate 51 Histology from a hot biopsy of angiodysplasia lesion showing dilated thin walled ectatic superficial capillaries with effete red cells in the lumen.

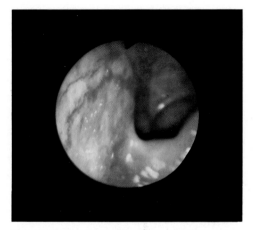

Plate 52 Linear telangiectasia seen in the caecum opposite the ileocaecal valve.

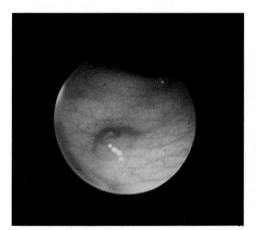

Plate 53 A cavernous haemangioma of 'blue rubber bleb' naevus type.

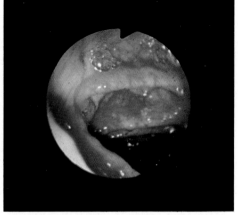

Plate 54 An extensive mucosal vascular malformation which extended from the splenic flexure to the hepatic flexure.

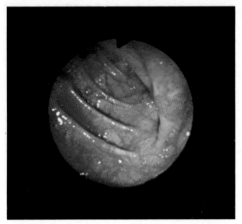

Plate 55 Another view of the same patient as shown in Plate 54.

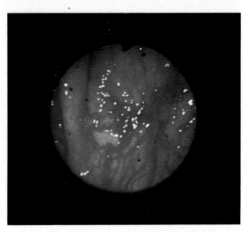

Plate 56 An extensive haemangioma of the colon.

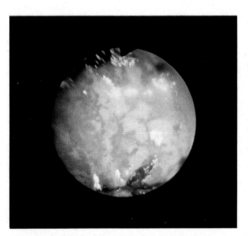

Plate 57 An extensive superficial vascular abnormality with areas of normal mucosa.

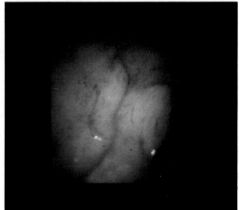

Plate 58 Colonic varices in a patient with splenic vein thrombosis.

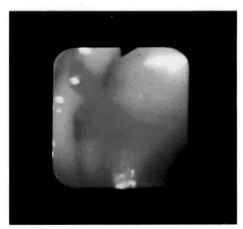

Plate 59 Bleeding from diverticular disease (by courtesy of Dr Harold Bernhard).

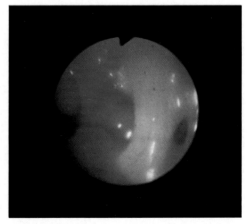

Plate 60 Fresh bleeding arising from a diverticulum.

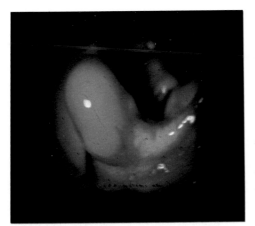

Plate 61 A small haemorrhagic colinic polyp.

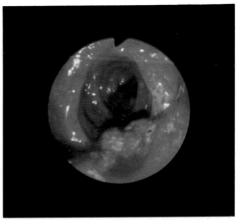

Plate 62 Torrential bleeding from multiple polyposis.

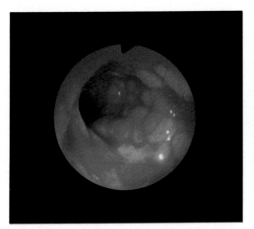

Plate 63 Massive haemorrhage from ulcerative colitis–a trickle of bright red blood is seen coming from the left colon.

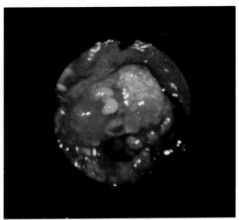

Plate 64 Bright red blood flowing from an ulcerated carcinoma at the hepatic flexure.

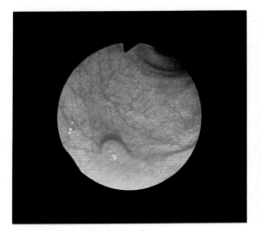

Plate 65 A small colonic adenoma.

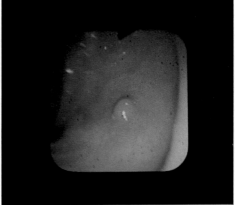

Plate 66 A small hyperplastic polyp.

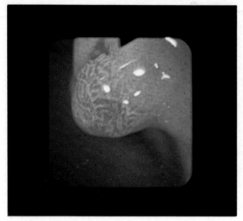

Plate 67 A small colonic adenoma.

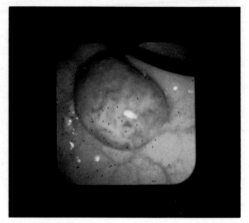

Plate 68 A 1.5 cm sessile hyperplastic polyp.

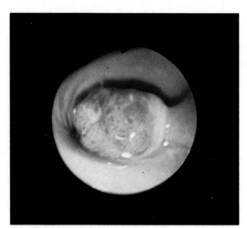

Plate 69 A pedunculated colonic adenoma.

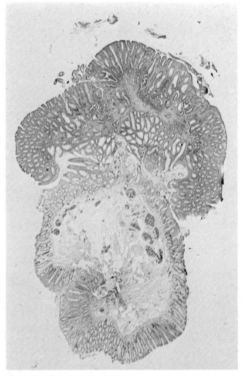

Plate 70 A tubular adenoma.

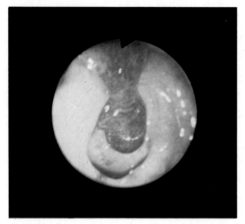

Plate 71 The reddened pedicle frequently seen with an adenoma but which will not reveal adenomatous tissue on histological section.

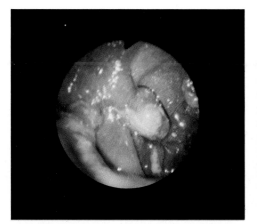

Plate 72 A pedunculated adenoma in melanosis coli showing the absence of coloration in the polyp tip but pigmentation of the stalk.

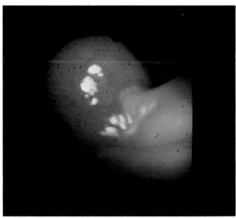

Plate 73 A benign-appearing smooth polyp with pedicle extending toward the right. This polyp had extensive cancer upon resection.

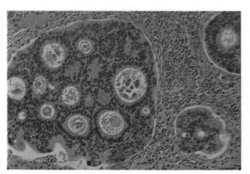

Plate 74 Nests of cancer in the head of the adenomatous polyp in Plate 73.

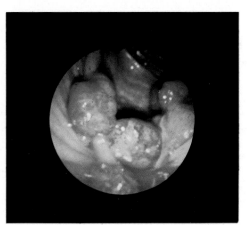

Plate 75 Multiple adenomatous polyposis coli.

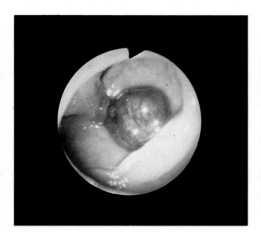

Plate 76 A pedunculated tubulo-villous adenoma.

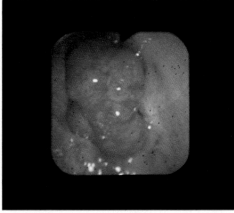

Plate 77 An irregular tubulo-villous adenoma in the sigmoid colon.

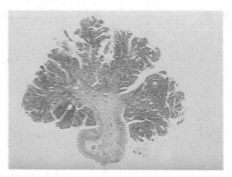

Plate 78 A tubulo-villous adenoma with histological structure intermediate between the typical tubular and villous adenoma.

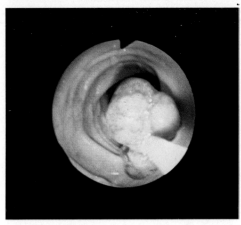

Plate 79 As with all polypoïd lesions it is not possible to distinguish histology without removal and retrieval.

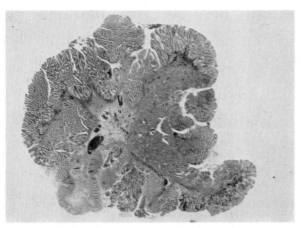

Plate 80 Tubulo-villous adenoma with a focus of invasive cancer.

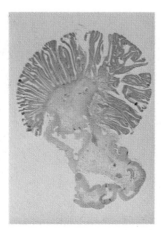

Plate 81 A villous adenoma which in this case is pedunculated.

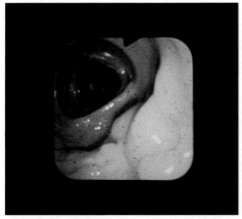

Plate 82 An irregular, pale, broad-based villous adenoma.

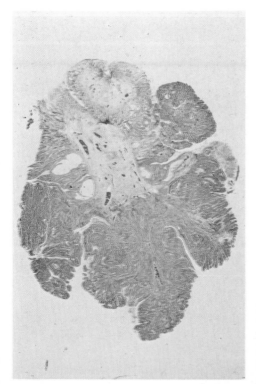

Plate 83 Adenoma with malignant change. A well differentiated carcinoma is seen arising in the head of a tubulo-villous adenoma but is well clear of the line of excision of the polyp.

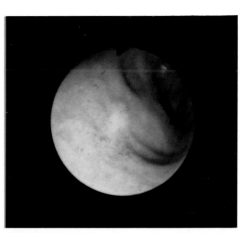

Plate 84 Post polypectomy scarring showing the flattened area of the scar.

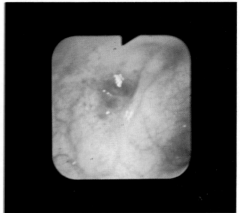

Plate 85 Post polypectomy scarring showing an involuting pedicle.

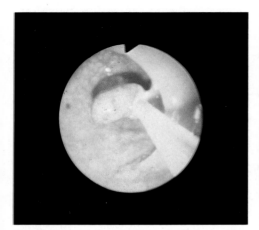

Plate 86 A vascular fibro-lipoma which must be removed like all polyps to determine the histology.

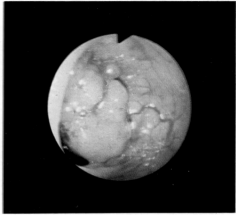

Plate 87 An unusually large juvenile polyp in a 47-year-old woman.

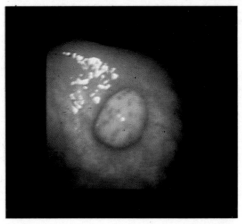

Plate 88 A juvenile polyp with a typical mottled surface.

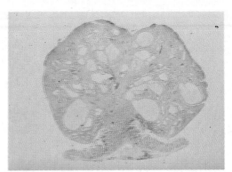

Plate 89 A juvenile polyp. The cystically dilated glands are separated by an excess of lamina propria.

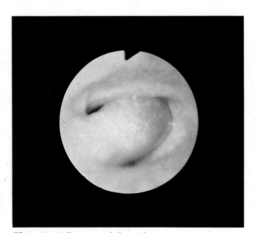

Plate 90 A lipoma of the colon.

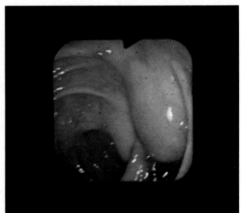

Plate 91 A colon lipoma lying in the caecum just above the ileocaecal valve.

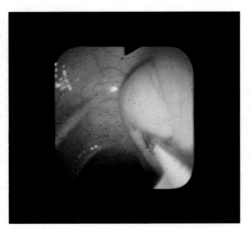

Plate 92 A colon lipoma showing compression with biopsy forceps – the 'pillow sign'.

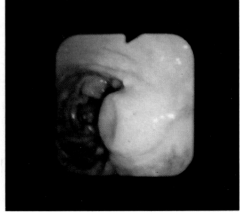

Plate 93 Sub mucosal leiomyoma showing the dimple in the head of the lesion.

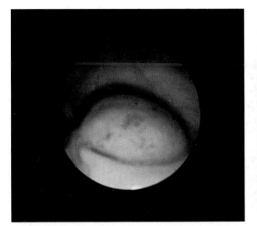

Plate 94 A leiomyoma of the caecum.

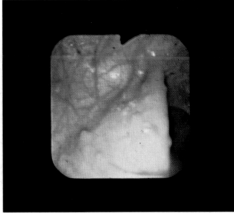

Plate 95 A number of small adenomas in a patient with early familial polyposis.

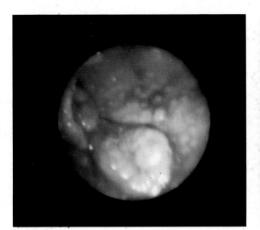

Plate 96 A carcinoma complicating polyposis coli.

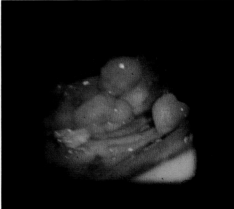

Plate 97 Multiple colon polyps in a case of Gardner's syndrome.

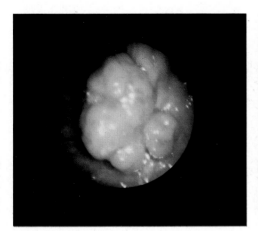

Plate 98 Peutz Jeghers polyp of the colon.

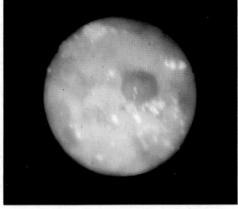

Plate 99 A sigmoid polyp in a patient with the Cronkhite Canada syndrome.

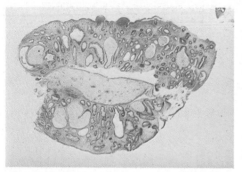

Plate 100 Cronkhite Canada syndrome. Many glands are dilated and some have ruptured.

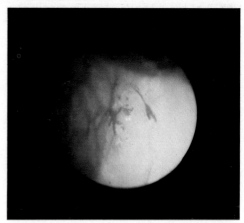

Plate 101 A small superficial colonic carcinoma.

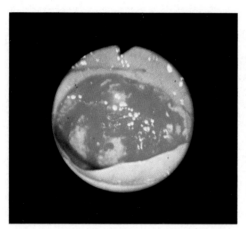

Plate 102 A haemorrhagic polypoid carcinoma.

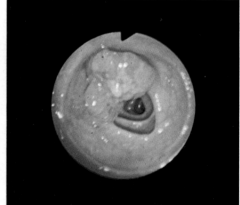

Plate 103 A polypoid carcinoma of the transverse colon.

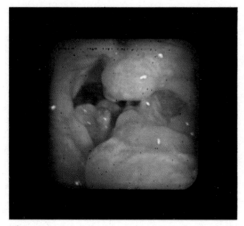

Plate 104 A polypoid carcinoma of the sigmoid colon.

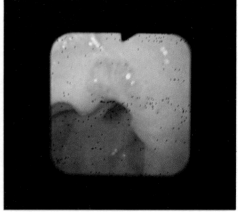

Plate 105 A small flat ulcerating carcinoma of the colon.

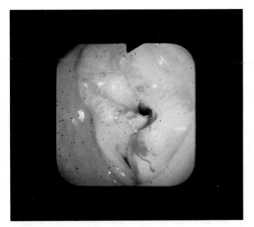

Plate 106 An obstructing ulcerated carcinoma of the sigmoid colon.

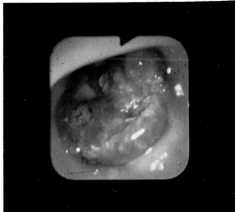

Plate 107 A flat ulcerated carcinoma in the sigmoid colon.

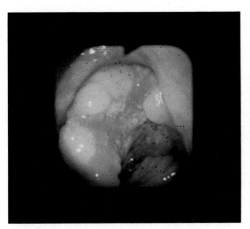

Plate 108 A small flat ulcerating cancer in the ascending colon.

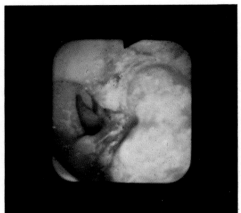

Plate 109 A fungating cancer in the sigmoid colon.

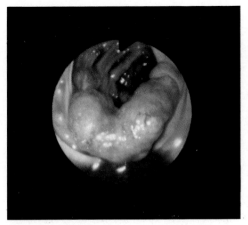

Plate 110 A flat carcinoma at the ileocaecal valve.

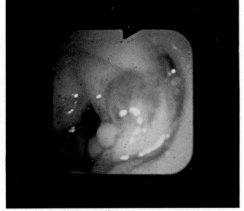

Plate 111 A recurrent carcinoma occurring at the suture line of the anastomosis.

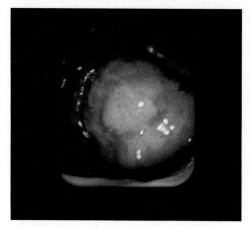

Plate 112 A large polypoid carcinoma of the splenic flexure.

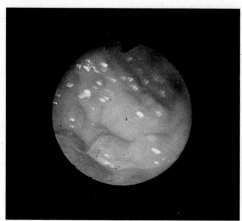

Plate 113 A lymphosarcoma of the colon. There are multiple small nodules, which appear submucosal.

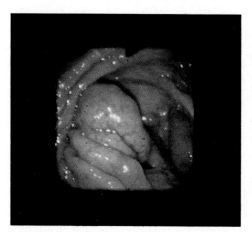

Plate 114 A polypoid lymphosarcoma of the ascending colon.

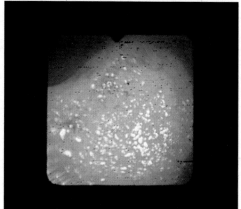

Plate 115 Granularity of the colonic mucosa in ulcerative colitis.

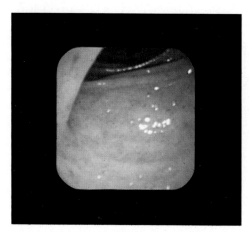

Plate 116 Erythema and loss of vascular pattern in early ulcerative colitis which showed no changes on the barium enema.

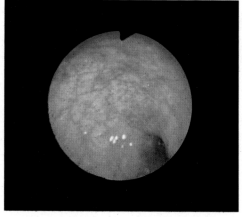

Plate 117 Early ulcerative colitis with mild vascular changes.

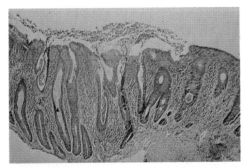

Plate 118 Surface inflammatory exudate over mucosa with crypt abscesses and goblet cell depletion.

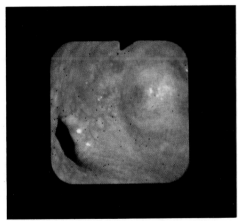

Plate 119 A gaping, non-functioning ileocaecal valve with caecal flattening in chronic ulcerative colitis.

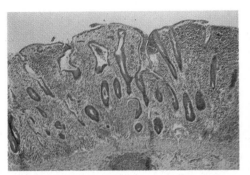

Plate 120 Irregular distorted crypt architecture with goblet cell depletion and crypt abscesses and heavy mucosal chronic inflammatory cell infiltrate in ulcerative colitis.

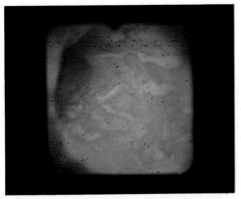

Plate 121 Typical bear claw ulcers in ulcerative colitis. Linear ulceration of this type should always be carefully differentiated from Crohn's disease.

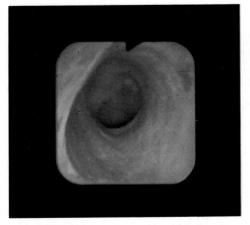

Plate 122 The appearances of inactive chronic ulcerative colitis.

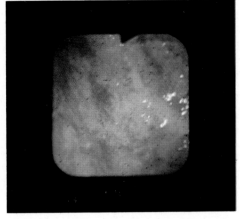

Plate 123 Vascular changes showing the erythematous changes of burnt out ulcerative colitis.

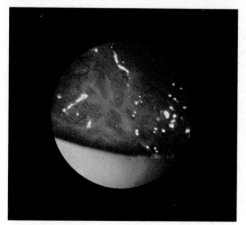

Plate 124 Post colitic scarring.

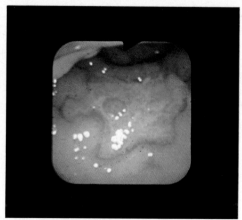

Plate 125 The genesis of a small pseudopolyp in an area of ulceration in ulcerative colitis.

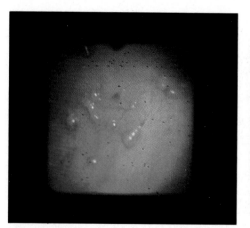

Plate 126 Multiple small pseudopolyps in ulcerative colitis.

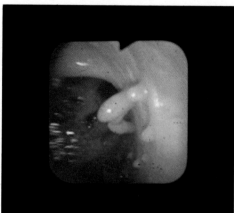

Plate 127 Finger-like pseudopolyps in an area of healed chronic ulcerative colitis.

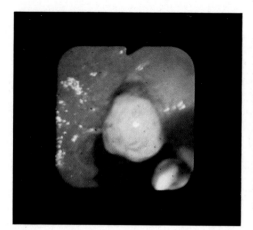

Plate 128 An inflammatory polyp of granulation tissue in chronic ulcerative colitis.

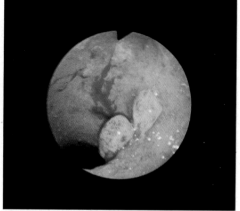

Plate 129 An inflammatory polyp composed of granulation tissue in chronic ulcerative colitis.

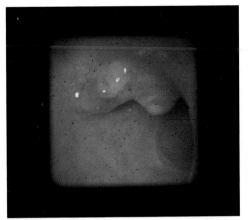

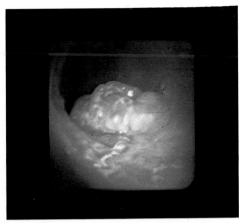

Plate 130 A pseudopolyp of granulation tissue in ulcerative colitis which is partly epithelialized.

Plate 131 A large irregular sessile pseudopolyp in chronic total ulcerative colitis which must be distinguished from a carcinoma.

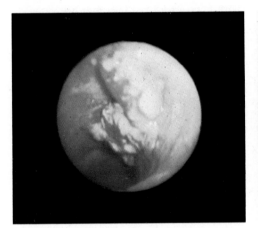

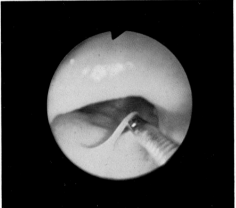

Plate 132 A solitary giant pseudopolyp in chronic ulcerative colitis.

Plate 133 A mucosal bridge in chronic ulcerative colitis.

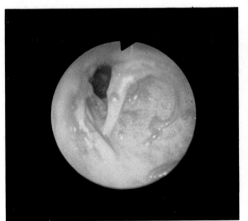

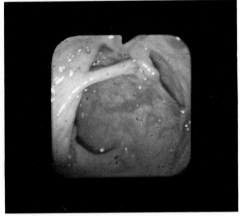

Plate 134 Inflammatory polyps and bridging in ulcerative colitis.

Plate 135 Mucosal bridging following severe chronic ulcerative colitis.

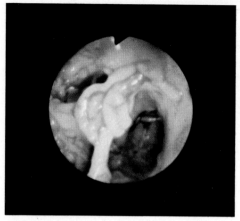

Plate 136 A 'knot' of pseudopolyps in chronic ulcerative colitis.

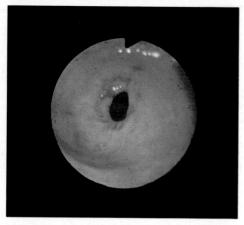

Plate 137. A benign fibromuscular stricture in chronic ulcerative colitis.

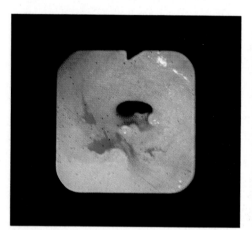

Plate 138 A benign fibromuscular stricture in chronic ulcerative colitis with small inflammatory polyps and trauma from attempts at intubation.

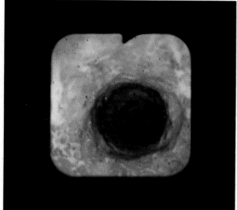

Plate 139 An inflammatory stricture in chronic ulcerative colitis.

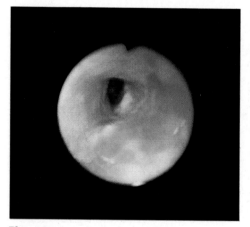

Plate 140 A carcinomatous stricture at the hepatic flexure complicating chronic total ulcerative colitis.

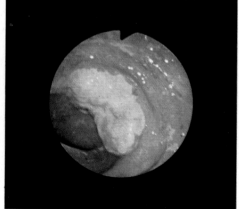

Plate 141 A carcinoma complicating asymptomatic chronic total ulcerative colitis.

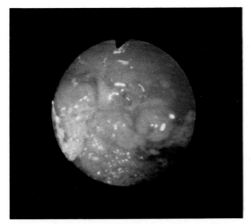

Plate 142 A flat villous adenocarcinoma in a patient with ulcerative colitis.

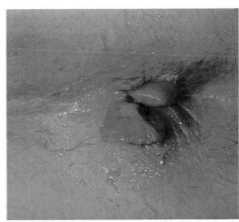

Plate 143 The typical anal lesions of Crohn's disease with a violaceous hue, skin tags, fissure and small fistula.

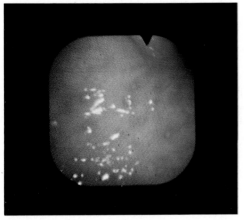

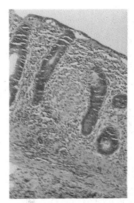

Plate 145 An intramucosal granuloma in Crohn's disease.

Plate 144 Typical aphthous ulcers in a patient with Crohn's disease.

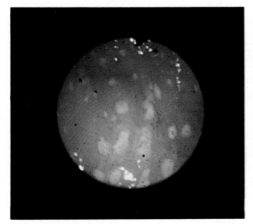

Plate 146 Micro ulcerations in Crohn's disease.

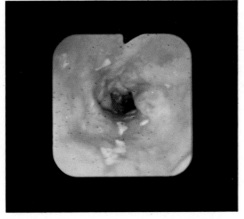

Plate 147 A benign stricture in active Crohn's disease.

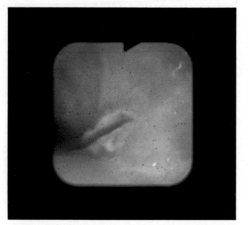

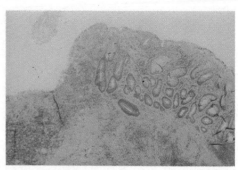

Plate 149 Mucosal cobblestoning with dense chronic inflammation adjacent to a linear ulcer.

Plate 148 A single linear ulcer in Crohn's disease.

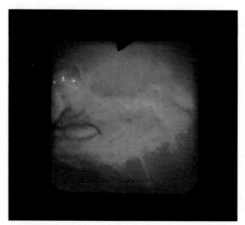

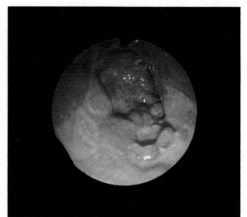

Plate 150 A deep ulcer with fistula in a patient with Crohn's disease at the splenic flexure.

Plate 151 Linear ulceration in colonic Crohn's disease.

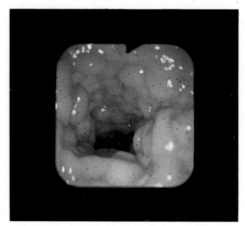

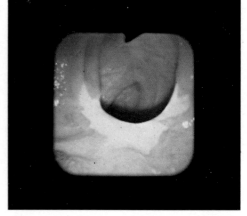

Plate 152 Cobblestoning in colonic Crohn's disease.

Plate 153 Recurrent Crohn's ulceration seen without narrowing at the ileo-colic anastomosis.

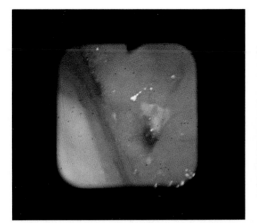

Plate 154 A narrowed ileo-colonic anastomosis with recurrent Crohn's ulceration.

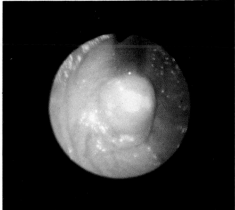

Plate 155 A Kock pouch, with U-turn during endoscopy. A normal nipple envelopes the instrument.

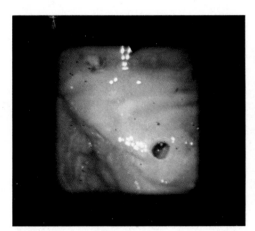

Plate 156 Nipple of Kock pouch with a fistula in the nipple causing incontinence.

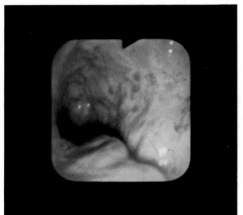

Plate 157 Ischaemic colitis. Pale mucosa with petechiael haemorrhages.

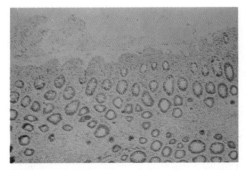

Plate 158 Early ischaemic colitis with superficial mucosal necrosis.

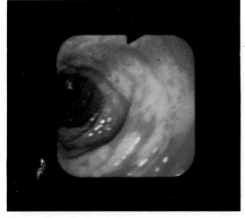

Plate 159 Ischaemic colitis. Serpiginous superficial ulceration.

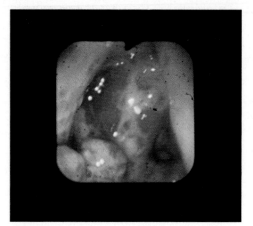

Plate 160 Edema and ulcerations in ischaemic colitis.

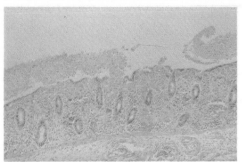

Plate 161 The surface pseudomembrane overlying focally ulcerated mucosa in which capillary micro-thrombi are present.

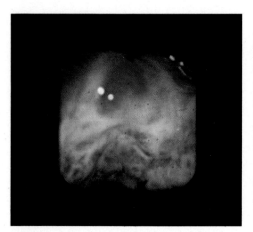

Plate 162 Advanced ischaemic colitis with greenish pseudomembrane and stenosis.

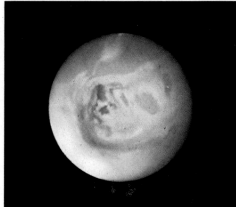

Plate 163 Ischaemic colitis with a pseudomembrane.

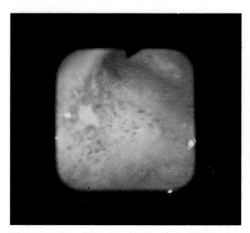

Plate 164 Petechiae surrounding a healing ischaemic ulcer.

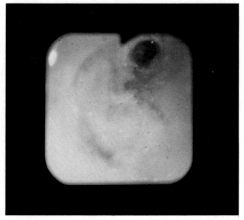

Plate 165 Healed ischaemic colitis with a smooth stricture.

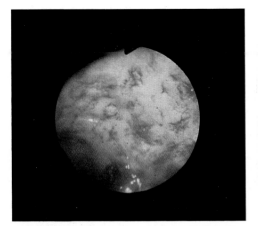

Plate 166 Radiation colitis with telangiectasia in the sigmoid colon.

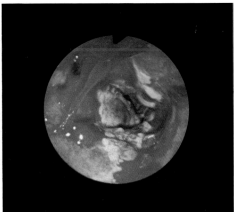

Plate 167 Acute ulcerating radiation proctosigmoiditis.

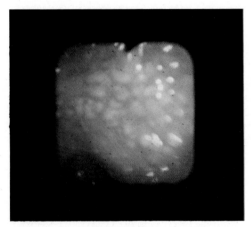

Plate 168 The pseudomembrane seen in a patient with antibiotic colitis (pseudomembranous colitis).

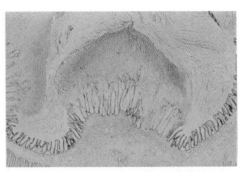

Plate 169 Pseudomembranous colitis. A full-formed plaque composed of a focal group of distended and disrupted crypts with an overlying pseudomembrane of mucin and polymorphs.

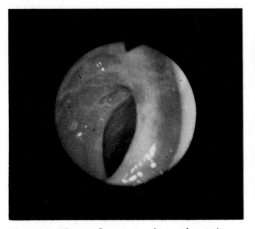

Plate 170 The confluent pseudomembrane in antibiotic colitis.

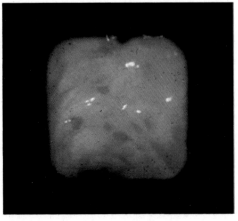

Plate 171 Early acute amoebic colitis.

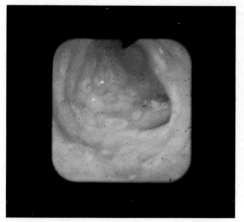

Plate 172 Characteristic punched out amoebic ulcers in the rectosigmoid region.

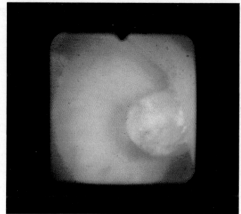

Plate 173 A calcified schistosome.

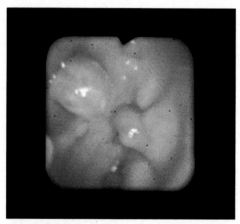

Plate 174 Bilharzial polyps at the splenic flexure.

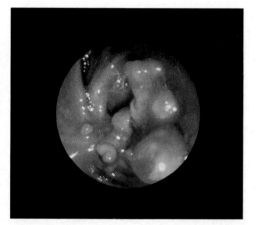

Plate 175 Bilharzial polyps in the caecum.

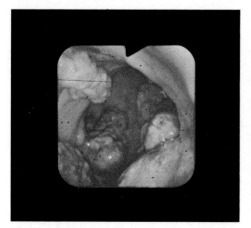

Plate 176 Schistosomal polyps in the colon.

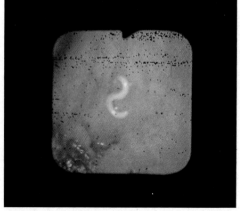

Plate 177 A trichuris worm in the right colon.

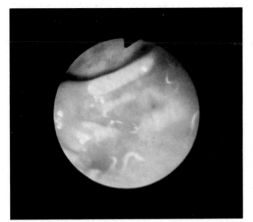

Plate 178 A trichuris worm in a pool of ileal fluid in the caecum.

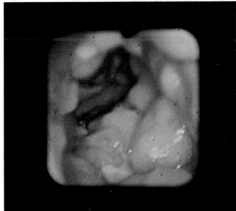

Plate 179 Tuberculosis involving the transverse colon. Note the similarity to the cobblestoning of Crohn's disease (Plate 152).

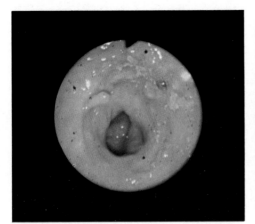

Plate 180 Tuberculosis of the caecum. Note the similarity to pseudopolyps in inflammatory bowel disease.

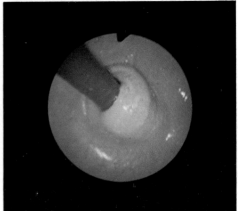

Plate 181 Megacolon shown with the colonoscope inverted in the dilated lumen.

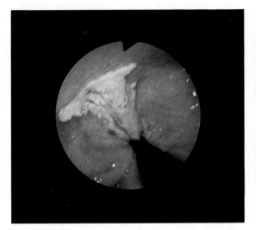

Plate 182 A solitary ulcer of the rectum seen with the colonoscope inverted.

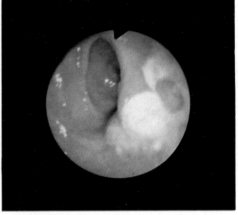

Plate 183 A solitary rectal ulcer.

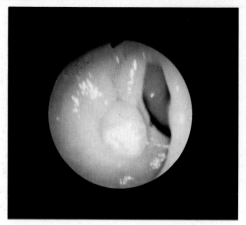

Plate 184 A healthy uretero sigmoidostomy.

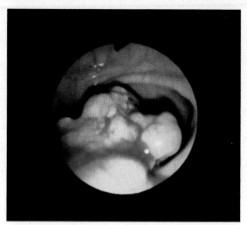

Plate 185 Carcinoma occurring in a uretero sigmoidostomy.

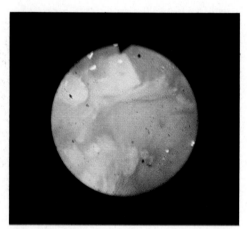

Plate 186 Colitis cystica profunda showing the typical cystic appearance.

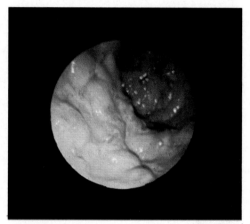

Plate 187 Air cysts seen in a patient with pneumatosis coli.

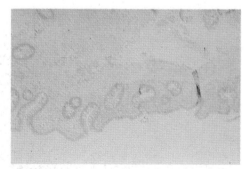

Plate 188 A submucosal gas-filled cyst with a lining of macronuclear and multinucleated macrophages from patient seen in Plate 187.

Index

Numbers in italics indicate plate numbers

Abdominal compression, 136, 143
Actinomycosis, 88, 366
Adenoma, 307–30, *36, 65, 67,*
  69–72, 74–83, 95
  see also Polyp
Air pressure hazard, 242, 273
Air insufflation, 157
Amoebic colitis, 88, 279, 345, 366,
  171, 172
Anaemia, 283
Anaesthesia
  general, 240
  paediatric, 385
Anatomy of colon, 112
  see also Colon
Anastomosis, 15, 376, *21–4*
  ileocolic, 15, 354, *24, 153, 154*
  stricture, 376
  recurrent Crohn's disease, *153,*
  154
  recurrent carcinoma, *111*
Angiodysplasia, 280, 291, 347,
  46–57
Angiography, 91, 102, 219, 252,
  281, 282, 290
  see also Radiology
Antibiotic colitis, 279, 323,
  168–70
Antibiotic prophylaxis, 191, 239
Anticoagulants, 20, 246
Aortic aneurysm, 247
Aphthous ulcers, 82, 348, 354, *144,*
  146
  see also Crohn's disease
Appendix, 143, *13, 15*
Aspirin, 20
Assistant, *see* Nurse/assistant
Arteriovenous malformation, *see*
  Vascular abnormality

Barium enema
  advantages, 63
  bowel preparation, 64
  bleeding, 91, 93, 290
  carcinoma, 99, 100
  complications, 74
  double-contrast, 65
  inflammatory bowel disease,
  75–88
  instant, 69
  neoplasia, 95
  polyps, 96
  single-contrast, 69
Beçhet's disease, 88
Biopsy, 57, 220, 221, 337–38, 344,
  350, 372
Bleeding, 267–300, *46–64*
  angiography, 91, 102, 219, 252,
  281, 282, 290
  approach, 12, 102, 269, 289
  cancer 15, 268, 272, *64*
  clinical experience, 274, 275,
  294–97
  colonoscopy indications, 12
  diverticular disease, 100, 277, 275,
  59, 60
  inflammatory bowel disease, 278,
  295, *63*
  intra-abdominal,
  post-polypectomy, 246
  intra-operative colonoscopy, 282,
  291
  massive, 91, 102, 282
  angiography, 282, 290
  barium enema, 91, 290
  colonoscopy, 12, 13, 195, 291,
  292, 293, 294, 297
  diverticular disease, 278, 282,
  283, 289, 291, 375–76

405

Bleeding (*continued*)
  paediatrics, 283, 388
  polyp, 276
  post-polypectomy
    delayed, 250
    primary, 250
    therapy, 219, 251, 252
  proctoscopy, 283, 289
  radiology, 270–72
    colonoscopy, 91–95
  radiation colitis, 88, 280, 346, *166,
    167*
  rectal, 91, 93, 102
  small bowel, 194
  solitary ulcer, 280, 346, *182, 183*
  technetium scan, 93
  unexplained, 274
  upper gastrointestinal, 289
  vascular abnormality, 280, 291,
    347, *46–57, 86*
  see also Colitis, Crohn's disease,
    Ulcerative colitis
Bowel preparation, *see* Preparation

Caecum, 113, 138, 143, *14, 17, 19,
    20, 46, 91, 175, 178, 180*
  see also Colon
Carbon dioxide (CO_2)
  distension, post-colonoscopy, 247
  diverticular disease, 373
  intra-operative colonoscopy, 191
  laser, 227
  mannitol, 21–23, 358, 385
  polypectomy, 203, 255, 256
Carcinoma, 327, *73, 74, 80, 83, 96,
    101–12, 185*
  bleeding, 274, *63*
  Crohn's disease, 328
  diverticular disease, 99, 374
  Dukes' staging, 186, 276, 333
  follow-up, 15, 100, 331
  high-risk groups, 15, 331
  inherited, 329
  metachronous, 277, 321, 331
  polyp, 215, 313, 316, 337
  radiology, 68, 69, 99
  recurrence, 336
  risk factors, 15
  screening, 186, 327
  synchronous, 14, 69, 233, 277,
    334
  ulcerative colitis, 81, 352

Cathartics, 21
  bisacodyl, 21, 24, 65, 385
  castor oil, 21, 24, 64, 358
  chemical, 21
  electrolyte imbalance, 237
  magnesium salts, 21, 24, 65, 358
  mannitol, 21–23, 255, 358, 368,
    385
    explosion hazard, 23, 255
  osmotic, 21
  senna, 21, 358
  Senokot, 21, 24
  sodium sulphate, 385
  whole-gut irrigation, 21, 23, 65
CEA (carcinoma embryonic antigen),
    336
Colitis, *115–80*
  Crohn's disease, 343–62, *143–56*
  infectious 344–51, *168–80*
  inflammatory bowel disease,
    343–62
  ulcerative, 343–62, *115–42*
Colitis cystica profunda, *186*
Colon
  anatomy, 112, 117
  appendix, *13, 15*
  ascending, 113, 143, *12, 108, 114*
  caecum, 138, 143, *14, 17, 19, 20,
    46, 91, 175, 178, 180*
  descending, 113, 116, *4*
  flexure
    hepatic, 137, 169, *11, 29*
    reversed hepatic, 139
    splenic, 116, 130, 131, 166, *7, 8,
      112, 150*
  fold, 143, 157, 163
    caecal sling, 138
  highlights, 163, *5*
  ileocaecal valve, 143, 144, *14,
    16–18, 91, 110*
  ileum, terminal, 144, *25*
  landmarks, 174, *1–25*
  sigmoid, 121, 126, 157, *21, 30, 77,
    99, 104, 106, 107, 109*
  transverse, 131, 133, 137, *9, 10,
    103, 179*
  vascular pattern, *3*
Colonoscope, *see* Instrumentation
Colonoscopy
  colostomy, 15, 74
  contraindication, 16, 357, 367
  emergency, 289

Colonoscopy (*continued*)
  fluoroscopic, 109–46
  indications, 12, 13, 195, 212, 228,
    292, 344, 367, 384
  intra-operative, 189
  limitations, 16, 195, 282
  non-fluoroscopic, 147–78
  paediatric, 63, 69, 91–5, 107,
    195, 335, 377, 383–401
  radiology, 63–108, 270–72
  suite, 27–38
  team, 29, 148
  therapeutic, 199–236
Complications
  air pressure, 242, 273
  analgesia, 238
  aortic aneurysm, 247
  bacterial endocarditis, 239
  bleeding, 209, 217, 245, 250, 258
    post-polypectomy, 209, 217, 250
    management, 219, 251–52
  carbon dioxide, 247
  distension post-colonoscopy, 246
  diverticular disease, 373–74
  explosion, 23, 203, 219, 254–56
  flexible sigmoidoscopy, 258, 259
  general anaesthesia, 240
  hypotension, 237, 238
  incomplete polypectomy, 243, 253
  infection, 239
  laceration, serosal, 240, 244
  miscellaneous 247, 248
  myocardial infarction, 246
  paediatric, 387
  perforation, 219, 241–44, 248,
    257, 373
    concomitant disease, 245, 373
    delayed, 249
    free, 241
    management, surgical, 242
    mechanical, 241
    polypectomy, 248, 249
    pneumatic, 242, 243
    site, 245
  pneumoperitoneum, 243, 373
  post-polypectomy syndrome, 217, 250
  premedication, 237, 238
    apnoea, 238
  prevention, 53, 57, 58, 220, 256
  preparation
    electrolyte imbalance, 237
    hypotension, 238

Complications (*continued*)
  rate, 218, 220
  thrombophlebitis, 238
  transmural burn, 217, 250
  vasovagal reflex, 246
  viral hepatitis, 240
Contraindications, 16, 213, 292, 357,
  367
Crohn's disease, *143–56*
  anal lesions, *143*
  aphthous ulcers, 82, 248, 254, *144,*
    146
  carcinoma, 328
  cobblestoning, 349, *149, 152*
  extent of disease, 87
  granuloma, 350, *145*
  Kock ileostomy, 74, 355, *155, 156*
  paediatric, 392
  pre- and post-operative evaluation,
    354, *153, 154*
  radiology, 82–8
  recurrence rate, 86
  ulceration, 348, *148–51, 153*
Current, *see* Therapeutic colonoscopy
Cytology, 53, 57, 239, 328, 338, 340,
  372
Cronkhite-Canada syndrome, 323,
  99, 100

Diazepam, 152, 237, 368, 386
Diet, 22, 64
Dilators, Eder–Puestow, 371, 372,
  378
Dilatation, 371, 378
Disinfection, 46, 58, 239
  cleaning room, 35
  ethylene oxide, 48, 240
  glutaraldehyde, 47–9, 58, 239
  iodophor (Hibitane), 47, 239, 240
  pHisoHex 239
  procedure, 48 58
Diverticular disease, 363, *30–5*
  bleeding, 277, 363, 364, 375, *59,*
    60
    massive, 278, 375–76
  carcinoma, 99, 364, 374
  clinical experience, 374
  diverticulitis, 16, 375, *35*
  false lumen, 369
  polyps, 374
  preparation, 25
  stricture, 100, 363, 371, 376, 378

Index

Dysplasia
  in adenomatous polyp, 310–13
  in ulcerative colitis, 328

EHT probe, 219
Electrosurgery, *see* Therapeutic
    colonoscopy
Emergency colonoscopy, 289–300
  see also Bleeding
Enema, cleansing, 24, 26, 181, 358,
    367
  barium, *see* Barium enema
Endometriosis, 322, 366
Endoscopy suite, 27–37
  cleaning room, 35
  colonoscopy room, 27–29
  conference room, 35
  position
    colonoscopy team, 29, 56, 57
    equipment, 31, 53, 54
    nurse/assistant, 30, 150
    patient, 120, 137, 140, 149, 191
  records, 58–60
  resuscitation equipment, 34, 58
  secretarial support, 36
  supplies, 34, 60
  trolley, 54
Epinephrine, 219, 252
Equipment
  ancillary, 34, 53
  electrocautery, 223
  snare 55, 208, 212
  trolley, 54
  see also Instrumentation
Ethylene oxide, 23, 48, 240
Explosions, 23, 203, 219, 254–56

Flexible Sigmoidoscopy, *see*
    Sigmoidoscopy, flexible
Fluoroscopy
  equipment, 33, 109
  technique, 109–46, 371
  radiation risk, 33
Foreign body, removal, 222
Forms, report, 59

Gardner's syndrome, 15, 330, *97*
Gas
  explosion, 23, 203, 219, 254–56
  hydrogen, 23, 203, 254, 255
  methane, 23, 203, 254, 255
  sterilization, 23, 48, 240

General anaesthesia, 240, 385
Glucagon, 66, 67, 368
Glutaraldehyde, 47–49, 58, 239

Haemorrhoids, 267, *1, 2*
Hamartomatous polyp, 302, 303,
    330, *98*
Hepatitis, viral, 240
Highlights, 163, *5*
High-risk groups, 15, 331, 356
Hot-biopsy, 221, 281, *36, 51*
  see also Therapeutic colonoscopy
Hydrogen, 23, 203, 254, 255

Ileocaecal valve, 143, 144, *14, 16–18,*
    91, 110
Ileocolic anastomosis, 15, 354, *24,*
    153, 154
Ileostomy
  radiology, 74
  Kock (continent), 74, 355, *155,*
    156
Indications, 12
  bleeding, 12, 195, 281, 292
  electrocoagulation, 219, 223, 281
  inflammatory bowel disease, 13,
    344
  intra-operative, 195
  laser, 228
  paediatric, 384
  polypectomy, 14, 212
  sigmoidoscopy, flexible, 179–80
  therapeutic, 179
Infective colitis, 344–51
  actinomycosis, 88, 366
  amoebic, 88, 279, 345, 366,
    171–172
  antibiotic, 279, 323, 345, *168–70*
  lymphogranuloma venereum, 88,
    366
  pseudomembranous, 323, *168–70*
  salmonella, 88, 344
  schistosomiasis, 279, 345, 366,
    173–76
  shigella, 88, 344
  staphylococcal, 88
  strictures, 366
  tuberculous, 88, 345, 366, *179,*
    180
  Yersinia enterocolitica, 88, 345

Inflammatory bowel disease, 13,
    343–62
  antibiotic colitis, 279, 323,
    168–70
  bleeding, 278, 295
  carcinoma, 51, 81, 84, 328, 352,
    356, *140–42*
  colonoscopy
    contraindications, 357
    indications, 13, 344
  differential diagnosis
    endoscopic, 344, 348, 351
    radiologic, 88
  extent, 351
  ischaemic, 88, 279, 295, 346, 365,
    157–65
  preparation, 357
  pseudomembranous colitis, 279,
    323, *161, 162*
  radiological features, 88
  radiation colitis, 280, 295, 346,
    166, 167
  solitary ulcer, 280, 346, *182, 183*
  stoma, 354
  strictures, 13, 353, 366, *162, 165*
  ulcers in, *159–64*
  see also Crohn's disease, Infective
    colitis and Ulcerative colitis
Inherited carcinoma, 329
Instrumentation
  accessories, 31, 34, 53, 54, 205
  cleaning, 46, 48, 58
  colonoscope, 39–42, 204, 292
    double-channel, 194, 204, 212
    floppiness, 152, 369
    paediatric, 369, 371, 384
    prototype, 5
    shaft, 41
    stiffness, 153, 369
    tip deflection, 154, 155, 369
  flexible sigmoidoscope, 179–80
  forceps, 45, 205, 221
  laser, 207, 225–30
  lecturescope, 147, 209
  lens system, 42
  light source, 43, 44
  intra-operative colonoscopy, 191
  maintenance, 46–49
  snare, 5, 45, 55, 201, 207, 208,
    212, 221
  stiffening sleeve, 45, 56, 128, 129
  television, 31

Intra-operative colonoscopy, 189–98,
    291
  bleeding, 194
  indications, 195
  instrumentation, 191
  limitations, 195
  position of patient, 191
  preparation, 190
  technique, 193, 291
Intubation of colon, *see* Technique
Iodophor, 47, 239, 240
Irritable bowel syndrome, 347
Iron, 20
Ischaemic colitis, 88, 279, 295, 346,
    365, *157–65*

Landmarks, colon, 174, *1–25*
  see also Colon
Laser
  argon ion, 202, 207, 225–30
  clinical experience, 225–30
  indications, 228
  limitations, 228
  neodymium–YAG, 202, 207, 225,
    230
  photocoagulation, 202, 281
  physical principles, 202
Limitations of colonoscopy, 16, 143,
    145, 195, 212, 283
Lipoma, 321, *86, 90–92*
Loops
  abdominal compression, 136, 143
  alpha, 116, 126, 183
  formation, 118, 120, 121, 159
  gamma, 116
  N-loop, 121–25
  push-through, 124, 141, 161
  reformation, 126, 136
  resolution, 125, 141
  right colon, 141
Lymphoid hyperplasia, 88, 90, 349,
    391
Lymphogranuloma venereum, 88,
    366

Magnesium salts, 65
Mannitol, 21–23, 255, 358, 368, 385
  explosion hazard, 23, 203, 219,
    254–56
Meckel's diverticulum, 268, 390

Medication
  anaesthesia, general, 240, 385
  antibiotic prophylaxis, 191, 239
  anticoagulants, 20, 246
  aspirin, 20
  diazepam, 152, 237, 368, 386
  flexible sigmoidoscopy, 181
  glucagon, 66, 67, 368
  hyoscine-*N*-butyl bromide, 66, 67, 144, 368
  iron, 20
  meperidine, 152, 368, 386
  metoclopramide, 21, 386
  metronidazole, 23
  naloxone (Narcan), 238
  paediatric, 386
  pethidine, 152, 368, 386
Megacolon, *181*
Melanosis coli, 365, *26–29, 72*
Metachronous lesion, 16, 277, 321, 331
Methane, 23, 203, 254, 255
Myocardial infarction, 16, 246

Nurse/assistant, 51–62
  check list, nursing, 54
  duties during examination, 56, 58, 120, 136, 150, 168, 209
  position, 30, 150
  tissue handling, 57, 301
  see also Endoscopy suite

Occult bleeding, 13, 283
Occult blood test, 13, 16, 101, 186, 333
  Hemoccult, 13, 16, 186, 333

Pacemaker, cardiac, 53, 213, 254
Paediatric colonoscopy, 46, 63, 69, 91–95, 107, 195, 335, 373, 377, 383–401
  clinical experience, 395–98
  complications, 387
  polypectomy, 387
  technique, 385–86
Patient, 19–26, 51–53
  paediatric, 373
  position, 120, 137, 140, 149, 191
  preparation, 19–26
Perforation, *see* Complications
Peutz-Jegher polyp, 302, 303, 330, *98*

Photography, 42
Pneumatosis coli, 322, *187, 188*
Pneumoperitoneum, 243, 373,
Polyp, *65–100*
  adenomatous, 213–16, 307–30
    tubular, 215, 309
    tubulo-villous, 215, 309
    villous, 215, 309
  bleeding, 276, *61, 62*
  carcinoma sequence, 215, 277, 313–16
  classification, 214, 301
  distribution, 214, 308
  diverticular disease, 374
  familial, 15, 330, *62, 75, 95, 96*
  follow-up, 15, 100, 215, 216, 330
  Gardner's syndrome, *97*
  hamartomatous, 302, 303, 330, *98*
  inflammatory, 84, 304, *125–32, 134, 136*
  juvenile, 302, 388, 389, *87–89*
    autoamputation, 303, 389
  lymphoid, benign, 306
  malignant, 215, 316
    policy, 215, 337
    potential, 310, 315
  metaplastic, 307, *66, 68*
  non-neoplastic, 321
  Peutz-Jegher, 302, 303, 330, *98*
  prevalence, 308
  pseudo-invasion, 317
  radiology of, 96
  retrieval, 211, *41*
  size, 209
  size and malignancy, 210, 214, 215, 315
Polypectomy, 14, 208–12, *36–45, 85, 86*
  bipolar technique, 212
  bleeding, 209, 217–19, 250–53, *44, 45*
  clinical experience, 212–16, 249
  contraindications, 213
  hot-biopsy, 211, 258, *36, 51*
  incomplete, 253
  indications, 14, 212
  marking of site, 196
  paediatric, 387
  piecemeal, 210, 249, *42, 43*
  power setting, 211
  retrieval, 211, *41*
  scarring, *85, 86*

Polypectomy (*continued*)
  size of polyp, 209, 212
  snare, 5, 45, 55, 201, 207
    biopsy, 221
    position, 208, *37–40*
  technique, 208–12, *37–45*
  see also Complications
Post-colonoscopy distension, 246
Post-operative colon, 14, 376
  anastomosis, 15, 376, *21, 22, 23,
    24, 111, 153, 154*
  barium enema, 74
  defunctioning colostomy, 15, 74
Preparation
  anticoagulants, 20
  aspirin, 20
  bleeding, 293
  bowel preparation, 20
  complications, 237
  dietary, 22, 64
  electrolyte imbalance, 237
  flexible sigmoidoscope, 25, 181
  general, 19
  iron therapy, 20
  patient, 19–26, 51
  saline lavage, 23, 65
  special, 24, 74, 75, 357, 367
  Vivonex, 25
Pseudopolyps
  inflammatory bowel disease, 349,
    351, 352, *125–32, 134, 136*

Radiation
  colitis, 88, 280, 346, *166, 167*
  stricture, 280, 366
Radiology
  angiography, 91, 102, 219, 252,
    281, 282, 290
  and colonoscopy, 63, 69, 91–95,
    195, 335, 337
  dosage, 75
  equipment, 33, 109
  errors, 95, 107
  instant enema, 69
  per oral pneumocolon, 72
  plain abdominal X-ray, 65
  see also Barium enema, Fluoroscopy
Rectal bleeding, 267–88
  see also Bleeding
Rectum, inversion in, 145, *2*
Report form (colonoscopy), 59
Resuscitation, 34, 53, 58

Salmonella, 88
Schistosomal colitis, 279, 345, 366,
  173–76
Screening for cancer, 186, 327, 333
Shigella, 88
Sigmoid colon, 121, 126, 157, *21, 30,
  77, 99, 104, 106, 107, 109*
  see also Colon
Sigmoidoscopy, flexible, 179–89,
  270, 339
  bleeding, 283
  clinical experience, 184–86
  cost benefits, 179, 186, 187
  complications, 258
  indications, 179
  instrumentation, 180
  preparation, 181
  screening, 180, 333
  technique, 182–84
  training, 180, 181
Sigmoidoscopy, rigid, 189, 270, 293,
  339
Snare, 5, 45, 55, 201, 207, 208, 212,
  221
Solitary ulcer, 280, 346, *182, 183*
Splenic flexure, 130, 131, 166–68,
  112, 150
Stiffening sleeve, 45, 56, 128, 129
Strictures, 364–66
  anastomosis, 15, 376
  diverticular disease, 100, 277, 363
  inflammatory bowel disease, 366
  ischaemia, 365, *165*
  management, 366, 367
  radiation, 366
  ulcerative colitis, 13, 329, *137–40*
Surveillance for cancer, 15, 330,
  356
Synchronous lesions, 14, 69, 277,
  320, 333

Technique
  abdominal compression, 136, 143
  air insufflation, 157
  ascending colon, 113, 143, *12,
    108, 114*
  caecum, 113, 138, 143, *14, 17, 19
    20, 46, 91, 175, 178, 180*
  descending colon, 113, 116, *4*
  difficulties, 125
  emergency colonoscopy, 289–300
  flexible sigmoidoscopy, 182

Technique (*continued*)
  flexure
    hepatic, 137, 169
    reversed hepatic, 139
    splenic, 116, 130, 131, 166
  fluoroscopic, 109–46
  folds, 143, 157, 163
  highlights, 163, *5*
  hooking, 135, 166
  ileum terminal, 144
  intra-operative, 193
  inversion at rectum, 145
  loops, *see* Loops
  lumen location, 163, *5*
  non-fluoroscopic, 147–78
  options, 148, 170–74, 176
  paediatric, 385, 386
  paradoxical motion, 160
  position
    change of 120, 121, 386
    hands, 120, 148
    paediatric, 385, 386
    patient, 120, 137, 140, 149, 191
    see Endoscopy suite
  shaft of colonoscope
    handling, 120, 151
    jiggle, 125
    rotational stability, 41
    stiffness, 152, 153
    straightness, 126–31, 156, 158
    torque, 41, 125, 131, 143,
      157–58, 370
  sigmoid colon, 121, 157, *21, 30,
    77, 99, 104, 106, 107, 109*
  sigmoid stiffening 'sleeve', 128,
    129
  'slide by', 45, 55, 118, 126, 370
  strictures 368–72, *137–40*
  team 29, 56, 148
  'tips' for colonoscopy, 170
  transillumination, 143, 175, *20*
  transverse colon, 133–38, 168, *9,
    10, 103, 179*
Television (closed-circuit), 31
Therapeutic colonoscopy, 199–236,
  377
  current, type, 200–01, 211, 224,
    250, 254
  dilatation, 371, 378
  electrocoagulation, 56, 57,
    222–25, 281
  electrode, button, 223

Therapeutic (*continued*)
  electro-hydro-thermal probe, 207,
    219, 224, 230
  equipment, 56, 205–07, 251
  explosion, 23, 203, 219, 254–56
  fulguration of angiodysplasia, 222,
    281
  hot-biopsy, 221, 281, *36, 51*
  perforation, 219, 257
  power setting, 211, 250, 253
  thermal energy, principles,
    199–203
Tissue sampling, 57, 301, 337, 372
Torque, *see* Technique, shaft
Training in colonoscopy, 147, 180,
  181
Transillumination, 143, 175, *20*
Transmural burn, 217, 250
Transverse colon, 131, 133, 137, *9,
  10, 103, 179*
Trichuris infestation, *177, 178*
Tuberculous colitis, 88, 366, *179,
  180*
Tumour, *see* Carcinoma and Polyp

Ulcerative colitis, *1, 115–42*
  bleeding, *64*
  carcinoma, 81, 328, 352, *140–42*
  differential diagnosis (Crohn's),
    348
  dysplasia, 328, 348, 353, 356
  extent of disease, 87, 351
  follow-up, 13
  indication for colonoscopy, 13
  mucosal bridging, *133–35*
  paediatric, 391
  preparation
    barium enema, 75
    colonoscopy, 357
  pseudopolyps 349–52, *125–32,
    134, 136*
  radiology, 76–80
  stricture, 13, 353, *140*
  ulceration, 348, *121*
  vascular pattern, *3, 116, 117*
Ureterosigmoidostomy, 256, *184*
  carcinoma in, *185*

Varices of colon, 282, *58*
Vascular abnormality, 222, 280, 281,
  291, 295, 347, *46–57, 86*

Yersinia enterocolitica, 88